D1330227

Oxford Handbook of
Pain Management

Published and forthcoming Oxford Handbooks

Oxford Handbook of
Pain
Management

Edited by

Peter Brook

Consultant in Pain Management
Pain Management Service
Bristol Royal Infirmary
Bristol
UK

Jayne Connell

Principal Clinical Psychologist
Bristol Royal Infirmary
Bristol
UK

Tony Pickering

Wellcome Senior Clinical Research Fellow
and Honorary Consultant Senior Lecturer in Anaesthesia
School of Physiology & Pharmacology,
University of Bristol,
Bristol

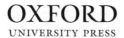

OXFORD
UNIVERSITY PRESS

OXFORD
UNIVERSITY PRESS

Great Clarendon Street, Oxford OX2 6DP.

Oxford University Press is a department of the University of Oxford.
It furthers the University's objective of excellence in research, scholarship,
and education by publishing worldwide in

Oxford New York

Auckland Cape Town Dar es Salaam Hong Kong Karachi
Kuala Lumpur Madrid Melbourne Mexico City Nairobi
New Delhi Shanghai Taipei Toronto

With offices in

Argentina Austria Brazil Chile Czech Republic France Greece
Guatemala Hungary Italy Japan Poland Portugal Singapore
South Korea Switzerland Thailand Turkey Ukraine Vietnam

Oxford is a registered trade mark of Oxford University Press
in the UK and in certain other countries

Published in the United States
by Oxford University Press Inc., New York

© Oxford University Press, 2011

British Library Cataloguing in Publication Data
Data available

Library of Congress Cataloging-in-Publication-Data
Data available

Typeset by Glyph International, Bangalore, India
Printed in China
on acid-free paper through
Asia Pacific Offset

ISBN 978–0–19–929814–3

10 9 8 7 6 5 4 3 2 1

Foreword

The prevalence of pain in the population is high and management may often be deficient, achieving an unsatisfactory outcome in terms of both inadequate pain relief and adverse events. Basic scientists have developed a wealth of knowledge of pain mechanisms and possible modalities that may modify these to achieve relief of pain. However, it remains frustrating that translation from laboratory experimentation to human therapy leaves many potential treatments wanting.

In part, the relative failure of putative treatments results from the complex biopsychosocial aetiology of pain, of suffering and of interpersonal response differences in humans. Thus effective clinical management of pain requires skilled assessment of each patient, often by a multidisciplinary team, good communication, evidence based knowledge and experience.

Papers reporting scientific advances and results of therapeutic trials, as well as systematic reviews, provide tools for management of pain. These tools require skilled application by a broad range of experienced practitioners to achieve optimal results for patients. An essential resource is an up to date textbook written by experienced scientists and clinicians which may also be used as a 'bench book'. To be effective, such a volume must be broad ranging, clearly written and offer excellent indexing and bibliography. The Oxford Handbook of Pain Management provides just such a resource.

Robert W. Johnson, MD.,FRCA.,FFPMRCA.
University of Bristol, UK.

Preface

Pain remains an all too common feature of our lives and its alleviation represents a 'Grand' challenge for healthcare practitioners. Although we have limited diagnostic tools, imperfect treatment options and flawed structures for their delivery there is much that can be achieved through multidisciplinary and holistic practices which can achieve the best outcomes in the treatment of both acute and chronic pain. This book stemmed from our mutual perception that too few people working in healthcare were privy to the broad range of approaches that were useful in the management of pain.

There will never be enough pain specialists and practitioners to meet the needs of all the patients who suffer in this way, thus for this knowledge to be effective it must be disseminated beyond 'centres of excellence' down to the shopfloor. As we have noted, effective pain management often requires a multidisciplinary approach yet the time spent learning about pain in medical school and nursing, physiotherapy, and clinical psychology training is limited and is often limited to a narrow perspective. So it seemed appropriate that we should attempt to collect and share current knowledge about the management of pain from a broad range of viewpoints to support new clinicians, and other colleagues across the world.

We felt that to be most useful this information source needed to be concise, to be quick and accessible, something that could sit in a pocket or on a nearby shelf. It is intended to be a pointer to good practice, giving key, immediate guidance. Practitioners have cannot hope to craft effective management plans based on the avalanche of information pouring daily through their letter boxes and in trays, rather they need distilled wisdom from a range of sources. In an attempt to meet this need we conceived the *Oxford Handbook of Pain Management*.

In places this book provides more than most clinicians will need at the coalface, and there is inevitable repetition of some common themes, but we hope that the core information is presented in a way that will encourage thought, help with decision making and provide starting points for more detailed consideration. We all continue to learn (often from our patient's experiences) and the field of Pain Management is constantly evolving. We have enjoyed collating our author's insightful contributions that have provided many different perspectives, and take this opportunity to thank them for their patience. This book has been a long time coming but, hopefully, is all the better for it.

'*The greatest mistake in the treatment of diseases is that there are physicians for the body and physicians for the soul, although the two cannot be separated*'. Plato

Contents

Contributors

Jonathan Anns

Sir Humphry Davy Department of Anaesthesia
Bristol Royal Infirmary
Bristol

Polly Ashworth

Pain Management Service
Gloucester Royal Infirmary
Gloucester

Michael Basler

Department of Anaesthesia and Pain Medicine
Glasgow Royal Infirmary
Glasgow

Andrew Beacham

Fairfield Health Centre
Bath

Marie Besson

Centre Multidisciplinaire d'étude et de traitement de la douleur
Hôpitaux Universitaires de Genève
Genève
Switzerland

Peter Brook

Pain Management Service
Bristol Royal Infirmary
Bristol

Angela Burnett

Medical Foundation for Victims of Torture
London

Nilesh Chauhan

Sir Humphrey Davy Department of Anaesthesia
Bristol Royal Infirmary
Bristol

Jayne Connell

Bristol Royal Infirmary
Bristol

Jo Daniels

Department of Psychology,
University of Bath
^{2}gether NHS Foundation Trust
Gloucester

Jonathan Gatward

Sir Humphrey Davy Department of Anaesthesia
Bristol Royal Infirmary
Bristol

Martin Gargan

Bristol Royal Hospital for Children
Bristol

CE Gilkes

Department of Neurosurgery
National Hospital for Neurology and Neurosurgery
London

Tim Gould

Sir Humphry Davy Department of Anaesthesia
Bristol Royal Infirmary
Bristol

Siobhan Grimes

Sir Humphry Davy Department of Anaesthesia
Bristol Royal Infirmary
Bristol

Grant Haldane

Anaesthetic Department
Hairmyres Hospital
Glasgow

Ewan Jack

Department of Anaesthesia
Stirling Royal Infirmary
Stirling

Stephanie Keel
Sir Humphrey Davy
Department of Anaesthesia
Bristol Royal Infirmary
Bristol

Simon Kelley
Division of Orthopaedic Surgery
The Hospital for Sick Children
Toronto
Canada

Lucy Kirkham
Sir Humphry Davy Department of
Anaesthesia
Bristol Royal Infirmary
Bristol

Murli Krishna
Pain Clinic
Frenchay Hospital
Bristol

Gill Lauder
Department of Paediatric
Anaesthesia
Bristol Royal Hospital for Children
Bristol

Christina Liossi
School of Psychology
University of Southampton
Southampton

Sarah Love-Jones
Pain Clinic
Frenchay Hospital
Bristol

Francis Luscombe
Department of Anaesthesia
Plymouth Hospitals NHS Trust
Derriford
Plymouth

Cattherina Mattheus
Sir Humphry Davy Department of
Anaesthesia,
Bristol Royal Infirmary,
Bristol

Steve Meek
Frenchay Hospital
Bristol

Janine Mendham
Pain Clinic
Macmillan Centre
Frenchay Hospital
Bristol

Heather Muncey
Service Improvement Manager
for Orthopaedics
Finance and Service Development
King Square House
Bristol

Steve Nichol
Department of Trauma and
Orthopaedic Surgery
Bristol Royal Infirmary
Bristol

Jonathon Oates
Department of Anaesthetics
Victoria Infirmary
Glasgow

Hazel O'Dowd
Pain Management Service
Frenchay Hospital
Bristol

Margaret Owen
Glasgow Pain Service
Western Infirmary
Glasgow

Nik Patel
Department of Neurosurgery
Frenchay Hospital
Bristol

Tony Pickering
Departments of Physiology and
Pharmacology
University of Bristol
Bristol

Colin Rae
Department of Anaesthesia
Stobhill Hospital
Glasgow

Mark Scrutton
Sir Humphry Davy Department of
Anaesthesia
Bristol Royal Infirmary
Bristol

Nicolas Snelling
Whiteladies Medical Centre
Bristol

Cathy Stannard
Pain Clinic
Macmillan Centre
Frenchay Hospital
Bristol

Charlotte Steeds
Pain Management Service
Bristol Royal Infirmary
Bristol

Les Shutt
Sir Humphry Davy Department of
Anaesthesia
Bristol Royal Infirmary
Bristol

Pete Stoddart
Department of Paediatric
Anaesthesia
Bristol Royal Hospital for Children
Bristol

Amanda C de C Williams
Research Department of Clinical,
Educational & Health Psychology
University College London
London

Lars Williams
Department of Anaesthesia
Southern General Hospital
Glasgow

Hannah Wilson
Sir Humphry Davy Department of
Anaesthesia
Bristol Royal Infirmary
Bristol

Symbols and abbreviations

📖	cross reference
▶	important
⚠	warning
♂	male
♀	female
>	greater than
<	less than
~	approximately
ACC	anterior cingulate cortex
ACE	angiotensin-converting enzyme
ACR	American College of Rheumatology
ACTH	adrenocorticotropic hormone
ADH	antidiuretic hormone
AMPA	α-amino-3-hydroxyl-5-methyl-4-isoxazole-propionate
APS	Acute Pain Service
ASIC	acid-sensitive ion channel
ATLS	Advanced Trauma Life Support
bd	twice a day
BDI	Beck Depression Inventory
BPI	Brief Pain Inventory
Ca^{2+}	calcium
CAD	coronary artery disease
CBT	cognitive behavioural therapy
CFS	chronic fatigue syndrome
CNMP	chronic non-malignant pain
CNS	central nervous system
CP	central pain
CPP	chronic pelvic pain
CRA	chronic refractory angina
CRP	C-reactive protein
CRPS	complex regional pain syndrome
CSE	combined spinal epidural
CSF	cerebrospinal fluid
CT	computed tomography
CTG	cardiotocograph
CTS	carpal tunnel syndrome

CVS	cardiovascular system
DBS	deep brain stimulation
DH	dorsal horn
DIC	disseminated intravascular coagulation
DMARD	disease-modifying antirheumatic drug
DVT	deep vein thrombosis
EA	electroacupuncture
EEG	electroencephalogram
ESR	erythrocyte sedimentation rate
FAPS	functional abdominal pain syndrome
FAQ	frequently asked question
FBC	full blood count
FBSS	failed back surgery syndrome
FD	functional dyspepsia
FGID	functional gastrointestinal disorder
fMRI	functional magnetic resonance imaging
g	gram(s)
GA	general anaesthetic
GI	gastrointestinal
GnRH	gonadotropin-releasing hormone
GP	general practitioner
HAD	Hospital Anxiety and Depression Scale
HSAN	hereditary sensory and autonomic neuropathy
HSV	herpes simplex virus
IASP	International Association for the Study of Pain
IM	intramuscular
INR	international normalized ratio
IT	information technology
ITU	Intensive Therapy Unit
IV	intravenous
K^+	potassium
L	litre(s)
LA	local anaesthetic
LBP	low back pain
mcg	microgram(s)
ME	myalgic encephalopathy
MEAC	minimum effective analgesic concentration
mg	milligram(s)
MI	myocardial infarction
mL	millilitre(s)
MRA	magnetic resonance angiography

MRI	magnetic resonance imaging
ms	millisecond(s)
MS	multiple sclerosis
MTC	minimum toxic concentration
MTrP	myofascial trigger points
MUA	manipulation under anaesthesia
MVD	microvascular decompression
N_2	nitrogen
N_2O	nitrous oxide
NA	noradrenaline
Na^+	sodium
NAPQI	N-acetyl-p-benzoquinone imine
NBM	nil by mouth
NCA	nurse-controlled analgesia
NMDA	N-methyl-D-aspartate
NNT	number needed to treat
NRS	numerical rating scale
OA	osteoarthritis
OCP	oral contraceptive pill
OT	occupational therapist
PAG	periaqueductal grey
PASS	Pain Anxiety Symptom Scale
PCA	patient-controlled analgesia
PCEA	patient-controlled epidural analgesia
PDPH	postdural puncture headache
PE	pulmonary embolism
PHN	postherpetic neuralgia
PICU	paediatric intensive care unit
PLP	phantom limb pain
PO	by mouth
PONV	postoperative nausea and vomiting
PPI	proton pump inhibitor
PR	rectally
PRN	as needed
PTSD	post-traumatic stress disorder
PVG	periventricular grey
qds	four times a day
QST	quantitative sensory testing
RA	rheumatoid arthritis
RCT	randomized controlled trial
REM	rapid eye movement

RF	radiofrequency *or* rheumatoid factor
RVM	rostroventromedial medulla
s	second(s)
SAH	subarachnoid haemorrhage
SC	subcutaneous
SCS	spinal cord stimulation
SF-36	Short Form-36 Health Survey
SNRI	selective noradrenaline reuptake inhibitor
SSRI	selective serotonin reuptake inhibitor
STD	sexually transmitted disease
SUNCT	short lasting unilateral neuralgiform headaches with conjuctival injection and tearing
$t_{1/2}$	half-life
TAP	transversus abdominus plane
TCA	tricyclic antidepressant
tds	three times a day
TENS	transcutaneous electrical nerve stimulation
TFT	thyroid function test
TMS	transcranial magnetic stimulation
TN	trigeminal neuralgia
TRP	transient receptor potential
U&E	urea and electrolytes
US	ultrasound
VAS	visual analogue scale
VPL	ventral posterior lateral
VRS	verbal rating scale
WBC	white blood cell
WFSA	World Federation of Societies of Anaesthesiologists
WHO	World Health Organization

Section 1

Acute pain

Basic principles of acute pain

Introduction

Pain is defined as 'An unpleasant sensory and emotional experience associated with actual or potential tissue damage, or described in terms of such damage' (International Association for the Study of Pain, 2007).

Acute pain can be defined as having been present for a short period of time (typically <3 or 6 months), or perhaps more usefully as pain that is biologically appropriate (in contrast to chronic pain), that is to say, associated with a healing injury or pathology.

Acute pain is most commonly nociceptive (response to a noxious stimulus) and can be thought of as an evolutionarily conserved set of defensive responses and behaviours whose purpose is to detect and protect the organism from harm. Indeed inherited defects in this system, which cause congenital pain insensitivity, are associated with a shortened life-expectancy, probably because of the increased frequency and severity of injuries that go undetected.

Acute pains play a key role in medical diagnosis with particular characteristic types of pain signifying the onset of organ damage (central crushing chest pain—heart attack, etc.) and the absence of such pains (as in 'silent' myocardial infarction (MI)) may be associated with worse outcomes.

Importantly, however, acute pain causes much suffering and since the earliest recorded times efforts have been made to provide relief through the use of analgesics (i.e. poppy extracts) and this remains a key humanitarian goal. Beyond such laudable ethical goals there are also many, apparently paradoxical, detrimental physiological processes that accompany the acute pain response that impair healing, cause morbidity, and slow recovery. Thus much of modern medical practice focuses on reducing or blocking the acute pain response to improve patient comfort and promote well-being.

Acute pain assessment

There is no objective measure of pain and all assessments attempt to quantify the subjective nature of a person's pain experience. The immediacy of acute pain enables simple rating scales to be reliable measures when used chronologically (see 📖 Self-report measurements of acute pain p.6). This is in comparison to the multitude of instruments used to measure chronic pain.

Frequent assessment of the intensity, time course, and type of pain is essential. It has been shown that such simple measures can significantly improve acute pain treatment and as such they should be recorded alongside other vital signs. As with any clinical symptom or sign, the assessment of pain should not be taken in isolation from other clinical features and the development of new pain should signal a need for re-evaluation of the patient.

Pain characteristics

Generally, most acute pain, particularly in the postoperative period, is nociceptive in nature and either somatic or visceral in origin. These pains may be discriminated on the basis of their different characteristics (see Table 1.1).

Table 1.1 Features of nociceptive pain

	Somatic nociceptive pain	Visceral nociceptive pain
Distribution	Well localized site with dermatomal radiation	Often vague distribution with a diffuse radiation
Character	Variable ranging from aching to sharp	Dull, cramping
Duration	May be constant but have 'incident' breakthroughs, e.g. on movement	Colicky and periodic
Autonomic features	Few autonomic associations	Often associated with autonomic symptoms e.g. sweating, palpitations

Much less commonly, acute pain can arise following damage to nerves (neuropathic). Specific signs and symptoms suggestive of neuropathic pain, such as shooting pains or allodynia, should be sought as these may require alternative treatment strategies.

It is important to note that patients may have more than one type of pain, e.g. somatic pain from a drain site as well as deeper visceral pains. It is also important to assess both pain at rest and on movement. Pain relief that allows movement is often described as 'dynamic analgesia'—of particular importance for procedures such as thoracotomy.

Conclusion

Acute pain can take many forms and can be the sentinel signal of organ pathology. It can respond well to analgesics but there is still evidence of undertreatment. Routine assessment of pain intensity is effective in improving the delivery of analgesic measures.

Measurement of acute pain

Measurement of pain in the postsurgical or trauma patient is essential both to aid diagnosis and to guide analgesia. The most accurate tools for measuring pain are those which rely on patients' reports of their pain level. One of these self-report tools should routinely be used for all post-surgical and trauma patients along with measurements of other vital signs. However, pain is not a sign which can be objectively measured, but is an internal, subjective experience, and consequently pain measurement depends on the patient's ability and willingness to report their pain accurately. It is essential that patients, who may find it bewildering to be asked to rate their pain, are given a clear explanation of what is being asked of them and in particular understand that pain *intensity* is being measured, rather than their overall level of distress or other sensory symptoms.

As well as regular assessments of the patient at rest, it is important that measurements are performed on movement (e.g. deep breathing or coughing), both before and after analgesic administration. The location of the pain and how it varies over time should also be recorded. If the patient has more than one pain, then each site should be measured separately. Pain cannot be measured while the patient is asleep; although a slumbering patient may be comfortable they may, by contrast, be oversedated from their analgesic, therefore they should be periodically roused for assessment.

Self-report measurements of acute pain

Numerical rating scale (NRS)

These usually use an 11-point integer scale (Fig. 1.1), asking the patient to rate their pain between 0 (no pain) and 10 (worst pain imaginable). An NRS is simple and quick to use, easy to understand, and gives reasonably accurate, repeatable data.

Visual analogue scale (VAS)

This consists of a 100-mm horizontal line, with the left-hand end representing no pain and the right-hand end representing the worst pain imaginable (Fig. 1.2). The patient is asked to mark a point on the line to represent their pain. The distance from the left-hand edge to the mark in mm gives a score out of 100. In theory this should produce a continuous variable, in practice VAS has a similar accuracy to NRS, but is more difficult to explain, time consuming to use, and requires a degree of manual dexterity on the part of the patient. There are a number of devices available which use a ruler with a slider to make the process easier.

Verbal rating scale (VRS)

This involves giving the patient a choice of words to describe their pain (e.g. 'none', 'mild', 'moderate', 'severe'). Although simple to understand, there is significant variability between individuals in interpretation of the words, and NRS or VAS is preferable because of greater accuracy and repeatability.

Self-report pain scales for young children

For younger children from about 3 years, pain scales with happy and unhappy faces can be used which represent how much hurt or pain the child is feeling. There are a number of validated scales available (e.g. the

Wong-Baker faces scale Fig. 1.3). The child should be asked to point to the face that best represents how much pain they feel. It is important that the child understands that the face on the left shows no pain or hurt and the face on the right shows very bad pain or hurt and that you are asking about pain, and not about how happy or sad the child feels, or what their face looks like.

Observation of pain behaviour

If the patient is an infant, or unable or unwilling to report their pain, then objective observation of pain behaviour must suffice. There are a number of pain scales, such as the CRIES[1] scale, which are validated for infants. These rely on observed parameters such as facial expression, crying, physical movement, and vital signs. It is important to remember that these are indirect measures, as pain cannot be objectively observed, and they are not as accurate as the self-report measures described earlier. The COMFORT[2] scale is a tool to assess pain in critically ill adults and children in the intensive care or peri-operative setting which uses 8 parameters: alertness, calmness, respiratory distress, crying, physical movement, muscle tone, facial tension, and vital sign measurements.

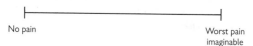

No pain   Worst pain
                                     imaginable

Fig. 1.1 Numerical rating scale (NRS).

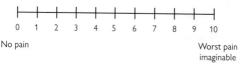

No pain   Worst pain
                                     imaginable

Fig. 1.2 Visual analogue scale (VAS).

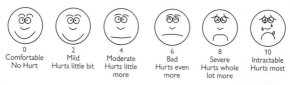

| 0 | 2 | 4 | 6 | 8 | 10 |
| Comfortable No Hurt | Mild Hurts little bit | Moderate Hurts little more | Bad Hurts even more | Severe Hurts whole lot more | Intractable Hurts most |

Fig. 1.3 The Wong–Baker faces pain scale.

References

1 Krechel SW and Bildner J (1995). CRIES: a new neonatal postoperative pain measurement score. Initial testing of validity and reliability. *Pediatric Anesthesia* **5**(1):53–61.
2 Ambuel B *et al.* (1992). Assessing distress in pediatric intensive care environments: the COMFORT Scale. *J Pediat Psychol* **17**(1):95–109.

Examination of the acute pain patient

Patients in pain whether in hospital, the GP surgery or in their own home will be particularly anxious and vulnerable. Thus the clinician should give due consideration for the comfort of the patient, who will be concerned that examination will exacerbate their pain. Respect privacy, confidentiality and modesty.

The pain examination will form a common component of a more general medical/surgical assessment and may provide important diagnostic clues. A change in pain may indicate the onset of new pathology (e.g. compartment syndrome). In some clinical settings the need for urgent treatment of the pain may mean that examination takes place at the same time as the history is taken. You may get little time for a thorough examination.

General observations

These typically increase in pain but also may indicate underlying illness, trends can be more important than spot values and can give an indication of timescale.
- Pulse
- Blood Pressure
- Heart Rate
- Respiratory Rate
- Temperature
- Pain score—should be recorded as a vital sign
- Other signs of pain and distress e.g. grimace, sweating

Specific examination of affected area

This may be a limb or a whole system e.g. respiratory system or CVS for chest pain. Don't forget to examine and document neurological findings carefully in any patient with back or neck pain and limb symptoms.

Look for signs of infection
- Erythema
- Swelling
- Skin temperature changes
- Pus or subcutaneous collection

Look for signs of injury
- Cuts
- Haematoma
- Deformity

Remember your 'surgical/medical sieves' during examination
Exclude causes other than infection and injury such as
- Inflammatory conditions
- Malignancy
- Ischaemia
- Nerve damage
- Metabolic disorder
- Vitamin deficiency

Look for signs of neuropathic pain

While nociceptive pain typically predominates in the acute setting, patients may also experience neuropathic pain. Try to decide whether pain seems neuropathic or nociceptive in origin as this will indicate the need for different treatment strategies. Sensory testing may reveal features that suggest neuropathic origin. Look for:

- Quantitative abnormalities—hyper/hypoaesthesia, hyper/hypoalgesia
- Qualitative abnormalities—paraesthesia, dysaesthesia, allodynia
- Spatial abnormalities—poor localization, abnormal radiation
- Regional autonomic features—colour, temperature and sweating
- Examine for other features associated with neuropathic pain—muscle cramps, motor paresis
- Be aware of phantom phenomena

Note: Allodynia can occur in both neuropathic and nociceptive pain

Definitions

- Hypoesthesia—Decreased sensitivity to stimulation
- Hyperesthesia—Increased sensitivity to stimulation
- Hypoalgesia—Diminished pain response to a normally painful stimulus
- Hyperalgesia—Increased response to a stimulus that is normally painful
- Allodynia—Pain due to a stimulus that does not normally cause pain
- Paresthesia—abnormal sensation. Spontaneous or evoked
- Dysesthesia—Unpleasant sensation. Spontaneous or evoked

Psychological aspects of acute pain examination

Full biopsychosocial assessment is time consuming and not usually peformed as part of the examination in the acute setting but try to make a simple assessment as to whether patient's psychological response is appropriate to clinical situation as well as looking at physiological and biological factors. Look for verbal and non-verbal clues. Watch the way the patient moves and their facial expressions. Make a note of patient's mood and behaviour if relevant.

Pain Scores

An important part of the examination of the acutely painful patient will include a measurement of the patient's pain scores. (See Measurement of acute pain p6 for more details.)

Treatment plan

The end goal of the acute pain examination is not just diagnostic but includes empathetic acknowledgement and the prompt implementation of an appropriate treatment plan.

Detrimental consequences of acute pain

Postoperative pain is often poorly managed and it is increasingly appreciated that this inadequacy in pain control can have a number of significant detrimental effects on patients. A greater awareness of these phenomena should help to motivate staff to provide better analgesia.

Outcomes

Patient suffering and distress

Recurrent publications still highlight an ongoing inadequacy in modern acute pain management with up to 30% of patients suffering moderate to severe pain following elective surgery.

Physiological derangement

Severe pain produces a neurohumeral response with activation of the sympathetic nervous system and the release of catecholamines. This results in a number of physiological changes:

- *Cardiovascular (CV)*: tachycardia, hypertension, increased myocardial oxygen consumption, myocardial ischaemia, impaired peripheral perfusion because of vasoconstriction.
- *Respiratory*: decreased lung volume, atelectasis, decreased cough, sputum retention, infection, hypoxia.
- *Gastrointestinal (GI)*: decreased gastric and bowel motility. Ileus.
- *Genitourinary*: urinary retention.
- *Metabolic*: increased catabolic hormones, e.g. cortisol, glucagon, growth hormone and reduced anabolic hormones, e.g. insulin, testosterone promote loss of muscle mass and a catabolic state.

Psychological

Depression, anxiety, fear, and sleep disturbances.

Chronic pain after surgery

Many patients develop prolonged and problematic pain following elective surgery as a direct result of the surgical intervention. The incidence varies but certain surgical procedures such as thoracotomy (>50%) or hernia repair (>10%) have a particularly high incidence. Surgical, patient, and anaesthetic factors are thought to be important in the development of this complication. It is axiomatic that patients with difficult to manage acute pain are often those who go on to develop chronic pain. It is believed that more aggressive acute pain management immediately postoperatively can reduce the incidence of chronic pain even in high-risk patients (however, robust evidence is lacking at present to support this hypothesis).

Postoperative morbidity and length of stay

Deranged postoperative physiology as a result of uncontrolled postoperative pain can ultimately lead to patient morbidity and delay postoperative recovery. At the very least, patients who are sore are more likely to remain in bed and not be capable of following postoperative regimens such as chest physiotherapy or deep breathing exercises. This can lead to postoperative complications such as chest infection, deep venous thrombosis and coronary events.

Acute pain services

History

Deficiencies in the management of pain following surgery were first high-lighted in the United Kingdom (UK) following the publication of a joint report from the Royal College of Anaesthetists and Royal College of Surgeons in 1990.[1] This suggested that up to 70% of patients were experiencing severe pain on UK wards following elective surgery and led to the introduction and development of acute pain services (APSs) in the UK. Unfortunately, despite an increase in numbers of APSs since that time, ongoing deficiencies in the quality of postoperative pain control continue to be documented.[2] It is thought that a lack of formal teaching about pain management in undergraduate medical and nursing programmes has contributed to this problem.

Structure

An APS should be multidisciplinary with representation from nursing and medical staff, physiotherapy, pharmacy, and secretarial support. The standard model in the UK is a nurse-delivered service which is supported by a doctor, usually a consultant anaesthetist.

Function

The APS carries out daily ward rounds to review postoperative patients and deals with any new patient referrals. This will also often extend to liaison with intensive care outreach for patients with pain that signals a medical deterioration. Although most APSs predominantly deal with surgical patients there is also evidence supporting a role of the APS in providing input to pain management on medical wards and in emergency departments.[2] Provision for out-of-hours cover should also be developed, particularly to cover problems associated with neuraxial blockade.

In addition to managing patients with pain problems, a major role of the APS is education. This involves both the provision of preoperative information for patients and the education of all staff members involved in the management of postoperative pain. The APS should develop and audit evidence-based, standardized protocols for patient care to ensure continuity of practice and the optimum treatment of pain.

Standardized care

Assessment of pain should be built into care pathways and staff should be taught to assess and document pain frequently and to offer analgesia regularly. Pain management strategies are also usually standardized to improve care, often involving the use of multimodal techniques. This standardized approach improves patient management and also tends to reduce the side effects of the intervention through greater familiarity with the techniques and chosen drug regimens. This standardized approach is often reinforced by written guidelines providing a resource for patient care available 24h a day.

Quality control

Most APSs will have an internal audit programme to ensure that practice is reviewed and updated regularly. Research is encouraged to help develop the service. The APS has a pivotal role in developing best practice locally and feeding back information on the efficacy of the service provided. Useful educational resources should be highlighted and examples of excellent practice promoted.

Conclusion

The modern APS is a multidisciplinary team using standardized approaches to assess and manage patients in pain. The service should be evidence-based, frequently audited and reviewed to ensure optimum patient care while endeavouring to limit the side effects of the analgesia used. A properly resourced and motivated acute pain service can have a major positive impact on recovery after elective surgery by reducing suffering and optimizing short- and longer-term outcomes following an acute surgical insult.

References

1 Royal College of Surgeons/College of Anaesthetists (1990). *Report of The Working Party on Pain after Surgery*. Royal College of Surgeons/College of Anaesthetists, London.
2 Acute Pain Management: Scientific evidence (3rd edn) (2010). Australian and New Zealand College of Anaesthetists & Faculty of Pain. Available at http://www.anzca.edu.au/resources/books-and-publications/acutepain.pdf

Anatomy of the pain network

The detection of noxious stimuli is a specialized role of the somatosensory system, which includes multiple sensations such as touch and temperature. The organization of the sensory pathway for all modalities is similar, comprising:

- A receptor, responsible for signal transduction.
- A primary afferent neuron from periphery to ipsilateral spinal cord (or brainstem).
- A second-order neuron which decussates as it ascends to integrative centres in the thalamus.
- Third-order neurons projecting from the thalamus to higher centres.

Pain, however, is something more than just a sensation—it is an experience with both a sensory and an emotional dimension. The strongly aversive nature of pain is important—pain acts as a warning system, which helps prevent tissue damage, or limits damage following injury.

Although we talk loosely of the 'pain pathway', there are actually multiple tracts that carry signals between primary afferent inputs and the brain. Together, these pathways can be considered a pain matrix and can be grouped into two discrete systems: a phylogenetically modern system carrying sensory/discriminative information to higher brain centres; and a more ancient medial system projecting less directly to deep brain centres associated with emotion and arousal. It is this latter pathway that mediates the diffuse, aversive component of the pain experience.

Nociceptor and primary afferent neuron

Nociceptors are the free nerve endings of finely-myelinated A-delta (Aδ) and unmyelinated C-fibres. They belong to primary afferent neurons whose cell bodies lie in the dorsal root ganglion. Nociceptors can be polymodal, i.e. they respond to a variety of stimuli, mechanical, thermal and chemical, but often they will respond preferentially to a limited repertoire of stimuli. Many are apparently dormant (particularly in the viscera) until sensitized by local inflammatory mediators. Aδ fibres carry the initial, sharp 'first' pain felt on mechanical or thermal insult, while C-fibres carry the dull, diffuse ache that follows.

Dorsal horn

Both Aδ and C primary afferents synapse with second-order neurons in the dorsal horn (DH) of the spinal cord—Aδ fibres on laminae I and V and C-fibres on lamina II (the substantia gelatinosa). Aδ fibres synapse directly with the second order neurons that make up the ascending tracts, while C fibres often synapse indirectly via interneurons. Inhibitory connections between the neurons within the DH make it an important site for modulation of the pain signal (see 📖 Endogenous mechanisms for control of pain p.17).

Ascending tracts

After crossing to the contralateral cord (decussation), secondary afferents ascend the spinal cord in several tracts, the most important of which are the spinothalamic and the spinoreticular tracts.

Spinothalamic tract

This arises from laminae I and V of the DH, and ascends anterolaterally in the white matter of the cord. The lateral spinothalamic tract ascends directly to the ventral posterior lateral (VPL) nucleus of the thalamus, subserving the sensory-discriminative aspect of pain perception. This is the phylogenetically modern part of the spinothalamic tract, also known as the neospinothalamic tract.

The older medial spinothalamic tract (or paleospinothalamic tract) is a polysynaptic pathway which sends collaterals to the periaqueductal grey (PAG) matter, hypothalamus, and reticular system in the midbrain before reaching the medial thalamus. This is thought to be responsible for mediating the autonomic and unpleasant emotional component of the pain experience.

Spinoreticular tract

The spinoreticular tract is phylogenetically older than the spinothalamic, arising from the deeper DH laminae VII and VIII and terminating in the reticular formation of the medulla and pons. Diffuse projections via thalamus and hypothalamus subserve the aversive component of pain.

Pain in the brain

The thalamus acts as an integration and relay centre for the pain pathway. From the VPL and medial nuclei, third-order neurons project to higher cortical and to midbrain centres.

The sensory–discriminative component

Third-order neurons project from the thalamus to the primary somatosensory cortex (SI) and secondary somatosensory cortex (SII). SI projections mediate localization of the pain stimulus, with somatotopic representation as for touch sensation (larger areas mapped for more densely innervated areas such as hands and lips). The role of SII is not so clear, though it may play a role in localization, and possibly encoding of stimulus intensity.

The affective–aversive component of pain

The most important projections are those to the limbic system, the insula and anterior cingulate cortex (ACC). The limbic system consists of a series of functionally related, phylogenetically ancient structures, associated with emotion, behaviour, and memory (e.g. amygdala, hippocampus, and hypothalamus). The ACC has a number of functions, including attention and response selection.

Descending pathways

In addition to the ascending tracts, the spinal cord also carries descending pathways that serve to modulate onward transmission of the pain signal at the DH, so called 'descending control systems'. Both inhibitory and facilitatory signals are carried from the integrating centres in the PAG via brainstem relays in the rostroventromedial medulla (RVM) and the pontine tegmentum (noradrenergic neurons) (see 📖 Physiology of pain transmission, p.16) to the DH.

Physiology of pain transmission

Pain warns us of impending or actual tissue damage, but the relationship between the severity of tissue injury and the magnitude of the pain response is non-linear and often unpredictable. Soldiers on the battlefield often report feeling no pain at the time of serious trauma, and most of us will be familiar with the surprisingly painless sporting injury that only begins to hurt some hours after the event. Conversely, skin may be rendered exquisitely tender by sunburn, and anticipation of pain can make insertion of an intravenous (IV) cannula an excruciating experience for the anxious patient. These discrepancies arise because the pain signal is subject to modulation at every level, from the periphery to the brain.

Physiology of nociceptors and peripheral sensitization

Nociceptors express receptors for a variety of molecules that activate and/or sensitize the receptor. This field has exploded recently with the discovery of classes of molecules expressed on primary afferents that are able to transduce physical and chemical stimuli; such as TRP (transient receptor potential) channels and the ASICs (acid-sensitive ion channels). Indeed the TRP channels have been identified as being the receptors for capsaicin (the hot component of chilli peppers, TRPV1), menthol (TRPM8), and garlic (TRPA1), accounting for the thermal sensations evoked by these chemicals. These polymodal sensors also detect changes in pH, temperature, and mechanical stretch. The nociceptor endings also contain receptors for classic inflammatory substances such as 5HT (5-hydroxytryptamine, serotonin), bradykinins and histamine (resulting in direct activation), substance P, leukotrienes, and prostanoids (producing sensitization). The nociceptor primary afferents also express specialized Na^+ channels, the tetrodotoxin-resistant NaV1.8 and NaV1.9 channels.

Following tissue injury, inflammatory mediators cause the skin surrounding the injured area to become hot and red, and an area of lowered threshold to mechanical and thermal pain can be mapped around the injury site. This phenomenon is known as primary hyperalgesia, and represents peripheral sensitization of local nociceptors.

Physiology at the dorsal horn and central sensitization

While most of the special senses adapt to an ongoing stimulus (e.g. accommodation to bright light or loud noise), thereby reducing perception, repeated noxious stimulation leads to enhanced perception of pain, known as hyperalgesia. This can happen in the periphery, as described earlier, or centrally, for example at the DH.

Under normal circumstances, a transient noxious stimulus at the periphery generates an action potential that propagates to the termination of the afferent fibres in the DH. Depolarization of the terminals leads to release of glutamate, which crosses the synaptic cleft to activate the postsynaptic AMPA (α-amino-3-hydroxy-5-methyl-4-isoxazole-propionate) glutamatergic receptors. Na^+ influx and postsynaptic depolarization follows, and the impulse propagates along second-order neurons.

Following sustained noxious input, neuropeptides (such as substance P and neurokinins A and B) are released along with glutamate. These produce sustained postsynaptic depolarization, permitting NMDA (N-methyl-D-aspartate) glutamatergic receptor activation. NMDA activation results in a large Ca^{2+} influx, initiating a biochemical cascade that eventually results in the hyperexcitable state of central sensitization. This is responsible for a secondary area of hyperalgesia around an injury site. This can be a transient phenomenon (hours), but ongoing noxious input can result in neuroplastic changes, including gene induction and synaptic strengthening. These mechanisms may be important in chronic pain states.

Endogenous mechanisms for control of pain

Melzack and Wall's gate control theory

The activation of nociceptors by a noxious stimulus does not invariably result in the perception of pain. Gate control theory postulates that onward transmission of noxious afferent signals can be blocked at a spinal level by inhibitory interneurons—specifically, large A-fibre input (proprioceptive touch) can decrease the response of DH projection neurons to C-fibre nociceptive afferents. This is probably the reason why we instinctively rub an injured extremity and forms the basis of TENS (transcutaneous electrical nerve stimulation) therapy.

The exact neurophysiology behind this phenomenon is controversial, but the principle is a useful one that applies to the pain system as a whole—onward transmission depends on the balance of inhibition and facilitation at various points of integration along the path from transduction to perception.

Segmental inhibition at the dorsal horn

Non-opioid inhibitory neurotransmitters at the DH include GABA, glycine, and monoamines such as noradrenaline and 5-HT. These can act presynaptically on primary afferents, reducing glutamate release, or postsynaptically, limiting postsynaptic depolarization.

Inhibitory interneurons within the DH are normally activated to attenuate incoming pain signals, prevent uncontrolled spread of pain impulses, and block cross-talk between nociceptive and other afferent inputs.

Supraspinal inhibition—the PAG-RVM system

Electrical stimulation of the grey matter surrounding the cerebral aqueduct of the third ventricle—the PAG—produces profound analgesia with no effect on non-noxious touch or thermal sensation. The PAG is an integrating centre for a supraspinal inhibitory pathway, receiving inputs from higher centres, such as the amygdala, hypothalamus, and forebrain, and sending inhibitory projections to the DH via the pons and medulla. As well as opioids, 5-HT and noradrenaline are important neurotransmitters in this system.

Endogenous opioids

Opioid receptors (mu, delta, and kappa) are inhibitory, and can be activated by both their respective endogenous ligands (the endorphins, enkephalins and dynorphins), or exogenous opioids (see 📖 p.20). Opioid receptors are found in high concentrations at the DH and throughout the higher pain matrix.

Attention, emotion, and pain

Pain perception can be reduced by the performance of cognitively demanding tasks (attentional modulation), and by inducing high levels of emotional arousal. These effects may be mediated by the descending control systems. Conversely, a descending activating pathway can enhance transmission at the DH. Inputs to this pathway from limbic system structures may explain some of the lowered pain threshold associated with anticipation and anxiety.

Pharmacology: opioids

An opioid is a chemical substance that has morphine-like action in the body. The term opiate refers to the natural opium alkaloids and their semi-synthetic derivatives.

Opioid receptors

Opioids bind to specific opioid receptors (mu, kappa, and delta; see Table 1.2) located in the central nervous system (CNS), spinal cord, and the periphery. Opioid receptors are G-protein coupled receptors which have similar inhibitory actions. It appears that most of the beneficial and detrimental effects of therapeutically used opioids are mediated by actions at mu receptors.

Endogenous opioid peptides

These are opioid peptides produced naturally in the body and include B-endorphins, enkephalins, dynorphins, and endomorphins. The most widely distributed opioid peptides possessing analgesic activity are met-and leu-enkephalin. The basic structural unit of all endorphins includes the following amino-acid sequences:

- Met-enkephalin: Tyr-Gly-Gly-Phe-Met.
- Leu-enkephalin: Tyr-Gly-Gly-Phe-Leu.

Mechanism of action

All opioids act at opioid receptors which are predominantly located at presynaptic sites and their stimulation leads to inhibition of neurotransmitter release. The receptors are linked to $G_{i/o}$-proteins, which inhibit adenylyl cyclase and decrease the production of cAMP, and lead to activation of K^+ channels and blockade of Ca^{2+} channels.

Classification

Opioid analgesics can be classified on the basis of their actions at opioid receptors.

- **Full agonists**: these agents produce the maximum possible effect upon binding to the receptor, if given at a high enough dose. Morphine, fentanyl, alfentanil, diamorphine, and pethidine are all classed as full agonists.
- **Partial agonists**: these agents produce a submaximal effect even in high dose. In the presence of high concentrations of full agonists, they effectively act as competitive antagonists and some can even precipitate withdrawal. Buprenorphine, pentazocine, nalbuphine, and butorphanol are examples of partial agonists.
- **Antagonists**: these agents exhibit high affinity but no intrinsic activity at the receptor site. Opioid antagonists include drugs like naloxone and naltrexone.

Table 1.2 Opioid receptors

Receptor	Agonist	Location	Function
Mu (OP3)	β-endorphin Endomorphin Morphine Pethidine Methadone Fentanyl	Brain: • Cortex (laminae III, IV) • Thalamus • PAG Spinal cord: • Substantia gelatinosa	Supraspinal and spinal analgesia Dependence Respiratory depression Constipation Euphoria
Delta (OP1)	Leu-enkephalin Met-enkephalin	Brain: • Pontine nucleus amygdala • Olfactory bulbs • Deep cortex	Analgesia Respiratory depression Euphoria Dependence
Kappa (OP2)	Dynorphin Morphine Pentazocine Nalorphine Nalbuphine	Brain: • Claustrum • Hypothalamus • PAG Spinal cord: • Substantia gelatinosa	Analgesia Sedation Meiosis

Pharmacological effects

Analgesia

Opioids are used for treatment of moderate to severe pain from all sources. Poorly localized visceral pain is relieved better than sharply defined somatic pain. Likewise, nociceptive pain is more responsive to opioids than neuropathic pain. The other dimensions of pain (apprehension, fear, autonomic effects) are also suppressed.

Sedation

Drowsiness and indifference to surroundings occurs initially without motor incoordination and ataxia. Higher doses progressively cause sleep and coma.

Respiratory depression

This is a dose-dependent effect by a direct action on the respiratory centre; both rate and tidal volume are decreased. The central neurogenic, hypercapnoeic, and hypoxic drives are suppressed in succession at increasing doses.

Cardiovascular effects

Morphine usually causes a mild bradycardia, probably as a result of decreased sympathetic drive. Vasodilatation occurs due to depression of vasomotor centres, by histamine release, and by a direct action on vascular tone.

Gastrointestinal effects

Constipation is a prominent feature of opioid use and tolerance does not develop. Decrease in propulsive contractions and secretory activity occurs throughout the gut. The resting tone in smooth muscles, particularly the sphincters, is increased. This causes delayed gastric emptying.

Mood and subjective effects

Patients in pain and anxiety may experience euphoria, while in the absence of pain, dysphoria may occur. There is usually a loss of apprehension, a feeling of detachment, mental clouding, and an inability to concentrate.

Nausea and vomiting

This occurs predominantly through an action at the chemoreceptor trigger zone in the medulla. But there is also a peripheral effect on delayed gastric emptying. Tolerance may develop on repeated dosing.

Histamine release

Morphine causes release of histamine from mast cells and produces bronchospasm and hypotension in susceptible individuals. Localized pruritus is common and it can become widespread.

Ocular effects

Meiosis is caused by stimulation of the Edinger–Westphal nucleus.

Hormonal effects

The release of adrenocorticotropic hormone (ACTH) and gonadotrophic hormones is inhibited by morphine, while antidiuretic hormone (ADH) secretion is increased.

Muscle rigidity

Rigidity of the thoracic wall or generalized muscle rigidity can occur with morphine and other opioids. It is typically related to bolus administration of potent opioids (e.g. remifentanil). The effect is mediated centrally and can be reversed with naloxone or overcome with muscle relaxants (in the perioperative setting).

Tolerance and dependence

Tolerance results from reduced drug effects through receptor desensitization. Many effects of opioid receptor activation show rapid tolerance including mood, itching, urinary retention, and respiratory depression. However, tolerance to analgesia occurs more slowly and constipation never shows tolerance. There is evidence that tolerance may be attenuated by co-administration of NMDA antagonists such as ketamine.

Dependence is characterized by unpleasant withdrawal symptoms that occur if opioid use is abruptly discontinued after tolerance has developed. This dependence makes patients unwilling to discontinue opioids. The withdrawal symptoms include dysphoria, sweating, nausea, depression, severe fatigue, vomiting and pain.

Rules for safe use of opioids

- Starting dose: should be small and titrated to response.
- Titration: should be done incrementally and patients should be monitored closely for the development of side effects.
- Patients on opioids will require vigilant long-term follow-up.
- Anticipate side effects and prophylactically administer laxatives and antiemetics (depending on the setting).

Opioid-induced hyperalgesia

Opioid-induced hyperalgesia is a recently described phenomenon associated with the long-term use of opioids. Individuals taking opioids can develop increasing sensitivity to noxious stimuli or evolve a painful response to non-noxious stimuli. This phenomenon may result from changes in NMDA receptors in the DH of the spinal cord. It should be suspected in patients whose pain changes in nature while on opioids or whose pain intensifies as the dose of opioid is increased. Treatment is by withdrawal of opioids (gradually).

Summary

Opioids are proven strong analgesics which can be used to treat moderate to severe pain. They have a well characterized side-effect profile and their dosing should be tailored to minimize side effects often through the coadministration of opiate-sparing adjuncts or with antiemetics and laxatives.

Pharmacology: non-steroidal anti-inflammatory drugs

Non-steroidal anti-inflammatory drugs (NSAIDs) have analgesic, anti-inflammatory, and antipyretic properties. At lower doses, NSAIDs are good for mild to moderate pain and higher doses have an anti-inflammatory effect. The analgesic property has a ceiling effect (higher doses do not result in enhanced pain control) unlike the incidence of side effects.

The classification of NSAIDs is shown in Table 1.3.

Table 1.3 Classification of NSAIDs

Group	Class	Drug
Non-specific COX inhibitors	Salicylates	Aspirin
	Acetic acid derivatives	Diclofenac, ketorolac, indometacin
	Anthralinic acids	Mefenamic acid
	Proprionic acids	Ibuprofen, naproxen
	Oxicams	Piroxicam, tenoxicam
Specific COX-2 inhibitors	Pyrazoles	Celecoxib, rofecoxib

Mechanisms of action

Peripheral mechanism

Cellular damage results in the production of prostaglandins, which sensitize afferent neurons (nociceptors) to noxious stimuli such as chemical, heat, and mechanical pressure. NSAIDs work, at least in part, by inhibiting cyclo-oxygenase, the enzyme that converts arachidonic acid to prostaglandins. Two subtypes of cyclo-oxygenase enzyme have been identified: COX-1, the constitutive form and COX-2, the inducible form. The various physiological roles of prostaglandins including gastric mucosal protection, renal tubular function, bronchodilatation, and production of endothelial prostacyclin and platelet thromboxane are mainly mediated by COX-1. Tissue damage induces COX-2 leading to production of prostaglandins that cause pain and inflammation. Conventional NSAIDs inhibit COX-1 and COX-2 with varying degrees of selectivity. COX-2 selective drugs (coxibs) were developed in an attempt to preserve the analgesic effects of COX antagonism without the detrimental effects on homeostatic processes.

Central mechanisms

There is evidence for an action of NSAIDs at a number of different central sites where the blockade of prostaglandin synthesis is analgesic. In particular, there is evidence of NSAIDs blocking the increased transmission of repetitive noxious inputs at a spinal level. They block a type of sensitization known as wind-up at doses much lower than those required for systemic effects through an indirect action on NMDA receptors.

Efficacy

NSAIDs are effective in treatment of mild to moderate acute pain. The number needed to treat (NNT) of diclofenac 50mg is 2.7, ibuprofen 200mg is 2.7, and intramuscular ketorolac 10mg is 2.6. COX-2 inhibitors are equally effective; the NNT of parecoxib 40mg IV being 2.2. They are also useful adjuncts in the management of severe pain of acute onset and have an opioid-sparing effect. NSAIDs are an integral component of multimodal analgesia. They can be equally effective in the management of chronic pain but their prolonged use is limited by side effects.

Adverse effects

NSAIDs have a number of major and minor side effects at recommended doses.

Renal effects

NSAIDs can precipitate acute renal failure with acute as well as chronic use. Prostaglandins are important for maintenance of renal blood flow and glomerular filtration. Inhibition of prostaglandins by NSAIDs can impair renal perfusion and cause renal failure. In hypovolaemia and dehydration, acute renal failure can occur even with a single dose, especially in the elderly. The risk increases with pre-existing renal impairment, hypovolaemia, hypotension, and use of other nephrotoxic agents and angiotensin-converting enzyme (ACE) inhibitors. COX-2 inhibitors have similar adverse effects on renal function.

Long-term use of NSAIDs is associated with interstitial nephritis, manifested as nephritic syndrome (oedema, proteinuria, haematuria and pyuria).

Gastrointestinal effects

NSAIDs cause a wide range of GI problems including dyspepsia, oesophagitis, gastritis, peptic ulceration, haemorrhage, and death. These complications are predominantly due to inhibition of COX-1 enzyme. The risk increases with higher doses, previous history of peptic ulceration, use for >5 days, concomitant use of aspirin, and age. COX-2 inhibitors have a better safety profile but their use is still relatively contraindicated in patients at risk of ulcers.

Cardiovascular effects

NSAIDS can precipitate cardiac failure, especially in the elderly and those with a prior history of heart disease. This is more likely with drugs like naproxen and piroxicam, which have a longer half-life ($t_{1/2}$). NSAIDs can raise blood pressure in some individuals to a variable extent and hypertensive patients are more susceptible to this side effect.

Antiplatelet effects

Aspirin irreversibly inhibits platelet function for the duration of their lifespan, whereas other NSAIDs reversibly inhibit platelet aggregation. Single doses of NSAIDs do not significantly increase surgical blood loss. However coadministration with aspirin or anticoagulants or the presence of a bleeding diathesis can increase the risk of significant blood loss.

Bone healing

Prostaglandins influence the balance of bone formation and resorption and are essential for bone repair. NSAIDs inhibit prostaglandin formation and experimental studies have implicated them as slowing bone healing. As yet there are no randomized control trials that show this is a clinically relevant problem. However it would seem wise to exercise caution when prescribing NSAIDs in patients at risk of malunion.

Respiratory effects

NSAIDs can precipitate asthma and should be avoided in any patient who has had exacerbation of asthma while taking aspirin or any other NSAID. Patients with allergic rhinitis, nasal polyps, and/or history of asthma are at increased risk of anaphylaxis due to NSAIDs.

COX II inhibitors and cardiovascular effects

Clinical trials like VIGOR[1] and APPROVe[2] have raised questions regarding the CV safety of selective COX-2 inhibitors. An increase in thrombotic events including MI and stroke were seen in patients on rofecoxib. The likely cause is an imbalance in production of prostacyclin and thromboxane A_2 due to selective inhibition of COX-2. Non-selective NSAIDs like diclofenac and ibuprofen have also been shown to have adverse CV effects. In light of these findings it is advisable to avoid both selective and non-selective NSAIDs in patients with risk factors for ischaemic heart disease.

Further reading

Bandolier. Available at: ♒ http://www.medicine.ox.ac.uk/bandolier/

References

1 Bombardier C et al. (2000). Comparison of upper gastrointestinal toxicity of rofecoxib and naproxen in patients with rheumatoid arthritis. *N Engl J Med* **343**:1520–8.
2 Bresalier RS et al. (2005). Cardiovascular events associated with rofecoxib in a colorectal adenoma chemoprevention trial. *N Engl J Med* **352**:1092–102.

Pharmacology: paracetamol

Uses

- Antipyretic.
- Primary simple analgesic (step 1 of WHO ladder, Fig. 2.1).
- Component of multimodal analgesia (e.g. opiate-sparing effect).

History

Discovered by the Bayer company in Germany 1883 but not commercially available until 1947 when the GI side effects of aspirin necessitated a different simple analgesic.

Mode of action

Potent inhibitor of prostaglandin E synthesis in anterior hypothalamus (hence central antipyretic effect) but also appears to block afferent transmission from peripheral nociceptors. The actual mechanism is poorly understood and may involve the inhibition of the recently described cyclo-oxygenase-3 enzyme.

Presentation

Tablets and capsules (dispersible, effervescent, and solid) and suppositories as well as an IV preparation. Often found in compound formulations with codeine (co-codamol), dihydrocodeine (co-dydramol), tramadol, caffeine, or methionine (Paradote®). These compound preparations provide little in the way of improved analgesia or safety above paracetamol alone. Care must always be taken in the prescription of the correct strengths of compound preparations e.g. co-codamol 8/500, 30/500. A compound preparation with dextropropoxyphene (co-proxamol) is available on a named patient basis only because of increased toxicity in overdose.

An IV formulation of paracetamol (propacetamol) has been available in Europe for some time but only recently has an IV paracetamol preparation (Perfalgan®) become available in UK.

The paracetamol dose is a standard 1g every 6h for adults with normal renal and hepatic function. In children, the oral dose is 15–20mg/kg body weight every 4–6h (to a maximum of 4g/day). It is also licensed for neonates at a dose of 20mg/kg loading and then 10–15mg/kg every 6–8h. As with all analgesics it is more effective when given regularly regardless of perceived pain.

Pharmacokinetics

Oral bioavailability is 70–90%, however with rectal administration this falls to 40%. This is mostly due to first-pass metabolism in the liver. It is rapidly (~30min) absorbed from the GI tract. As it is non-ionized and lipid soluble it crosses the blood–brain barrier easily. Less than 5% is excreted unchanged in the urine. The elimination $t_{\frac{1}{2}}$ is nearly 2h. The major route of elimination is by hepatic metabolism to a mix of glucuronide and sulphate conjugates with a small proportion (<5%) to N-acetyl-p-benzoquinone imine (NAPQI) which is a highly toxic by-product. This is conjugated with glutathione to become inactive. Glutathione can become exhausted in paracetamol overdose—with consequent NAPQI hepatotoxicity.

Side effects

Paracetamol has few significant effects on the CV, respiratory, renal, or GI systems when taken in recommended doses, giving it a good safety profile and accounting for its popularity. However, in overdose there is a real risk of delayed hepatic failure. Fatalities have been described with as little as 3g of paracetamol.

Safety

Hepatic damage typically occurs with doses in excess of 15g where NAPQI accumulation causes eventual irreversible centrilobular necrosis. In suspected overdose, plasma levels can be measured and related back to a time nomogram to estimate the risk of toxicity. If the risk line is approached within 10–12h of ingestion then the 'antidotes' N-acetylcysteine or methionine can be given which act as alternative sources of glutathione. Liver function tests are *not* that useful in assessment but it is known that an international normalized ratio (INR) of >2.2 and/or a bilirubin >40mg/L are associated with a very poor outcome. Fulminant hepatic failure because of paracetamol overdose is an indication for super-urgent hepatic transplantation.

Summary

Paracetamol is a safe and effective drug when used within its recommended dosage. It should always be considered as a regular adjunct postoperatively. It reduces opiate requirements hence limiting the unwanted side effects of these drugs. Although its mechanism of action is poorly understood it has reliable pharmacokinetics when given orally or intravenously. In overdose there is a specific antidote which is effective if given within a tight time window.

Pharmacology: local anaesthetics

Uses
- Local analgesia
- Local anaesthesia
- Antiarrhythmics.

History
Topical anaesthesia was first used clinically by the administration of cocaine to the eye for a cataract operation in 1884 by Karl Koller (its effects on sensation had been described by Niemann as far back as 1860.)

Due to the addictive nature of cocaine the synthetic procaine was introduced in 1905 by Einhorn. The first non-ester (i.e. amide) local anaesthetic (LA) was lidocaine introduced in 1943 by Lofgren.

Mechanism of action
All LA agents act in a similar way by blocking the conduction of action potentials in excitable tissues. They produce a reversible blockade of voltage-gated Na^+ channels from the intracellular side of the cell membrane.

LAs are weak bases and exist in an equilibrium between the free base (uncharged) and the protonated form. To reach the internal binding site on the Na^+ channel, the drug must cross the cell membrane (and any layers of insulating myelin). Only the free base is membrane permeant. On crossing the cell wall the LA becomes protonated in the acidic intracellular milleu which allows blockade of the Na^+ channels.

This equilibrium between the free base and the charged protonated state follows the Henderson Hasselbach equation:

$$pKa - pH = \log_{10} \frac{[BH^+]}{[B]}$$

where BH^+ is the ionized form and B is the unionized form of the drug.

As can be seen, the quantity of unionized drug varies with the surrounding pH (increased by alkalosis) as well as the pKa of the drug.

Systemic absorption or administration of LAs results in a predictable cascade of toxicity. This progresses from initial mild CNS symptoms such as perioral tingling, through convulsions, unconsciousness, and coma. These are paralleled by increasing cardiac toxicity resulting in dysrhythmias and subsequent refractory cardiac arrest. Such cardiac arrests are typically refractory to resuscitation because of trapping of LA within rapidly acidifying myocytes. The use of Intralipid® in cases of LA toxicity has shown some promise for recovering such refractory situations.

Chemical structure
Local anaesthetics are either:
- Ester structures (including cocaine, procaine, and amethocaine) are rapidly broken down by local and circulating non-specific esterases giving them a short duration of action. These have a high incidence of allergic reactions (probably due to the metabolite para aminobenzoic acid).

- Amides which typically have a longer duration of action (including lidocaine, bupivacaine, and prilocaine) and very rarely exhibit allergy (often due to the preservative vehicle).

Administration

LA drugs can be given by a myriad of routes: topical, mucosal, infiltration, single nerve block, plexus block, neuraxial block (the last three as a single shot or with a continuous infusion via a catheter). They can rarely be used as an IV preparation for some chronic pain conditions and as a treatment for persistent ventricular tachycardia.

Side effects

Many side effects are predictable (and should be anticipated) as a consequence of the dose of drug administered; e.g. hypotension due to blockade of sympathetic fibres resulting in vasodilatation, and paralysed limbs due to blockade of motor fibres following neuraxial blockade. In systemic toxicity, CNS symptoms (convulsions followed by coma) and cardiac dysrhythmias are most feared.

Prilocaine and benzocaine can cause methaemoglobinaemia although this is usually not symptomatic.

Pharmacokinetics

Local factors

The characteristics, speed of onset, and duration of nerve blockade depend crucially on the pharmacokinetics of the drug in its site of injection. The speed of onset of block depends on the proportion of free base and the lipophilicity of the LA as these facilitate the penetration of lipid membranes. The duration of block relates to both the degree of intracellular trapping and also to effects on local blood flow (vasoconstriction/vasodilation). These factors can be manipulated to speed and prolong the block by choosing the correct agent, warming, adding bicarbonate or vasoconstrictors such as adrenaline.

A selective block of sensory nerve fibres can be produced by careful LA dosing. Because small fibres (C and Aδ) have less myelin they are more susceptible to block by LA. This can produce a sensory block that spares motor function (as in ambulatory labour epidurals).

Absorption

This is directly related to:
- The site of administration—i.e. the higher the associated blood flow then the quicker the systemic absorption.
- The dose of the drug in a relatively linear relationship.
- Any coadministered vasoconstrictor e.g. adrenaline . This will slow the systemic absorption.

Elimination

As mentioned earlier, esters are metabolized in the plasma and liver by non-specific esterases. Amides are hepatically metabolized. There are no active metabolites. Very small amounts of LA are excreted unchanged in the urine.

Common preparations

Lidocaine

- 1% or 2% liquid for injection.
- 4% and 10% for topical/mucosal administration, commonly used for airway anaesthesia.
- Premixed with adrenaline (1 in 80,000 for dental work).
- 5% patches for some chronic pain conditions.

Bupivacaine

- 0.25% and 0.5% for injection (racemic mix of stereoisomers).
- With glucose 80mg/mL = 'heavy' bupivacine used for spinal anaesthesia (the higher baricity gives a postural effect).

Levobupivacaine

- 0.1–0.75% for injection. The levo (S) isomer of bupivacaine—this has a similar profile of action but with less avid binding to cardiac Na^+ channels so may be safer in inadvertent overdose.

Ropivacaine

- 0.2%, 0.5%, 0.75%, and 1.0% for injection. Similar to bupivacaine but slightly less potent. Racemically pure so may have less cardiac toxicity.

Prilocaine

- 1% for injection. Most commonly used for IV regional anaesthesia (Bier's block)
- 4% (or 3% with felypressin) for dental work.

EMLA® cream–eutectic mixture of local anaesthetic—lidocaine + prilocaine. Used for skin analgesia prior to IV cannulation. Especially in paediatrics and for needle phobics. Needs 30–40min of application before anaesthesia is established.

Ametop® gel–tetracaine gel with similar use to EMLA®. Has a faster onset of action.

Safe doses

The maximal safe dose of the commonly used LAs:

- Lidocaine: 3mg/kg (or 7mg/kg with adrenaline).
- Bupivacaine: 2mg/kg.
- Levobupivacaine: 2mg/kg.
- Ropivacaine: 2mg/kg.
- Prilocaine: 5–8mg/kg.
- Amethocaine: 1.5mg/kg.

Summary

LA drugs can provide excellent analgesia and anaesthesia. Effective local/regional block can negate the need for opiates and their associated side effects. Many surgical procedures can be done without the need for general anaesthesia. However, they are intrinsically all potentially dangerous and a good knowledge of their side effects and how to manage and avoid them is mandatory.

General pain management techniques

WHO analgesic ladder

Background

The World Health Organization (WHO) introduced the analgesic ladder in 1986 to provide a global guideline for the treatment of cancer pain (Fig. 2.1). It provides a framework for the use of oral analgesic medications with the aim of achieving adequate pain relief for varying degrees of pain. It has subsequently been adopted by many APSs as providing a model for the treatment of a range of different pains.

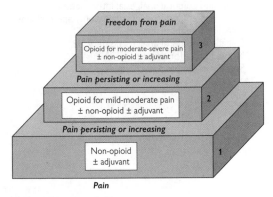

Freedom from pain

Opioid for moderate-severe pain
± non-opioid ± adjuvant **3**

Pain persisting or increasing

Opioid for mild-moderate pain
± non-opioid ± adjuvant **2**

Pain persisting or increasing

Non-opioid
± adjuvant **1**

Pain

Fig. 2.1 The WHO analgesic ladder.

The analgesic ladder suggests the following drugs for use at each level:
• **Level 1:**
  • NSAIDs (aspirin, ibuprofen)
  • Paracetamol.
• **Level 2:** weak opiates for mild to moderate pain (codeine, tramadol).
• **Level 3:** opiates for moderate to severe pain (morphine, oxycodone, fentanyl and methadone).

The WHO coined 5 phrases to emphasize the correct use of analgesics:
• **'By mouth':** oral is the preferred route of administration.
• **'By the clock':** regular administration of analgesics as determined by the pharmacokinetics rather than 'on demand'.
• **'By the ladder':** such that the drugs employed should be escalated in line with the pain reported such that for each patient the pain should be treated with level 1 drugs before escalating to add drugs from level 2 or 3.

- *'For the individual'*: the dose of drug, particularly opiates, should be tailored to the individual.
- *'Attention to detail'*: the effectiveness of the analgesic regimen depends on accurate prescription, administration, and monitoring of analgesic drugs in relation to both effect and side effects.

Adjuvant drugs

At all levels adjuvant drugs can be used to improve analgesia and minimize side effects.
- **Antiemetics**: particularly with opioids.
- **Laxatives**: to alleviate opioid-induced constipation.
- **Corticosteroids**: useful to reduce pain associated with nerve compression or raised intracranial pressure.
- **Psychotropic drugs**: to aid with anxiety, sleep, mood, spasm, and also analgesia.

Successes and limitations

The WHO ladder has been very effective in providing a global guide to the administration of analgesics for cancer pain. It has been shown to be effective and provides a useful political tool to leverage improvements in palliative care. Using the ladder it has been reported that 70–90% of the cancer pain population achieve good pain relief.

The extrapolation of the ladder to other settings has perhaps been less successful, particularly in the acute pain setting.

Examples of common alternative strategies:
- For postoperative pain, the ladder is inverted to start at rung 3 alongside LA techniques before tapering off as healing occurs.
- In acute pain it is less likely to be acceptable to gradually increase the potency of the analgesics in a stepwise fashion. Rather there will be titration of a strong opioid along with non-opioid analgesics to obtain rapid control of pain.
- There is also a trend away from the partial opiate agonists (such as codeine) used in level 2 towards smaller doses of full agonists such as oxycodone. This is because there is little evidence to support the analgesic benefit of combinations of partial opiate agonists with NSAIDs/paracetamol.

Routes of administration

There are many possible routes of administration and clinicians have been imaginative in the ways that they have administered analgesic drugs. Despite this plethora of available routes, oral administration remains by far the most common mode of administration and in general should therefore be considered the standard against which other routes are compared. However, in terms of speed of onset and bioavailability the reference comparison is against IV administration.

Oral

In terms of patient acceptability, simplicity, cost, and convenience, the oral route is the preferred route of administration for analgesics. However, drugs must be absorbed from the GI tract and also withstand first-pass liver metabolism after portal transit. This usually means a delay between administration and onset of analgesic effect as well as reduced bioavailability of drug. Absorption from the gut is variable and may be affected by food, beverages, gastric pH, time of day, and GI pathology such as vomiting or diarrhoea. Most drugs are absorbed in the small intestine and thus gastric stasis can delay absorption considerably. Some formulations are designed to provide a sustained release of their active constituent through enteric coatings and matrix carriers (e.g. prolonged release opiate preparations), thus smoothing peaks and troughs in blood levels. Some analgesics also alter GI function (e.g. opioids—slowed GI transit plus nausea and vomiting; NSAIDs—erosions and ulceration) thus affecting their own absorption. The oral administration of morphine is a good example of a drug that shows large variability between individuals in its absorption, first-pass metabolism, and bioavailability, making it necessary to titrate doses in each patient.

Rectal

The rectal route of administration is a commonly used alternative when oral administration is impractical, unpleasant, or a local effect on the lower GI tract is required (laxatives). Absorption is typically slower than oral as the surface area of the rectum is comparatively small and is markedly affected by faecal loading. The rectum has two routes of venous drainage systemic (inferior) and portal (superior) and thus some of the drug will avoid first-pass metabolism; this can be significant for drugs like morphine, requiring altered dosing compared to oral. It was hoped that rectal administration might reduce the GI side effects of NSAIDs; however, these effects are mediated by systemic drug and thus are found with all routes that provide equivalent plasma levels. Explicit consent is required prior to rectal administration, particularly when given to anaesthetized or sedated patients. The rectal route is contraindicated in patients with diarrhoea or neutropenia (risk of sepsis).

Intravenous

Usually provides the fastest onset of drug action and optimal bioavailability. This therefore represents the most certain way to administer a drug in order to test or establish its effect. However, along with these benefits come drawbacks:

- Worse side-effect profile because of the rapid rise in plasma drug concentration.
- Need for experienced trained staff.
- Increased risk of severe allergic reactions and anaphylaxis.
- Problems with IV access itself—infection, thrombosis, air embolism.
- Phlebitis, pain on injection, and local irritation.

Thus this route of administration is often reserved for care of patients in secondary care (e.g. hospitals) with immediate access to resuscitation teams and equipment.

Because of the rapid peak of plasma drug concentration there is often a similarly steep fall off in effect as the drug is metabolized or redistributed from the circulation. This is particularly the case for opioids and has prompted the introduction of continuous and patient-controlled infusions (see 📖 Patient-controlled analgesia p.40).

Intramuscular

This has been seen as a technique requiring less skill than IV administration yet still allowing parenteral access. With good technique and clear protocols intramuscular (IM) administration can produce effective analgesia. As a consequence, it is commonly employed in settings with lower levels of staffing and monitoring; however, there is a misleading implied assumption of greater safety inherent in this practice. There are a number of potential difficulties with IM injection that make it hazardous and the most common is variable drug absorption. The rate of drug uptake from tissues is dependent on the blood flow. The blood flow within any given muscle is inhomogenous and this varies with time and cardiovascular status. The injection may also be placed either close to (or within) a vessel or in associated adipose tissue with a poor blood supply. Thus absorption is variable and inherently unpredictable, so if an injection of drug proves ineffective it is difficult to decide whether to repeat the injection or wait until absorption is complete. This increases the potential risks of over- and underdosing.

Other risks associated with intramuscular injection include:

- Infected or sterile abscesses (i.e. diclofenac).
- Pain on injection.
- Haematoma (thus contraindicated in the presence of coagulopathy).
- Scaring, fibrosis and necrosis.
- Sciatic nerve injury—following wrong site gluteal injection.

To minimize these risks requires careful attention to technique, appropriate choice of drugs (non-irritant and small volume), and patient selection.

Subcutaneous

The subcutaneous (SC) route has gained favour largely through the administration of opioids and adjuncts using syringe drivers for palliative care. This allows parenteral administration of potent opioids while permitting considerable freedom of daily activity. A SC needle (butterfly) is sited (typically over the abdomen, upper chest, or lateral thigh) and the pump rate adjusted (the starting rate typically based on a conversion of the previous oral opioid dose) with close monitoring. Once an effective dose is found then the patient can be allowed to continue with the infusion in the community. It tends to be used when the oral route is impractical and has the theoretical advantage that the continuous infusion (once equilibration has occurred) should provide a stable therapeutic dose without peaks and troughs (although bolusing is possible for breakthrough pain). In addition it is possible to mix analgesics with antiemetics, antisialogogues, or anxiolytics to enhance the therapeutic effect. The ideal analgesic for SC injection is lipid soluble to facilitate absorption, potent (minimizing the volume of injectate) and non-irritant (diamorphine is commonly employed).

Transdermal and topical

In order to cross the skin a drug must be lipophilic and remain in contact with the skin for a sufficient period of time to allow transfer. This mode of administration has been employed effectively for LAs such as EMLA® cream (eutectic mix of local anaesthetics) which after 20–40min produce a numb area of skin. It is also used for the topical application of NSAIDs to painful areas (although much of the analgesic effect is mediated by systemic drug).

There is a recent trend towards transdermal administration of opioid analgesics with the development of patch technologies that allow controlled release of drug (e.g. fentanyl/buprenorphine). These are preferred by some patients and are advocated as improving compliance and perhaps reducing side effects. They are certainly more expensive than other modes of administration and because of the slow onset of effect and difficulties with titration they should be reserved for patients that have already been stabilized on an opioid. A depot of active drug forms beneath the patch and thus patch removal does not immediately lead to cessation of effect. Hence it can be dangerous to use patches to treat acute pain as the depot may persist long after the pain has resolved leading to a risk of respiratory depression.

Intrathecal/epidural

see Spinal and epidural analgesia: introduction p.42.

Nasal and buccal

Both routes provide a rapid access to the systemic circulation via mucous membranes thus avoiding first-pass metabolism. Both opioids (e.g. buprenorphine) and NSAIDs may be administered by the sublingual route. A lozenge formulation of fentanyl has been introduced for breakthrough pain. The nasal administration of diamorphine has been used effectively in paediatric practice to administer opioids to frightened, uncooperative children especially in accident and emergency areas as an alternative to IV administration (see 📖 p.126 and p.88).

Inhalation

The most commonly used inhaled analgesic is Entonox® (see 📖 p.85). Although there are some advocates of nebulized opioids especially for chronic cough/dyspnoea, there is little evidence to support this practice as being better than systemic administration.

Patient-controlled analgesia

The concept of patient-controlled analgesia (PCA) has evolved to allow patients to directly control their analgesic consumption based upon their pain perception. Many patients prefer to be in control of their own pain relief and PCA allows them to be part of a short feedback loop that can produce better analgesia, with fewer side effects, as compared to more conventional analgesic administration regimens (e.g. IM; see Fig. 2.1). Furthermore, the PCA technique decreases the workload for ward staff and may limit the potential for drug administration errors. Only regional techniques such as epidural or spinal anaesthesia are rated superior to PCA in patient satisfaction surveys.

The term PCA has become synonymous with an IV electronic opioid pump with a patient-controlled bolus facility. However, the PCA principle can be applied to use other delivery routes such as intranasal, transdermal, or, indeed, epidural.

Determinants for use

- Awake, cooperative, and competent patient.
- Appropriate patient selection and education are paramount for success.
- Trained staff.
- Routine, frequent patient monitoring—using PCA-specific charts:
  - Respiratory rate
  - Sedation
  - Pain score (adequacy of analgesia)
  - Pump settings and running balance of volume of drug administered.

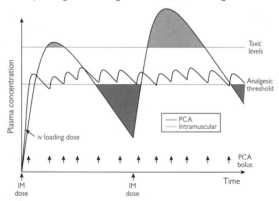

Fig. 2.2 Plasma pharmacokinetics of intermittent intramuscular and PCA dosing with morphine. Note that the IM dosing regime is associated with periods of under and overdosing leading to worse analgesia and side effects (respectively).

Standard PCA regimens and drugs used (Table 2.1)

Morphine is the drug of choice and is available as prefilled syringes, either commercially or prepared by pharmacy. Although other opioids can be substituted to accommodate interindividual differences in the reaction to

Table 2.1 Standard PCA regimens and drugs (all with a lock-out period of 5min)

Drug	Concentration	Bolus
Morphine	1mg/mL	1–2mg
Fentanyl	10mcg/mL	10–20mcg
Pethidine	10mg/mL	10–20mg
Tramadol	10mg/mL	10–20mg
Diamorphine	0.5mg/mL	0.5–1mg

opioids, there is little evidence for superiority of one drug against another across patient populations.

Practicalities of use

- All patients should receive an adequate loading dose of the chosen opioid prior to commencing the PCA.
- A multimodal regimen should be prescribed, including non-opioid analgesics (NSAIDs/paracetamol) to be given regularly wherever possible.
- Can be employed in conjunction with regional or local anaesthesia, such as nerve blocks or epidurals (infusion should not contain opioids).
- Background infusions are generally avoided (increased side effects), except in opioid-tolerant patients or young children (see 📖 Opioids p.126).
- Opioid-tolerant patients should have a background infusion based on their calculated daily intake of morphine or methadone:
  - Oral morphine: parenteral morphine = 2:1 (e.g. 20mg oral morphine = 10mg IV/SC/IM morphine).
  - Oral methadone: parenteral morphine = 1:1 (e.g. 20mg oral methadone = 20mg IV/SC/IM morphine).

Side effects and safety

- Nausea and vomiting:
  - Ensure antiemetics are prescribed.
  - Antiemetics such as droperidol, ondansetron, or cyclizine can be added to the PCA syringe but there is little evidence for efficacy.
- Respiratory depression: naloxone should be prescribed for use in the event of an overdose.
- Sedation:
  - Patients often drift off to sleep to be woken up in pain. Consider altering the bolus dose or ensure adequate rescue and regularly administered analgesia are available.
  - Supplementary oxygen is advisable in the perioperative period.
- Pruritus: oral antihistamines or small doses of naloxone (0–100mcg IV) can reverse problematic pruritis.
- Ideally a dedicated, separate IV lumen should be used for a PCA: alternatively a one-way valve should be employed to prevent opioid reflux into the IV fluid line should the cannula become blocked.
- Beware of norpethidine toxicity (with pethidine PCAs), especially in the parturient.
- Use tamper-free pumps with lockable settings/syringe.

Spinal and epidural analgesia: introduction

Central neuraxial blockade is widely used perioperatively either as the sole anaesthetic technique or in combination with general anaesthesia. These blocks are commonly continued into the postoperative period as they can provide an excellent quality of analgesia.

Intraspinal analgesia is an embracing term used to describe both epidural and intrathecal delivery of analgesics. Much of the discussion that follows is applicable to either route, but a clear distinction needs to be made between the two techniques. Intrathecal drug administration delivers analgesics directly into the cerebrospinal fluid (CSF) in the subarachnoid space producing a sensory level, whereas epidural delivery places the drug into the potential space outside the dural sac to provide a segmental block (see ⬚ Fig. 2.3, p.46). Both of these techniques can be done as single-shot injection for a short duration of action or can provide maintained analgesia via indwelling catheters.

Neuraxial techniques are also used in a variety of other settings:

• Preoperative/pre-emptive analgesia: advocated by some to decrease the severity of postoperative pain.
• For labour pains and procedures; e.g. instrumental deliveries (see ⬚ Neonatal pain: treatment p.114).
• Trauma pain such as rib fractures.
• Chronic pain: both malignant and non-malignant.

Known advantages of intraspinal analgesia

• Excellent quality of analgesia.
• Improved patient satisfaction.
• Prolonged duration via infusion or patient-controlled devices.

Putative benefits

• Reduced postoperative respiratory complications, particularly in patients with pre-existing respiratory disease.
• Increased oxygen delivery/demand ratio with less perioperative myocardial ischaemia.
• Attenuation of perioperative stress response.
• Improved peripheral flow (vasodilatation) with reduced vascular graft occlusion rates.
• Can facilitate bowel recovery after abdominal surgery.

Risks

Side effects

• Hypotension secondary to sympatholysis.
• Nausea and vomiting.
• Motor blockade (with higher concentrations of LA).
• Pruritus (commoner with opioids).
• Urinary retention (incidence higher with opioids).

Complications

• Failure of technique—inadequate analgesia (5%).
• Postdural puncture headache—after inadvertent dural tap with a Tuohy needle. Incidence 0.5–1% of all attempts. Headache in >50%.

- Subarachnoid headache following lumbar puncture (1:20–1:200 depending on needle diameter and profile).
- Neurological damage (1:10,000–1:200,000):
  - Spinal nerve root trauma.
  - Cauda equina syndrome (associated with hyperbaric 5% lidocaine and preservatives).
- Total spinal anaesthesia (CV collapse and respiratory arrest).
- Infection—abscess, meningitis, arachnoiditis.
- Epidural haematoma.
- Masking of limb compartment syndrome.
- Pressure sores secondary to inadequate patient care, peripheral hypoperfusion, immobility, and numbness.
- Drug-related adverse reactions, including LA toxicity (see ▢ Side effects p.31) and anaphylaxis.

Drawbacks

- Insertion requires technical expertise and aseptic technique.
- Patient requires IV access.
- Demand on APS:
  - Sufficient trained and competent nursing staff to monitor patients and manage/flag problems.
  - 24-h medical staff coverage with anaesthetist support.
  - Guidelines, protocols, and audit of complications.

Contraindications

Absolute

- Absence of patient consent
- Bleeding diathesis
- Local infection around injection site
- Allergy to LAs
- Psychosocial issues
- Hypotension and hypovolaemia.

Relative

- Systemic infection or bacteraemia
- Mild coagulopathy.

Patients on anticoagulants e.g. heparin/warfarin, should have their clotting corrected prior to central neuraxial blockade (or removal of catheter).

Spinal and epidural analgesia: anatomy and technique

Anatomy

The brain and spinal cord are covered by 3 meningeal layers; the dura, arachnoid, and pia. The spinal cord is ensheathed by the pia and surrounded by the CSF held within the arachnoid membrane. The arachnoid and the dura are closely apposed. Thus within the dural sac are found the spinal cord (above L2), nerve roots, and filum terminale. The epidural space is outside the dura; the subdural space is the potential space between the dura and the arachnoid; and intrathecal or subarachnoid injections are made direct into the CSF.

The epidural space surrounds the dural sac with the following borders:
- Superior: fused periosteal and spinal layers of dura at foramen magnum.
- Posterior: ligamentum flavum, vertebral laminae.
- Anterior: posterior longitudinal ligament.
- Lateral: medial vertebral pedicles and intervertebral foramina.
- Inferior: epidural space continues into sacrococcygeal ligament.

Contents of epidural space
- Exiting nerve roots
- Venous plexuses and arteries
- Fat, lymphatics, connective tissue.

Useful landmarks
- L3/4 intervertebral space at level of iliac crests ('Tuffier's line').
- T8 spinous process at tip of scapula.

The epidural space is at its widest in the lumbar region where it measures 5–6mm in depth at the L2/3 interspace, when the spine is flexed.

Technique for epidural injection (Fig. 2.3)

Requirements
- Aseptic technique.
- Trained assistant, monitoring and resuscitation equipment.
- LA for infiltration of skin.
- Epidural needle ± catheter: adult Tuohy needle (16G or 18G) has a blunt, contoured bevel with stylette and an 8-cm shaft.
- Catheter passed via needle into the epidural space (3–5cm in space).

Patient positioning
- Sitting or lateral.
- Fully flexed spine ('fetal' position, if lateral).
- Epidurals may be inserted in awake or anaesthetized patients. However it is considered better practice to have patients awake, to alert the operator to potential nerve damage or needle misplacement.

Approach

- Midline: care needed to identify midline accurately.
- Paramedian: useful at levels T3–9 (acute angle of spinous processes).
- Cervical: radiological imaging usually required.
- Caudal: between sacral cornua (can be done with patient prone).

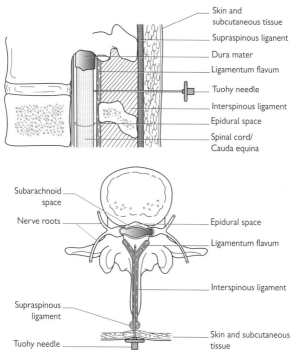

Fig. 2.3 Anatomical approach to the epidural space.

Loss of resistance principle

Employs a low resistance syringe, filled with saline/air, attached to epidural needle. When performing a midline lumbar epidural block, the needle will advance through:

- Skin and SC tissue.
- Supraspinous ligament—dense and offers some resistance.
- Interspinous ligament—often more laxity.
- Ligamentum flavum—increased resistance and more drag.

- A sudden loss of resistance signals entry into the epidural space.
- The drug or catheter should flow or feed freely into the epidural space.

Checks and precautions

- Intrathecal placement—aspirate to test for CSF flow, test dose.
- Intravascular placement—blood aspirated (beware false negative), test dose
- Brief paraesthesia is common; however, if prolonged then cease injection, remove needle/catheter, and suspect nerve injury. Unwise to continue with planned anaesthetic/procedure if pain persists. Make regular neurological assessment, consider need for imaging and/or referral.

Technique for spinal injection

Injections are made into the CSF below the level of the 2nd lumbar vertebra, to avoid damaging the spinal cord. A variety of different spinal needles are available but the incidence of post-spinal headache is reduced if a small diameter (e.g. 25G) needle with a pencil point tip is employed.

The same positioning and aseptic techniques are used, as described for epidurals (see earlier). The spinal needle is inserted via the midline or paramedian approach and a distinct 'pop' can often be felt as the needle passes into the dural sac. Clear CSF should be freely aspirated.

Single-shot spinal injections are not much used as an analgesic technique (except in the immediate perioperative period or labour). However, indwelling catheters have been used for continuous spinal analgesia and these can be tunnelled to a SC reservoir pump for long-term infusions (see 📖 Intrathecal and epidural drug delivery systems p.204).

Spinal and epidural analgesia: drugs

Local anaesthetic agents

These produce the characteristic nerve block by preventing action potential conduction along axons (see 📖 p.30)

Amide group

- Bupivacaine: in common use, supplied as 0.25% or 0.5% concentration, and as racemic mix or L-stereoisomer (less cardiotoxic). Intermediate duration of action.
- Ropivacaine: pure L-stereoisomer so greater cardiac safety than bupivacaine. Less potent but with otherwise similar properties.
- Lidocaine: shorter acting with best safety profile.

Ester group (higher incidence of allergic reactions)

- Procaine
- Amethocaine.

> Whenever LA agents are injected via the epidural route, it is recommended that an initial bolus test dose is administered. This is to check for inadvertent intrathecal (leading to high block) or intravascular placement.

Opioids

There is a high density of opioid receptors in the spinal cord, most being found in the DH where they are involved in nociceptive pathways. Thus intraspinal administration of opioids can have an analgesic effect which is synergistic with LAs. This synergy allows the dose of LA to be reduced, minimizing motor block and sympatholysis. Intraspinal opioids also have systemic and central actions producing complications:

- Nausea and vomiting
- Pruritus
- Sedation
- Respiratory depression
- Urinary retention and constipation.

Opioids in common neuraxial use include:

- Fentanyl
- Diamorphine
- Morphine.

The lipid-solubility of each agent determines their speed of onset and their redistribution both systemically and to higher centres.

Corticosteroids

These are used epidurally for their anti-inflammatory actions, especially in chronic conditions such as lumbar radiculopathy (e.g. triamcinolone). Care is needed to avoid intrathecal administration because of the risk of arachnoiditis. Repeated injections usually limited to 3/year to avoid systemic steroid side effects.

Others

- α-agonists: adrenaline or clonidine can act to both prolong duration of action by vasoconstriction and produce a synergistic analgesic action by a direct action on spinal α2 adrenoceptors.
- Ketamine: NMDA receptor antagonism.
- Baclofen: $GABA_B$ agonist, usually for spasticity.

Spinal and epidural analgesia: safety

These neuraxial block techniques are all intrinsically potentially dangerous and therefore should be administered with due care and attention by trained staff in a safe environment to minimize these risks.

Principles

- Clearly label all epidural giving sets and catheters; errors can be fatal.
- Only staff trained in the use of these devices should be allowed to operate them.
- Agents used in neuraxial blockade should ideally be preservative-free to avoid the risk of chemical arachnoiditis and neurotoxicity.
- Always cross-check all drugs given neuraxially, as certain drugs such as vinca alkaloids are fatal if given intrathecally. The connectors for neuraxial injections are being systematically redesigned to make interconnection with intravenous drug lines less likely.
- Never inject LA if pain is elicited during injection.
- Always aspirate from an epidural catheter prior to injecting any agent to identify intravascular or intrathecal migration of the catheter, also give divided doses to reduce risk.

Caution: Signs of local anaesthetic toxicity

- ***CNS:*** circumoral tingling, tinnitus, drowsiness, convulsions and coma.
- ***CVS:*** hypotension and bradycardia, refractory ventricular fibrillation, and tachyarrhythmias leading to cardiac arrest.

▶ Be aware and respect the maximum safe doses for each agent.

Management of local anaesthetic toxicity

- Awareness and prevention more effective than cure.
- Basic life support with advanced life support as indicated.
- Recent guidelines recommend the early use of IV high-concentration lipid (Intralipid®), which is reported to help reverse cardiac arrest secondary to bupivacaine toxicity.

Nerve blocks for acute pain

LA nerve blocks can be used in the acute setting to:
- Provide temporary pain relief whilst awaiting definitive procedure, e.g. femoral nerve block for fractured neck of femur.
- Decrease intraoperative analgesic requirements.
- Avoid the need for general anaesthesia altogether.
- Attenuate the surgical stress response.
- Reduce postoperative analgesic requirements.
- Speed discharge from hospital.

Advantages include:
- Usually simple to perform.
- Low rate of complications and thus relatively safe.
- High patient satisfaction.
- Decreased drug-related side effects, e.g. opioid-induced nausea and vomiting.

Disadvantages
- Acquired skill requires learning curve.
- Can sometimes be technically challenging, e.g. in obese patients.
- Some blocks require specialized equipment, e.g. nerve stimulator.
- Time-consuming.
- Often requires skilled assistant—impact on resources and manpower.

Risks include:
- Intravascular injection
- Agent toxicity
- Nerve damage
- Infection.

▶ **Caution**

It is recommended that regional blocks are performed in awake patients, particularly if a blind technique without the aid of a nerve stimulator or visual aid such as ultrasound (US) is used. This will facilitate the early recognition (and hopefully limitation) of complications such as nerve injury or intravascular injection.

General principles, technique, and requirements
- Informed consent.
- Appropriate clinical area, with adequate facilities including:
  - Oxygen
  - Resuscitation equipment
  - Standard monitoring equipment.
- Equipment check prior to use.
- Failsafe routine to avoid omissions.
- Aseptic, sterile technique throughout.
- Careful aspiration before LA injection—divided doses, injected incrementally.

Identification of the correct location

Most blocks are performed using body surface landmarks, bony promi-nences, and arterial pulsation to guide the initial needle placement. Some then rely on fascial or muscle plane 'pops' to direct the LA into the correct site (e.g. ilioinguinal nerve blocks or transversus abdominus (TAP) blocks). However, there are a number of other methods used to identify the correct location close to nerves:

- Paraesthesia—when elicited in the required territory is an excellent indication of correct needle placement. Patient must be warned in advance of the occurrence of paraesthesia.
- Nerve stimulators use the application of brief voltage or current pulses to elicit muscle contraction when the needle is in close to the nerve. The amplitude of the pulse can be adjusted to give an indication of the proximity to the nerve. Can be used in the unconscious patient.
- US-guided nerve blockade is a recent development driven by improvements in the quality and availability of readily portable US equipment:
  - Improved accuracy of targeting LA.
  - Fewer block failures.
  - Potentially decreased risk of inadvertent intravascular injection and nerve damage.

Specific nerve block techniques

There are countless described approaches to block peripheral nerves and a comprehensive lexicon is beyond the scope of this book. However, it is instructive to describe some representative examples of common plexus, peripheral nerve, and field blocks to illustrate the methodology.

Interscalene brachial plexus block

Indications

- Anaesthesia of whole arm, mostly for shoulder, arm, and forearm.
- Diagnostic tool for chronic pain conditions of shoulder/arm.
- Palliation in acute pain emergencies.

Anatomy

- Brachial plexus provides nearly entire somatic innervation of arm.
- Formed by union of ventral rami of C5–8 and T1.
- Occasionally receives minor contributions from C4 and T2.
- On exiting intervertebral foramina, the roots converge to form trunks, divisions, cords, and terminal nerves.
- 3 distinct trunks form behind and pass between anterior and middle scalene muscles: superior, middle, and inferior (vertical arrangement).
- Trunks run alongside subclavian artery:
  • Superior trunk: mainly from C5–6.
  • Middle: C7.
  • Inferior: C8 and T1.

Technique

- Patient positioned supine with head on pillow turned to opposite side.
- Identify interscalene groove at level of C6 (cricoid):
  • Best identified while sniffing or with head raised.
  • Often able to roll nerve bundle under fingertips.
- Enter skin with needle perpendicular to all planes—end up angled slightly caudad.
- Pop into nerve sheath:
  • Paraesthesia down arm.
  • Elicit deltoid or biceps motor response with nerve stimulator.
- Should be within 25mm of skin.
- 20–40mL of LA depending on block density required—should form a palpable rostrocaudal 'sausage'.

Complications:

- 10–20% fail to achieve full ulnar nerve blockade.
- Phrenic nerve block (up to 100%):
  • Avoid bilateral blocks.
  • Caution in patients with respiratory disease.
- Vertebral artery puncture or injection.
- Epidural, subdural, or intrathecal injection.
- Stellate ganglion block (30–50%), leading to Horner's syndrome.
- Recurrent laryngeal nerve block (30–50%), leading to hoarseness.

Femoral nerve (and '3 in 1') block

From the same injection site it is possible to block either just the femoral nerve or a '3 in 1' combination with the lateral cutaneous and obturator nerves (good for hip surgery).

Indications

- Anaesthesia of anterior thigh.
- Fractures of femoral shaft/neck or patella.
- Postoperative pain relief following thigh, patellar, or knee surgery.
- If combined with sciatic or popliteal nerve blocks, it provides anaesthesia for distal leg.
- Possible to insert a catheter for prolonged blockade.

Anatomy

- Femoral nerve is the largest branch of lumbar plexus—formed from L2–4.
- Descends between psoas and iliacus muscles.
- Passes under inguinal ligament, lateral to femoral artery—Nerve–Artery–Vein–Y-fronts (NAVY).
- Superficial branch is mainly sensory to anterior thigh with motor supply to sartorius.
- Deep branch mainly motor to quadriceps muscle with some sensory supply to knee joint and medial aspect of leg.
- Terminates as purely sensory saphenous nerve.

Technique

- Supine position leg abducted and slightly externally rotated.
- Entry site is 1cm lateral to femoral artery, 2cm below inguinal ligament.
- Using nerve stimulator needle, aim 45° cephalad:
  - Observe for quadriceps twitches (patellar dance).
  - Adjust stimulus intensity to optimize position.
- Inject LA after excluding intravascular placement:
  - 10mL for femoral block.
  - 30mL with inferior digital pressure for 3 in 1.

Complications

- Intravascular injection femoral artery and vein nearby.
- infection—groin crease area.

Intercostal nerve block

Indications

- Rib fractures, chest wall contusion, pleurisy, and flail chest.
- Postoperatively—pericardial window, thoracotomy (T10–2).
- Fractured sternum.
- Prior to chest drain insertion.

Anatomy

- Intercostal nerves are formed from ventral rami of T1–12.
- Usually run subcostally with intercostal vein and artery, in plane between internal and innermost intercostals—variations can occur; US may be a useful tool to aid correct needle placement
- Gives off lateral cutaneous branch before costal angle.
- Can be missed if block placed medial to mid-axillary line.

Technique

Classic approach
- Posteriorly at angle of the ribs, just lateral to sacrospinal muscles.
- With this approach, there is a 5-mm safety margin before the needle enters pleura.
- Usually performed with patient prone.
- Identify inferior border of rib at appropriate level to be blocked (7–8cm lateral to spinous process).
- After instilling local anaesthesia to skin, using fine-bore needle, 'walk' needle caudad off lower edge of rib.
- Whilst cautiously advancing needle, a slight loss of resistance is often encountered upon entering the correct space.
- After aspirating, inject 3–5mL of LA into space; repeat at required levels.

Midaxillary approach
- Increased likelihood of pneumothorax.
- Often misses lateral cutaneous nerve branch.
- Easier in patients unable to move due to pain.

Complications
- Pneumothorax: uncommon in trained hands, often subclinical or asymptomatic (varied estimates, from 0.1–2%).
- Systemic toxicity: large vascular supply means rapid absorption, especially a hazard when large volumes of LA injected.
- Hypotension: likely to occur if central neuraxial spread has followed.

Transversus abdominis block

Indications

Postoperative analgesia for any surgical procedures involving the anterior abdominal wall (e.g. open prostatectomies, appendicectomies, lower segment Caesarean section, and midline laparotomies).

Technique
- Can use blind landmarks and 'pops' or US-guided approach—US guidance reported to improve reliability.
- Entry point commonly at lumbar triangle (of Petit):
  - Anterior border formed by external oblique.
  - Posterior latissimus dorsi and inferiorly iliac crest.
  - Floor formed by internal oblique.
- Lumbar triangle is immediately posterior to midaxillary line—which means that lateral cutaneous branches of intercostal nerves are also blocked, providing full anaesthesia of anterior abdominal wall.
- Using blunt 22G needle, cross through external and internal oblique muscle planes (i.e. two 'pops') where the transversus abdominis plane will be encountered.
- Inject large volume of LA e.g. 20–30mL, after aspirating, on each side (titrate dose of LA depending on patient's size).

Complications

Relatively rare, no serious complications yet reported following the recent introduction of this approach to abdominal wall anaesthesia

Summary

Nerve blocks can offer many advantages in the treatment of acute pain (either before or after the noxious event). However, there are many pitfalls for the unwary so they should be performed in a safe environment according to accepted protocols and only undertaken by practitioners skilled in the recognition and treatment of complications.

Further reading

Allman KG and Wilson IH (eds) (2006). *Oxford Handbook of Anaesthesia*, 2e. Oxford University Press, Oxford.
Tsui B (ed) (2008). *Atlas of Ultrasound and Nerve Stimulation-Guided Regional Anesthesia*. Springer.

Specific clinical situations

Postoperative pain management: overview

Introduction

Postoperative pain continues to be a problem with significant numbers of patients experiencing moderate to severe levels of pain. In addition to being unpleasant for patients, pain is associated with many physiological changes that can adversely affect recovery following surgery. Thus optimal pain management can prevent or reduce many unwanted effects and speed recovery and discharge from hospital. However, this is difficult to achieve as:

- The amount of pain is not directly related to the severity of the procedure.
- Patients show considerable variation in their response to pain treatments.
- Preoperative anxiety, catastrophizing, neuroticism, and depression are associated with higher postoperative pain intensity

Because pain is an individual, multifactorial experience, good pain management often requires a multidisciplinary input from doctors, nurses, physiotherapists, pharmacists, and psychologists—working within the framework of an acute pain team.

A proactive approach to pain assessment and management can reduce pain, increase patient comfort and satisfaction, improve patient outcome, and reduce hospital stay.

The techniques employed during the operation, as well as analgesic medication delivered pre- and postoperatively, can have a major impact on patient outcomes by enabling fast-track care pathways.

Incidence of pain

- 70% of patients have moderate to severe pain at some time in their postoperative course.
- 1–3% experience acute neuropathic pain.
- The incidence of poor pain control appears to be highest following orthopaedic surgery.
- Inadequate postoperative pain control leads to severe pain at home for day case patients.

Pathophysiological effects of acute pain

- The release of catabolic hormones produces breakdown of proteins, muscle wasting, lipolysis, and insulin resistance.
- CV effects include hypertension, tachycardia, myocardial ischaemia, and a lowered ventricular fibrillation threshold.
- An increase in coagulability occurs because of immobility and epinephrine release and leads to an increased risk of deep vein thrombosis (DVT) and pulmonary embolism (PE).
- Abdominal pain produces splinting of the diaphragm and shallow breathing along with a reduced efficacy of coughing. This combination predisposes to hypoxia and an increased incidence of chest infections.
- GI dysfunction, such as ileus, can be induced by opioids but may also be a consequence of pain.

Goals of pain management

- To educate patients and carers about the anticipated pain, treatment strategies, and the techniques used to assess pain.
- To deliver optimal multimodal pain relief.
- To minimize the incidence of side effects and complications.
- To provide efficient, cost-effective pain relief.

Preoperative education

Information

- It is critical to ensure that the patient and the family have appropriate expectations of postoperative pain and the methods for relief.
- Patients given a description of the pain to be expected have less pain, use fewer analgesics, and a have a shorter length of hospital stay.
- Unrealistic expectations can lead to anger, disappointment, and the fear and anxiety that something has gone wrong.
- The total absence of any postoperative pain is not a realistic goal. Therefore the types of pain, their severity, and duration should be explained.

Assessment

It is axiomatic that regular assessment of pain inevitably leads to improved pain management.

- The methods of assessment should ideally be discussed with the patient preoperatively.
- The most reliable indicator of pain is a patient's self-report.
- Patients may be experiencing excruciating pain even while smiling, using laughter as a coping mechanism.
- The assessment of pain should be recorded on a bedside chart and treated as a vital sign.
- The degree of pain relief should be determined after each pain management intervention.

Patient choice

Pain management should involve an individual approach basing the choice of analgesia on the severity and type of pain, and the patient's wishes. It is important to involve the patient in discussions about the methods of postoperative analgesia, particularly where epidural analgesia and PCA are being considered. If the patient is not happy about a particular technique it is unlikely to be successful.

Use of guidelines and protocols

Specialized analgesic technologies, including systemic or intraspinal, continuous or intermittent opioid administration or patient-controlled dosing, LA infusion, and inhalational analgesia should be governed by policies and standard procedures that define the acceptable level of patient monitoring and appropriate roles and limits of practice for all groups of health-care providers.

Postoperative pain management: analgesics

Pre-emptive or preventive analgesia

Premedication

Analgesia can be given to patients prior to arrival in the theatre suite. The oral route is preferred unless there is a clinical contraindication.

Pre-emptive analgesia

This term refers to the delivery of analgesic intervention(s) before the first surgical incision. The rationale is to stop (or obtund) the transmission of the intense nociceptive barrage to the brain that occurs with the onset of surgery. In theory this should prevent sensitization of the neural pathways and reduce the requirement for subsequent postoperative analgesia. There is good evidence from animal studies that this can be effective. However, it has not been possible to unequivocally demonstrate that an analgesic intervention made before surgical incision significantly improves postoperative analgesia.

Preventive analgesia

Preventative analgesia aims to provide a longer duration of effective analgesia in the perioperative period (hours to several days). There is evidence that successful analgesic interventions in this initial perioperative window have a beneficial effect on postoperative pain or on analgesic consumption that exceeds the expected duration of action of the drug.

- NMDA receptor antagonist drugs show preventive analgesic effects. For some procedures the use of ketamine at induction reduces postoperative morphine consumption.
- The severity of pre- and postoperative pain influences the development of chronic postsurgical pain and there is evidence that early analgesic interventions reduce the incidence of chronic pain after surgery.

Pain management should therefore begin prior to surgery and be continued throughout the patient's hospital stay.

Intraoperative pain relief

Good intraoperative pain relief is often the key to success of postoperative pain control. Analgesic drugs should be given early enough (determined by their pharmacokinetics) to ensure sufficient analgesia when the patient is waking from the procedure. A multimodal strategy should be employed, including paracetamol +/– NSAIDs and either an opioid, LA block, or regional blockade.

The World Federation of Societies of Anaesthesiologists (WFSA) analgesic ladder

The WHO analgesic ladder was introduced to improve pain control in patients with cancer by employing a logical strategy to pain management (see 📖 WHO analgesic ladder p.34). The same principles have been adopted and modified by acute pain teams in postoperative pain management. One such scheme is the WFSA analgesic ladder (Fig. 3.1), which has been developed to guide the treatment of postoperative pain. Early postoperative pain can be expected to be severe and may need controlling with strong analgesics in combination with LA blocks and peripherally-acting drugs. As pain is easier to prevent than to bring under control once it has become entrenched then proactive early management is crucial to a good outcome.

The dose of opioid should be increased until pain relief has been

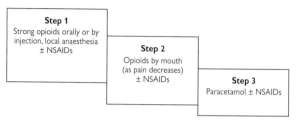

Fig. 3.1 WFSA analgesic ladder.

achieved or side effects prevent increasing the dose further. There is a very large variation in amount of opioid required between patients and because opioids have no ceiling effect they should provide effective analgesia for most surgical procedures. The opioid prescription should allow for the great variation in individual opioid requirements. If side effects prevent increasing the opioid dose further, a different opioid drug should be considered. When increasing doses of opioids are ineffective in controlling pain, a prompt search for new or residual pathology is indicated—also consider neuropathic pain.

Transition from parenteral to oral medication
As a general principle, oral analgesia should be favoured wherever possible. Parenteral injections can cause pain and local trauma that may prevent patients requesting analgesia. Further they increase infection risks for both patients and staff. However, in some instances, the oral route may not be possible because of the nature of the surgery. Rectal, IM, and SC administration all have a time delay and considerable variability in absorption to the circulation and the IV route is usually the most appropriate in the initial perioperative period, allowing rapid loading and titration against effect.

Typically, postoperative pain will decrease with time and the need for drugs to be given by injection should diminish. The second rung on the postoperative pain ladder is the restoration of the use of the oral route to deliver analgesia. Initially, strong IV analgesia may need to be replaced with strong oral opioid analgesia (e.g. morphine sulphate solution® and morphine sulphate (modified release)). The previous parenteral dose in 24h should be calculated and this dose should be given orally in divided doses of a long-acting opioid. A fast-acting opioid should be prescribed for breakthrough pain. This can subsequently be stepped down to combination preparations of weak opioids or smaller doses of strong opioids. Finally, as healing continues, pain may be controlled with simple analgesics such as paracetamol and NSAIDs.

Postoperative pain management: adjuvants

The conventional analgesics may be supplemented with adjuvant drugs that have different mechanisms of action. Postoperative pain management is often limited by side effects such as nausea and vomiting. These agents can act synergistically to improve analgesia and reduce the dose of conventional analgesic required.

Clonidine

α2 adrenergic agonist (oral, IV, epidural, or spinal—typically 1–3mcg/kg) is sometimes given preoperatively and has a number of useful actions including an opioid-like analgesia without some of the characteristic opioid-ergic side effects.

• Sedation and anxiolysis.
• Anaesthetic-sparing and opioid-sparing effect.
• Decreases arterial blood pressure and heart rate.
• Does not produce respiratory depression, itching, or urinary retention.
• Prevents postoperative shivering.
• Decreases nausea and vomiting.
• Lasting postoperative analgesic effect.
• Does prolong postoperative ileus.

Dexamethasone

A glucocorticoid which has been used extensively to reduce swelling following surgery and has been found to be analgesic for some procedures.

• Some types of postoperative pain are reduced, e.g. tonsillectomy.
• There is strong evidence for a reduction in postoperative nausea and vomiting (PONV).
• Reduced convalescence time.
• Attenuates inflammatory responses (C-reactive protein, interleukin-6).
• Opioid-sparing effect has been demonstrated.
• Although prolonged use of steroids is associated with morbidity, the available evidence suggests that a single dose is relatively safe.

Ketamine (IV, IM, or SC)

Ketamine is a NMDA antagonist with a useful pharmacodynamic profile as an anaesthetic or analgesic agent. The NMDA receptor is involved in sensitization of pain circuits and therefore the antagonist is rationally employed as an analgesic adjuvant. Ketamine in subanaesthetic doses is effective in reducing morphine requirements in the first 24h after surgery and also reduces PONV. Adverse effects are typically mild but can manifest as psychomimetic symptoms. The role of ketamine for postoperative analgesia can be useful for challenging cases (particularly by low-dose infusion) but its routine use is still debatable.

Gabapentin/pregabalin

These antiepileptic medications were initially only indicated for the treatment of pain with a neuropathic component. However, recent studies in the perioperative setting have demonstrated a consistent opioid-sparing effect with some reduction in side effects. There is also hope that there may be a corresponding reduction in chronic pain that accompanies their perioperative use but this has not yet been substantiated.

Muscle spasm

Muscle spasm may accompany postoperative pain and responds poorly to opioid analgesia. Diazepam, lorazepam, or baclofen are the agents of choice. Lorazepam may also be helpful when there is an overlay of anxiety that compounds the pain problem or in burns patients.

Smooth muscle spasm

This is a relatively common feature following GI, urological, or biliary surgery. These, characteristically colicky, pains may be eased by the administration of hyoscine (a muscarinic antagonist) to produce smooth muscle relaxation.

Acute neuropathic pain

Neuropathic pain is defined as 'pain initiated or caused by a primary lesion or dysfunction of the nervous system' (see 📖 Assessment of neuropathic pain p.150). Nerve injury occurring in the operative period may present as acute neuropathic pain postoperatively within hours of injury or may be delayed for days or even months. Many patients who develop these pains continue to experience pain at 12 months and early recognition and treatment of these symptoms may reduce the incidence of chronic pain.

Characteristics

Shooting, stabbing, or burning pain that is distinct from early pain and is particularly unpleasant.

Treatment

With neuropathic pain medications (see 📖 Antidepressants, Anticonvulsants p.170, 172) such as amitriptyline 10–30mg at night, or an anticonvulsant, usually gabapentin 300mg tds increasing to 800mg tds. Both of these drugs may also be useful when postoperative pain is poorly controlled.

Postoperative pain management: regional techniques

Regional analgesia

Epidural analgesia (see 🕮 Spinal and epidural analgesia p.42)

For many surgical procedures, particularly upper abdominal and thoracic, trials of epidural analgesia consistently demonstrate superior analgesia when compared to parenteral opioids.

Several benefits of epidural anaesthesia/analgesia in terms of reducing morbidity have been demonstrated in selected patient groups. They include:

- Reduced blood loss
- Improved bowel mobility and gut function
- Fewer cardiac ischaemic events
- Improved cough
- Reduced atelectasis and pulmonary infection
- Improved quality of life.

The effects of continuous postoperative LAs on the bowel may be particularly beneficial in terms of reducing ileus and hospital stay. The use of epidural analgesia improves graft survival in peripheral vascular disease and should be encouraged for the first 48h following surgery.

It is not possible to show the benefit of any anaesthetic or analgesic option in isolation in terms of its effect on mortality, given the safety of modern anaesthesia. This is due to the relative rarity of catastrophic outcomes and the role of integrated approaches to improving surgical outcome.

There are also well-established risks associated with epidurals including hypotension, infection, haematoma, and pressure sores. They impede mobilization when used for orthopaedic surgery. Furthermore, a significant proportion of epidurals do not function well and there is a relatively high failure rate (~5%).

The use of patient-controlled epidural analgesia (PCEA) reduces amount of drug given and minimizes side effects of epidural analgesia, but it does not provide as good analgesia as an infusion, particularly overnight.

Spinal analgesia (see 🕮 Spinal and epidural analgesia p.42)

Usually intrathecal LA or opioid is used as a single-shot technique but may be used as an infusion into the postoperative period.

Postoperative pain management: other techniques

There are many other approaches to control postoperative pain including:
- Intra-articular opioids and NSAIDs (see 📖 Pharmacology: non-steroidal anti-inflammatory drugs p.24)
- Peripheral nerve blocks, plexus blocks/infusions (see 📖 Specific nerve block techniques p.52)
- Intraoperative cryotherapy for thoracotomy.

Non-pharmacological methods

The techniques include reassurance, instruction in coughing, deep breathing, turning and ambulation, TENS, acupuncture, relaxation, psychology, and massage. These can be used to supplement conventional techniques in the following circumstances:
- Incomplete pain relief
- Fear and anxiety
- In those wishing to limit drug medication
- For those keen on the specific techniques
- Procedure related pain.

Transcutaneous electrical nerve stimulation (TENS)

TENS has been shown to reduce pain and improve mobility following orthopaedic, lower abdominal, and thoracic surgery. It reduces morphine requirements and therefore opioid side effects.

Acupuncture

Preoperative low and high frequency electroacupuncture reduces analgesic requirements after lower abdominal surgery.

Manual and massage therapy

There is relatively little evidence that these techniques are helpful with postoperative pain.

Postoperative pain management: summary

- Provide information for the patient and family.
- Base the choice of analgesia on severity and type of pain anticipated.
- Individualize therapy and respect patient choice.
- Make regular assessments of pain.
- Preferentially administer oral analgesics.
- Use non-opioid analgesics whenever possible.
- For moderate to severe pain, increase the opioid dose until pain relief is achieved or side effects occur.
- Use epidural LA and/or opioid for severe acute pain.
- Add NSAIDs for analgesia and opioid-sparing effects.
- All major hospitals performing surgery should have an APS using a multidisciplinary team approach with input of medical, nursing, pharmaceutical, and psychological expertise.
- A named member of staff must be responsible for the hospital policy on postoperative analgesia.

Increased pain in a previously comfortable patient

Be aware that any sudden increase in analgesic requirement postoperatively may be a warning that:
- There is a complication of surgery.
- There is a complication of pain relief technique, e.g. an epidural haematoma.
- The nature of pain has changed—neuropathic component, psychological, or environmental factors have assumed a greater importance.

Further reading

Royal College of Anaesthetists and The British Pain Society (2003). *Pain Management Services: Good Practice*. Royal College of Anaesthetists and The British Pain Society, London.
Royal College of Anaesthetists (2009). *Guidance on the Provision of Anaesthetic Services for Acute Pain Management*. Available at: ℳ http://www.rcoa.ac.uk/index.asp?PageID=477

Pain management in patients on long-term opioids: acute pain

Patients may take high doses of opioids over long periods of time to control pain from malignant disease or severe chronic pain. A further group of opioid-dependent patients may either be taking opioid recreationally or as part of a maintenance program. All these patients may have higher postoperative requirements for analgesia than opioid-naïve patients.

Incidence

In the UK, about 1.1% of males aged 16–24 and 0.5% of females receive opioids on prescription, a figure that is increasing year on year. There are an estimated 202,000 problematic users.

Acute pain management

The aim is to provide good pain relief and prevent opioid withdrawal during the postoperative period.

- Morphine sulphate (modified release) can be used in the postoperative period to provide a maintenance level and a short-acting opioid should be employed for breakthrough pain.
  - Prescribe an 'as required' 2-hourly oral morphine dose for 'breakthrough' pain at about 1/6 of the total m/r morphine dose: e.g. total dose m/r morphine per day = 120mg, then breakthrough dose should be 20mg morphine sulphate solution® 2-hourly.
- If the patient is nil by mouth, an IV infusion of morphine can be used in the immediate postoperative period. Calculate the daily oral dose of m/r morphine or equivalent and divide this by 2. This is the amount of morphine that should be given intravenously in a 24h period. This provides the background pain relief and prevents withdrawal symptoms.
- Patients can use a PCA pump for extra doses of morphine. The regimen should be initiated with a standard 1mg bolus/5min lock-out. They should be reassessed frequently and may require higher bolus doses.
- Opioid patches can be continued throughout the perioperative period to provide a maintenance level that can be topped up with a PCA for postoperative pain. A 25mcg fentanyl patch = 100mg oral morphine/24h = 50mg morphine IV/24h.
- Opioid Partial agonists should be avoided because they may precipitate withdrawal.
- Paracetamol and NSAIDs should be given regularly to all patients for their opioid-sparing effects.
- Regional analgesia should be used wherever possible.

Pain management in patients on long-term opioids: withdrawal

Additional considerations in opioid-dependent patients

- The perioperative period is not the time to treat addiction!
- There may be addiction to other drugs such as alcohol and benzodiazepines.
- Signs and symptoms of withdrawal must be sought (see Table 3.1).
- Withdrawal can occur after 2 weeks of opioid use. Severity *is not* necessarily related to the quantity of drug used.
- Untreated heroin withdrawal reaches its peak at 36–72h after the last dose and subsides substantially after 5 days. Methadone withdrawal peaks at 4–6 days, subsiding at 10–12 days.

Signs of opioid withdrawal
- Sympathoactivation
- Anxiety, craving, agitation
- Abdominal pains
- Hallucinations.

Table 3.1 Signs of withdrawal—A score of 4 or more indicates significant withdrawal and an opioid should be given

Signs	Positive		Negative
Pupils dilated ≥5mm	2	Pinned pupils ≤2mm	−2
Restlessness	1	Drowsy	−1
Sweating	2		
Skin goosebumps: Just palpable = Easily palpable =	1 2		
Pallor	1		
Yawning	1		
Runny eyes: eyes watery= eyes streaming=	1 2		
Runny nose: sniffing= profuse=	1 2		
Pulse rate >20 beats faster than baseline	1		
Pulse rate >30 beats faster than baseline	2	Pulse rate >20 beats slower than baseline	−2
BP >20mmHg above baseline	1		
BP >30mmHg above baseline	2	BP >20mmHg below baseline	−2
Tremors	1		

BP, blood pressure.

Pain management in patients on long-term opioids: opioid substitution

Opioid substitution

In order to avoid withdrawal symptoms, patients on long-term opioids must receive their usual opioid dose or an equivalent dose of another opioid.

Conversion from street heroin to morphine equivalents

Most bags of street heroin cost about £10 at present, and are packed as 0.2g; the majority of this weight is the other substances 'cut' with the diamorphine. Thus 1g of heroin is roughly equivalent to 60–80mg of methadone. However, it should be noted that the purity of street heroin varies greatly and up-to-date advice on conversion should be sought from the local drug and alcohol control unit.

Management plans

These patients can be very demanding and conflict often arises between staff and the patient. Drug and alcohol rehabilitation services should be contacted if difficulties arise.

Methadone

- If the patient is in a methadone maintenance programme, the current dose should be confirmed with the prescribing agency. If the methadone dose cannot be confirmed, an assessment of withdrawal symptoms should be made on the first day of admission and an appropriate amount of methadone prescribed.
- The prescribed methadone should not be considered part of the acute pain management as its slow kinetics prevents effective dose titration. It should only be used to prevent withdrawal. 40mg in the morning is sufficient for most patients but about a quarter will require a twice-daily dose of 20mg. It is unusual to need more than 60mg.
- The methadone must be consumed in front of the nurse who administers the drug.
- If there is any question that the patient is using street drugs while in hospital, the pathology lab can carry out a urine toxicology screen.

Buprenorphine

- Some patients are maintained on buprenorphine and it is seen as preferable by some users and is considered safer by some drugs teams.
- It is easier to continue buprenorphine than change to methadone when the patient becomes hospitalized.
- It is a partial opioid agonist and therefore higher morphine doses may be required for analgesia.

Naltrexone

- Naltrexone, a mu antagonist, is used to treat opioid or alcohol abuse in a dose of 25–50mg/day. It is also available as long-acting implants but the duration of action after removal of an implant is unknown.
- It is similar to naloxone but has a higher oral efficacy and a longer duration of action ($t_{1/2}$ = 14h).
- 100mg naltrexone will completely block the effect of 25mg diamorphine for 24h (still blocks 50% of action at 72h).
- There may be upregulation of opioid receptors so abrupt discontinuation of naltrexone may lead to a period of increased opioid sensitivity.
- For elective surgery, naltrexone should be discontinued for a minimum of 24h but preferably 48–72h preoperatively. There will be opioid resistance at first but as naltrexone levels decrease, the amount of opioid required will also decrease. Patients must be monitored for signs of overdose.
- In the event of an emergency, a similar approach should be used but pain relief may be less than optimal. The patient needs to be monitored closely while naltrexone levels fall.

Pain management in patients on long-term opioids: postoperative pain

Management of postoperative pain

- Agree a pain management plan with the patient in advance, including the choice and dose of the drug and timing.
- Regional analgesia should be used where possible to avoid the need for further opioid analgesics (NB withdrawal potential).
- Multimodal analgesia with paracetamol, NSAIDs, and a PCA with morphine is the next best approach.
- It may be helpful to add adjuncts such as clonidine or ketamine to improve analgesia and also to ward off withdrawal symptoms.

The use of patient-controlled analgesia

- The use of PCAs is advocated as the opioid requirements may be high and it reduces staff–patient confrontations about pain relief. These patients often have a fear of withdrawal and being without access to opioids can make them very agitated even though they are not experiencing withdrawal. Empowering them to decide on when they use the PCA can improve management of pain.
- PCA should be set up as normal, starting with a 1mg bolus and 5min lockout time. This will need frequent review. Patients often need a larger than average PCA bolus dose and they may benefit from a background infusion.
- Ensure the pump is tamperproof and use the minimum reservoir possible.

If a patient is a reformed drug abuser:

- He/she may tolerate a considerable amount of pain without opioid treatment in order to prevent relapse into dependency.
- Relapse to opioid abuse may result from opioid medication but this is rare and untreated pain may also lead to relapse.
- Use regional and local techniques where possible.
- If opioid drugs must be used they should be withdrawn as soon as possible.

Discharge from hospital

- If a patient is receiving methadone treatment from GP/specialist services it is essential they have early notification of the discharge date.
- Patients should not be discharged on combination analgesics because of the risk of potential paracetamol overdose.
- Where opioid intake has been reduced, warn the patient against returning to preadmission street drug dose. The tolerance to respiratory depression will have decreased.
- Methadone should not be prescribed for the patient to take home.

Pain management in patients on long-term opioids: summary

- Patient on long-term opioids have higher postoperative analgesic requirements than opioid-naïve patients.
- The perioperative period is not the time to treat addiction.
- The aim is to provide good pain relief and prevent opioid withdrawal.
- Background opioids need to be prescribed to prevent withdrawal.
- Addiction to other substances needs to be considered and substitutes prescribed if necessary.
- A pain management plan should be agreed in advance if possible.
- Paracetamol and NSAIDs should be prescribed for their opioid-sparing effects.
- Regional analgesia should be used whenever possible.
- Opioids for pain relief may need to be given in higher doses than usual.
- PCA opioids provide good postoperative pain management.
- Discharge from hospital should be notified to the GP/Specialist Drug Service and arrangements for continued prescribing made.

Pain control in the Intensive Therapy Unit

Pain and discomfort are common in the heterogeneous group of medical and surgical patients admitted to intensive care.

Pain results from:

- The primary insult (operation or trauma).
- Invasive medical interventions; monitoring and therapeutic devices (IV lines, urinary catheters, drains, endotracheal tubes).
- Routine care (suctioning, physiotherapy, dressing changes, turning).
- Chronic pain associated with comorbidities.

Patients are often unable to discuss or cooperate in the assessment of their pain. Poor control of pain leads to inadequate sleep, exhaustion, disorientation, and may contribute to respiratory complications. Unrelieved pain triggers the stress response—tachycardia, increased myocardial work, catabolism, hypercoagulability and immunosuppression—all of which are detrimental to patient outcomes.

Assessment of pain

The most appropriate method of assessment will depend on the individual patient, their ability to communicate, and the skill and experience of staff in interpreting pain behaviours or physiology. Up to 40% of patients discharged from intensive care can recall episodes of unrelieved pain. When possible, elective patients should be educated about the potential for pain and how to communicate their pain prior to admission to ITU.

In the awake intensive care patient, the unidimensional numerical rating score (NRS) is the most proven. Verbal rating score (VRS) and visual analogue score (VAS) can also be used (see ☐ Self-report measurements of acute pain p.6). Vocalization may not be possible and so pointing at clearly drawn scales or asking the patient to make some movement (e.g. nodding, blinking) in response to a specific question about their pain intensity can be useful.

There is a lack of satisfactory, objective measures of pain when communication with the patient is impossible. Behavioural–physiological scales have been used. These assess pain-related behaviours (movement, body posture, facial expression), and physiological indicators (heart rate, blood pressure, respiratory rate). However, these non-specific indicators may be misinterpreted and physiology may be modified by the underlying illness, independent of pain.

Methods of pain assessment (qualitative or quantitative) can easily be criticized, but many studies of acute pain team activity have demonstrated the importance of pain assessment and the value of educating staff. Measuring the magnitude of pain and repeatedly monitoring the response to analgesia are concepts basic to the practice of intensive care. Rational use of algorithms and protocols (often unique to individual units) is beneficial.

Analgesic therapy

Non-pharmacological strategies are essential; positioning, stabilization of fractures, modification of certain physical stimuli (e.g. traction on a drain catheter or endotracheal tube), massage, and even aromatherapy. Sedation may be helpful to cover brief periods of intensely painful stimulation.

The choice of analgesic drugs will vary from unit to unit and country to country. Drug choice is influenced by drug pharmacokinetics and pharmacodynamics, the predicted length of stay of the patient, local unit policies, and cost implications. The treatment of pain is also complicated by the parallel need for sedation. The actual combination of sedation and analgesia will be specific to each patient.

Considerations include:

- The reason for admission and whether analgesia is required at all.
- The stage of the illness (e.g. postoperative pain may be reduced by the time the patient is fit enough to wake and wean from ventilation).
- Associated organ dysfunction (liver, renal) can modify metabolism and modify the optimum choice of drugs.
- Previous drug therapies also have to be factored, to avoid drug interactions or make allowance for previous addictions.
- The possible route of administration—parenteral, enteral, regional.

Intravenous opioids

Opioids form the backbone of analgesic regimens in ITU, often combined with a sedative. Optimal characteristics for use in ITU include rapid onset, short $t_{1/2}$, no side effects or toxic metabolites, and low cost.

Morphine

Has relatively poor lipid solubility and slow onset of action. Its peak effect is at 20min after IV injection. Plasma levels decline rapidly (1–2h) due to redistribution. Its elimination $t_{1/2}$ is 3–7h via conjugated to inactive morphine-3-glucuronide and the more potent morphine-6-glucuronide. Both accumulate in renal failure. Extrahepatic sites for metabolism exist; hence, in cirrhosis clearance of morphine may be relatively normal. It is a popular choice, partly because of low cost, but it will accumulate. Hypotension can occur from histamine release.

Fentanyl

Has high lipid solubility (CNS levels parallel plasma levels) which accounts for its rapid onset (1–3min) and large volume of distribution. Redistribution to fat and skeletal muscle is fast (2min). Plasma elimination $t_{1/2}$ is 3–4h. Infusions will accumulate in the tissues. Fentanyl is metabolized by dealkylation and hydroxylation. Inactive metabolites are excreted in bile and urine. Decreased hepatic blood flow and plasma protein may prolong clearance in the elderly.

Remifentanil

Is a potent, selective, mu-opioid agonist with optimal characteristics. Rapid onset (1min), it has a predictable metabolism by non-specific esterases in blood and tissues, with a constant context-sensitive $t_{1/2}$ of 2–3min, meaning that independent of the duration of infusion it does not accumulate. The main metabolite, remifentanil acid, has weak opioid effects, is excreted in the urine, but is not obviously affected in renal impairment. Cost limits its widespread use. The fast offset can be a disadvantage requiring staff vigilance to avoid discontinuation of infusion as there is a risk of precipitant awakening.

Alfentanil

Is a good compromise. It has a rapid onset (1–2min), despite lower lipid solubility than fentanyl, it rapidly crosses the blood–brain barrier. It has a short duration of action ($t_{1/2}$ 70–90min) due to secondary redistribution and hepatic dealkylation to noralfentanil. The high protein binding and decreased lipid solubility result in a volume of distribution ¼ of fentanyl with much less accumulation. The metabolites have little opioid activity and are non-toxic. There are no problems in renal failure. Its short $t_{1/2}$ and small volume of distribution make it a useful drug for continuous infusions.

The opioids are commonly employed in combination with sedative drugs and the synergy reduces the relative dose required of each drug. This is often advantageous to counter the hypotensive effects of the sedative drugs.

- When a patient is to be kept sedated for long periods, morphine together with midazolam for sedation may be justified. However accumulation of both drugs is a problem and sedation/analgesia 'holds' are essential every 24h.
- If the period of sedation is to be short, allowing rapid awakening for weaning or neurological assessment, favour remifentanil or alfentanil, particularly in combination with propofol. The cost of these drugs may be offset by the shorter length of stay of the patient.
- If the patient does not need simultaneous sedation, relatively lower doses of opioids are necessary to prevent respiratory depression and sedation. In this situation, the potent, rapid onset opioids remifentanil and alfentanil have to be titrated with caution.

Side effects of opioids (and strategies to modify effects)

- Respiratory depression (early tracheostomy and stop drugs)
- Gastric stasis and ileus (prokinetics)
- Sympatholysis and vagally induced bradycardia (ino-/chrono-tropes)
- Depression of level of consciousness and hallucinations (limit dose)
- Dependence and withdrawal problems (limit duration, clonidine)

NSAIDs

Have a limited use in intensive care due to their side effects, which can often complicate the primary reason for admission. These side effects include:

- GI bleeding, increased incidence in intensive care patients often managed with early enteral nutrition and H2 antagonists.
- Platelet function modified within 6h of therapy.
- Renal failure, loss of the autoregulatory compensation of the kidney in hypovolaemia and hypotension via PGE and PGF2 vasodilation to improve medullary blood flow in the kidney.

Paracetamol

Is in common use, particularly intravenously. It can be used alone for milder pain, and is a valuable supplement to opioid analgesia. Its use should be modified (<2g/day) in patients with depleted glutathione stores (alcoholics), in hepatitis, and liver damage/failure.

Tramadol and weak opioids

Can fulfil a useful role, because of problems with NSAIDs and paracetamol, when analgesia is needed for mild to moderate pain.

Routes of administration

- Continuous IV infusion: problems of overdosage and accumulation occur unless optimal drug chosen. Algorithms with pain, sedation scores, and daily infusion holds are mandatory.
- PCA: reduces accumulation problems but patient needs to be alert and oriented.
- IM/SC: of no value in intensive care where IV access is prerequisite.
- Oral: gut absorption may be unreliable. Use of early enteral nutrition means staff usually aware of gut function.
- Transdermal: unreliable in this population as unpredictable absorption in low perfusion states.

Regional analgesia

There are many complications and risks associated with IV opioid therapy. These combined with the advantage of shorter periods of ventilation and faster weaning have led intensivists to include regional techniques, whenever appropriate to minimize systemic opioid use.

- Epidural: ideal for postoperative thoracic and abdominal surgery. Also of benefit postcardiac surgery. Caution in the septic patient and when coagulopathy occurs as a therapeutic manoeuvre (activated protein C, haemodialysis) or with liver failure/ disseminated intravascular coagulation (DIC). Beware particularly on insertion and removal of catheters. Also concern about insertion in the sedated patient.
- Regional nerve blocks: upper and lower limb blocks can be useful adjuncts when single-limb injury or multiple site injuries. Bolus injections are often too short acting for an intensive care patient. Catheter techniques are most valuable. Risks are duration of placement versus infection, LA toxicity, and coagulopathy.
- Peripheral nerve blocks: less useful other than short-term relief.
- Infiltration: short-term relief, e.g. for invasive procedures or drain sites.
- Topical: used for urinary catheter insertion, bronchoscopic intubation and endoscopy.

Summary

The majority of ITU patients will need an analgesic plan and successful analgesia will contribute to improved patient outcomes. All of the existing treatments have side effects and contraindications requiring careful monitoring to avoid patient harm. A significant proportion of ITU patients report episodes of poor analgesia that almost certainly contribute to post-ITU traumatic stress disorder.

Trauma

One of the commonest indications for analgesia in the hospital setting. It may be divided into minor (sprains, dislocations, fractures, and superficial wounds), major (involving severe injuries to chest, abdomen, or head), and polytrauma (involving combinations of all those listed for minor and major). Major trauma can affect all ages but most commonly involves the young (58%), males (73%), and often individuals under the influence of drugs or alcohol (51%).

Immediate management

Minor injuries

These can usually be adequately managed with combinations of simple analgesics (paracetamol ± NSAIDs) and weak opioids (tramadol or codeine), in addition to cold packs, strapping, and reassurance.

Major trauma

Victims of major trauma frequently present in a state of CV or respiratory instability requiring immediate life-saving procedures following ATLS guidelines such as endotracheal intubation, defibrillation, or chest drain insertion.

After this immediate assessment and resuscitation phase:
- Stabilize fractures, this will reduce pain.
- Provide the awake patient with information.
- Give analgesia, (with caution in the presence of cardiorespiratory instability).
- Continuously monitor:
  - Neurological status after a head injury.
  - Neurovascular status after limb injury.
- Surgical evaluation should take priority over analgesic titration in the face of sudden increases in pain (e.g. extremity swelling) or somnolence (e.g. from an expanding subdural haematoma).

Analgesics (see 📖 Fig. 3.1, p.61)

Opioids
- IV morphine titrated in increments (2–5mg) at 5min intervals with careful observation of vital signs should give adequate and rapid pain relief. This intervention may also facilitate patient assessment.
- PCA can be instituted preoperatively in the acutely injured patient.
- The IM route is dangerous in the trauma patient because of unpredictable absorption and should be avoided.

Entonox®
- Entonox® can provide good analgesia in both the immediate phase and over the longer term. Can be deployed at scene of injury or in ambulance.
- It has a maximum analgesic effect in 45s.

> Never deliver O_2/N_2O mix from anaesthetic machine as there is a risk of hypoxic mixture (deaths have occurred in Emergency Department setting).

Paracetamol
- IV paracetamol may reduce opioid requirements.

NSAIDs
The use of NSAIDs in the trauma patient remains controversial because of the risk of:
- Excessive bleeding
- Gastric stress ulcers
- Effect on renal function—contraindicated in shocked patient
- Concern about impairment of bone healing.

Regional anaesthetic techniques
- Regional anaesthetic approaches may be beneficial for particular sites:
  - The discomfort and splinting due to flail chest injury may improve with epidural analgesia.
  - Epidural infusions have a role to play in major lower limb trauma.
  - Borderline perfusion of an injured limb can increase with a sympathetic blockade by an epidural LA.
- Contraindicated in sepsis, coagulopathy, or cardiorespiratory instability.

Local techniques
Can be very useful in particular circumstances, e.g. femoral nerve block for patellar fracture.

Anxiety
Small doses of benzodiazepines such as lorazepam may help to control anxiety. Note potential for synergistic respiratory depression or sedation when used with opioids.
  Anxiety may be due to:
- Fear of pain
- Fears for the future
- Worries about others involved in the accident
- The possibility of prosecution or litigation.

Acute neuropathic pain
- Pain from damage to nerves can occur early in trauma and often responds poorly to opioid drugs.
- Antidepressants and anticonvulsants should be considered in patients who complain of shooting or burning pain (e.g. amitriptyline or gabapentin).
- Doses may need to be adjusted to achieve optimum pain management.
- Ketamine as an IV infusion 0.1–0.25mcg/kg/min can be used to reduce opioid requirement, but also to help neuropathic pain that is not well controlled with other medications.

Long-term management

Once the patient is stable and urgent management complete, they may face a long recovery period with multiple operations. Additionally, complications from the trauma and subsequent mobilization can be painful.

Development of chronic pain

- Patients who have severe prolonged acute pain may develop long-term chronic pain. Therefore good pain control in the acute period is very important.
- Trauma may trigger neuropathic pain due to nerve damage (e.g. complex regional pain syndrome—CRPS).
- Postsurgical pain is another type of chronic pain associated with trauma.

Prevention of complex regional pain syndrome

- Relatively minor injuries can be complicated by the development of CRPS (see ☐ Complex regional pain syndromes p.288).
- Physiotherapy with good pain relief and an early return to normal use is important in the prevention of this complication and early intervention should be sought if signs develop.

Pain management

- Individual patient analgesic requirements vary widely and must be titrated individually.
- The age of the patient is often a better guide to opioid dose than weight.

Trauma: management of specific injuries

Vertebral fractures

- Severe pain often requires hospitalization and bed rest which exacerbate the problem, i.e. muscle wasting and pressure sores.
- Paracetamol, NSAIDs, and opioids are often not helpful.
- Salmon calcitonin has been reported to reduce pain as early as 1 week into treatment with minor side effects:
  - Intranasal: 200IU for 28 days.
  - 100IU SC also reduces risk of new fractures.
- Vertebroplasty has been advocated for the treatment of vertebral fractures:
  - Involves image-guided, minimally invasive, injection of a cement mixture to the vertebrae.
  - Used to strengthen a fractured vertebra.
  - However, 2 recent controlled trials have failed to show a conclusive benefit.

Chest trauma

Chest trauma of any type can cause chest pain by causing rib fracture, or muscle strain, or contusion. Pain worsens prognosis through splinting, impaired coughing, and atelectasis.

Rib fractures can be managed with

- Regular paracetamol ± weak opioids.
- NSAIDs if not contraindicated.
- Opioids either via a PCA or orally for more severe pain.
- Intercostal nerve blocks may be appropriate in the acute phase but there is a risk of pneumothorax, toxicity, and these blocks have a relatively short duration of efficacy.
- Epidural/paravertebral LA.

Epidural or paravertebral analgesia after severe blunt injury to the chest significantly improves subjective pain perception and critical pulmonary function tests compared to IV narcotics and may decrease the length of hospital stay.

Fractured neck of femur

Muscles surrounding the femur are powerful and the spasm that occurs after femoral fracture can be very painful. Multimodal analgesia and PCA are effective. Femoral nerve block for pain relief for the immediate presentation followed by continuous infusion of LA 0.25% bupivacaine at 5mL/h can optimum analgesia in patients who often do not tolerate opioids well.

Fractured pelvis and lower limb injuries

- Pelvic fractures occur in 20% of polytrauma cases. Fractured pelvis is very painful and often requires traction or fixation.
- Morphine is the drug of choice in the acute phase unless the patient is haemodynamically unstable. PCA and continuous infusion methods provide more effective pain control than intermittent dosing.

Analgesic doses

The following are starting doses and need to be altered depending on the response.

>70 years old or very frail:

- Regular paracetamol 1g qds.
- Oral morphine 5mg 2-hourly as required or PCA.
- Tramadol infusion 600mg made up to 50mL with saline run at 1–2mL/h for patients unable to manage PCA.
- Cyclizine 50mg 6-hourly IM/orally as required for nausea.
- **Do not use** NSAIDs for patients >70 years of age unless very specifically indicated.
- Daily monitoring of urine output and renal function is required in patients >70 years of age.

<70 years, reasonably well:

- Oral morphine 10mg 1-hourly as required or PCA.
- Cyclizine 50mg 6-hourly as required for nausea.
- Paracetamol 1gm 4-hourly.
- Diclofenac 50mg tds (or up to 150mg/day by any recommended route).
- Ibuprofen 400mg tds.
- **Do not use** these NSAIDs in the presence of renal impairment, coagulopathy, severe asthma, or aspirin-induced asthma or serious upper GI pathology. Use for 48h only then review the prescription.

An unexpected increase in pain should be considered surgical until proved otherwise. It may also herald the onset of neuropathic pain.

- Epidural infusion of LA and opioid provides superior analgesia and can facilitate nursing care. It can be started during pelvic fixation under general anaesthetic (GA).
- Sciatic neuropraxia and axonotomesis is common and patients may require treatment for neuropathic pain.
- Almost half of patients with a pelvic fracture go on to have chronic pain that has both nociceptive and neuropathic elements.

Compartment syndrome

Orthopaedic or vascular procedures on a leg may result in a compartment syndrome which is often associated with a period of ischaemia or injury to the muscles. There is intracompartmental swelling with loss of function, often the earliest manifestation being loss of dorsiflexion of the foot and pain. If not treated promptly by decompression, a compartment syndrome may result in chronic postischaemic neuropathy. There is no good evidence that the use of PCA obscures signs of compartment syndrome.

▶Avoid epidural analgesia in patients at high risk of developing a compartment syndrome because of the possible risk of masking the pain that signals the onset of critical ischaemia.

Muscles surrounding the femur are powerful and the spasm that occurs after femoral fracture can be very painful. Multimodal analgesia and PCA are effective

Head injury and morphine

Morphine does not obscure signs of raised intracranial pressure but good observation is necessary. PCA is the optimum method. Codeine represents a poor choice in patients with head injury.

Amputation

- Preoperative epidural infusions of LA alone or LA with opiate and/or clonidine have been advocated to minimize postoperative phantom limb pain; however, as yet supportive evidence is lacking.
- Postoperative infusions of LA along the sciatic or posterior tibial nerve is a safe and effective method for the relief of postoperative pain but do not prevent residual or phantom limb pain.
- In those patients with a significant component of phantom limb pain, tricyclic antidepressants or anticonvulsant medications may need to be initiated in the postoperative period.

Entonox®

Uses

- MUA (manipulation under anesthesia) of fractures
- Extrication from vehicles
- Transportation (ambulances)
- Removal of drains/sutures
- Adjustment of orthopaedic appliances/traction/pins etc.

Complications

N_2O diffuses into a space 34x more quickly than N_2 comes out. Gas in an enclosed space will expand. Entonox should be avoided in:

- Air embolus
- Pneumothorax
- Air in the head
- Air in a viscus, e.g. gut
- Decompression sickness
- Fractured ribs (may be a pneumothorax).

Contraindications

In addition to those already listed:

- Where the patient's conscious state is impaired, e.g. head injury
- Vomiting
- Facial or jaw injuries.

Pain relief in the Emergency Department

Pain is the commonest reason for attendance at an Emergency Department, yet is commonly undertreated, often due to cursory assessment of pain level.

- Use a pain score or ladder (see 🕮 Measurement of acute pain p.6).
- Use visual clues (sweating, agitation, shaking).
- Consider likely diagnosis—analgesia may result from specific treatment, e.g. nitrates for cardiac pain.
- Consider possible side effects and allergies.
- Reassurance and calm explanation should always be used.
- More than one pharmacological approach may be indicated.

Specific clinical presentations

Fractures and soft tissue injuries

Pain is due to movement of fragments and pressure from haematoma.

- Always immobilize fractures.
- Consider aspiration of joint haematoma—especially elbow and knee.
- Elevation where possible assists in minimizing swelling.
- Long-bone fractures—neck or shaft of femur, tibia—start with IV morphine. There is no fixed upper limit for morphine—look for respiratory depression and drowsiness. 30–40mg may be required in some cases.
- Shaft of femur fracture—IV morphine, then femoral nerve block, then apply Thomas or Donway splint.

Non-steroidal anti-inflammatory drugs (NSAIDs)

- Should not be used routinely in early pain management of soft tissue injury—paracetamol is as effective with a better side-effect profile.
- Use short-term NSAIDs for inflammatory conditions such as bursitis, synovitis, in addition to paracetamol.
- A 'one off' dose of an IV agent such as ketorolac (30mg) is often useful in refractory cases.

Some distal limb fractures and dislocations are amenable to nerve block: digital or metacarpal blocks for finger injuries, ulnar nerve block for 5th metacarpal fractures. Ankle block can be useful in foot injury but success is more variable.

Reduction of dislocations and realignment of displaced fractures greatly reduces pain and should be carried out as soon as possible. Some dislocations require emergency relocation due to threats to tissue viability—e.g. ankle dislocations where skin viability may be threatened—relocation indicated prior to X-ray. In most cases X-rays are obtained first, necessitating IV morphine.

Rib fractures and sternal fractures are particularly painful for 2–3 weeks. Oral paracetamol with or without codeine, and NSAIDs are used: multiple fractures may require a thoracic epidural.

Burns
- Pain is reduced by cooling the affected area with running water initially then a cold wet towel: a cooling gel is sometimes used by paramedics.
- Covering the burn reduces pain by preventing airflow over it—clingfilm allows assessment without removing the cover.
- IV morphine in adults and nasal diamorphine in children are typically required for larger burns.

Cardiac pain
- Diamorphine or morphine IV reduces both pain and anxiety. Consequent reduction in catecholamine secretion may reduce risk of arrhythmias. Arterial and venous vasodilatation reduces both preload and afterload.
- Measures to minimize ischaemia by maximizing blood flow with nitrates, β-blockers, and antiplatelet agents will also contribute to pain relief.

Acute abdomen, renal and biliary colic
- Pain from an 'acute abdomen', e.g. peritonitis, is traditionally treated with IV opiates. **Do not** withhold opiates whilst awaiting a surgical opinion—although it can change the physical signs, this has been shown to be unnecessary and unkind.[1]
- Colic is due to smooth muscle spasm. Antispasmodics such as hyoscine butylbromide, anti-inflammatories such as ketorolac or diclofenac may be used with or without opiates.

Pleurodynia/pleurisy
- Pleuritic pain occurs with a range of conditions such as pneumonia, emboli, and viral illnesses such as coxsackie B ('devil's grip').
- NSAIDs and paracetamol in combination may be used: viral pleurodynia typically lasts 3–5 days.

Mechanical low back pain
- Patients presenting to Emergency Departments with non-traumatic low back pain are usually self-medicating and may already have consulted other clinicians. Complex psychological and social factors may be involved in long-standing cases.
- Emergency Department care does not attempt to be holistic or comprehensive in such cases. The reason for attendance is usually poor pain control and consequent loss of mobility.
- Typical management is concurrent administration of paracetamol, codeine, and NSAIDs, with diazepam for up to 7 days, with advice to seek therapy from a physiotherapist, osteopath, or chiropractor.

Paediatric pain

Assessment

- Pain in children is harder to assess and treat due to the difficulties in communicating with young children, fear, and cooperation problems. Specific training is useful in paediatric pain management.
- Assessment of paediatric pain involves careful observation of the child's behaviour and activity and listening to the parents as well as the child. Children often deny pain out of fear of treatment.
- Pain scoring in young children is assisted by the use of the Wong–Baker faces pain scale (see 📖 p.7).

Treatment

- Treatment of pain in children (as in adults) is greatly helped by addressing fear and anxiety, though this is time consuming. A nurse with paediatric training may be able to spend time with the child and parents building up trust through play: if time allows, this can be very effective.
- Distraction therapy, such as story telling, kaleidoscopes, or other methods may be used to hold the child's attention whilst potentially painful treatments are carried out. Though rarely sufficient alone, when used in addition to pharmacological approaches such as LA cream, cannulae can be inserted with minimum distress for child, parent, and doctor.
- Nasal administration of diamorphine is now 'first-line' treatment of severe pain in children in UK Emergency Departments.

Nasal diamorphine—strong pain relief without needles[2]

Diamorphine is extremely water soluble and is rapidly absorbed from the nasal mucosa: A fixed volume of 0.2mL of variable concentration is administered via a 1ml syringe with the child's head tipped back. Dose is 0.1mg/kg.

Easily achievable with minimum cooperation: children find it only mildly unpleasant and may have a salty taste at the back of the throat. 0.1mg/kg is given and analgesia equivalent to 0.2mg/kg of IM morphine but with quicker onset of action. In children expected to require further opiate doses, the initial nasal dose may be followed by application of LA topical cream and subsequent cannulation 30min later.

References

1 Ranji SR, *et al.* (2006). Do opiates affect the clinical evaluation of patients with abdominal pain? *JAMA* **296**:1764–74.
2 Kendall JM, *et al.* (2001). Multi-centre randomised controlled trial of nasal diamorphine for analgesia in children and teenagers with clinical fractures. *BMJ* **322**:261–5.

Management of burn pain

Incidence of burns

In the UK about 250,000 people are burnt each year. 13,000 of these are admitted to hospital and 1,000 patients have severe enough burns to warrant formal fluid resuscitation. Half of these are aged under 12.

The most common cause of burns is flame injuries followed by liquid scalds. Less common causes are electrocution and chemical injuries. There is a male predominance except in elderly people.

Compromising factors

Burn victims' health is often compromised by some other factor, such as alcoholism, epilepsy, drug abuse, or chronic psychiatric or medical illness.

Pathophysiology of burn pain

Pain starts immediately after the injury to the tissues. Nerve endings that are completely destroyed will not transmit pain, but those that remain intact along with regenerating nerves will trigger pain throughout the course of treatment.

▶It is important to remember:
- The pain is not proportional to the degree of tissue damage.
- The degree of pain relief is not proportional to the dose of analgesic medication administered.
- Pain from burn wounds does not necessarily decrease with time. They remain painful until they are fully healed.

Primary hyperalgesia

Burns wounds are very sensitive to both mechanical and chemical stimuli. Any pressure on the wound, especially debridement, or the application of topical preparations, will cause pain. This is due to the sensitization of peripheral nociceptors secondary to the intense inflammatory response.

Secondary hyperalgesia

There is an increase in the sensitivity of the DH neurones caused by prolonged stimulation of the primary afferent neurons known as 'wind-up'. Upregulation of NMDA receptors in the spinal cord is responsible for this. Hypersensitivity is seen in the surrounding tissues which may result in an increase in opioid requirement during dressing changes over time.

Psychological factors affecting pain control

Fear, anger, anxiety, sorrow, depression, irritability, and fatigue are all common feelings that may exacerbate, or be exacerbated by, the patient's pain response.

If severe pain is experienced from the initial treatments, the experience of pain leads to worry about the next, leading to a vicious circle of anxiety/pain/anxiety. Feelings of animosity may then develop between the patient and medical personnel.

Phases of burn wounds

Emergency phase

This phase starts immediately after the accident and lasts a few hours or days and is due to stimulation of skin nociceptors.

Pain management in the emergency phase

Analgesics should be administered intravenously. Morphine is the drug of choice in the acute phase. This should be titrated in increments every 5min until the patient is comfortable. If the patient is able to cooperate, a PCA machine should then be used. If the patient is unable to cooperate morphine should be given as an IV infusion adjusted as necessary. Paracetamol can be given intravenously, but NSAIDs should be avoided until resuscitation is complete and renal function is normal.

Around 48h after a burn injury a hypermetabolic state usually occurs. There is increased blood flow to the tissues and organs. Changes in plasma proteins such as albumen result in alteration of drug pharmacokinetics. This may result in altered efficacy of analgesics.

Healing phase (after 72h)

This stage may last days or months. Continuous background pain is often of low intensity but therapeutic procedures including dressing changes and physiotherapy can cause severe pain lasting for several hours.

Pain management in the healing phase

Background pain

Patients should be given information about the pain of burns and analgesic methods available. It should be made clear that the total absence of pain following a burn is normally not a realistic goal. Pain intensity and pain relief should be recorded on the bedside vital sign chart.

Non-opioid analgesics

Unless contraindicated, every patient should receive regular paracetamol with the addition of an NSAID. For patients unable to take medications by mouth, it may be necessary to use the parenteral or rectal route.

Opioid analgesics

Failure to provide adequate pain relief is often due to the following:
- Fear of patient addiction: in a study of over 10,000 cases in 33 burns centres, not a single case of iatrogenic addiction to opioids occurred.
- It is wrongly believed that over-frequent administration of analgesics will cause a decrease in the patient's response to the drugs.

In the early stages, an IV morphine infusion may be necessary with PCA. Later, a PCA alone may be adequate and this can be either IV or SC. Sepsis is a constant problem in burn patients and it is better to avoid indwelling cannulae. Oral analgesia should be introduced as soon as possible using a slow-release opiate for background pain, such as MST®, and a quick-acting preparation, such as Oramorph®, for breakthrough pain.

High doses of opioids are often required to bring pain under control.

Benzodiazepines

Fear and anxiety are common with burn injury. A benzodiazepine such as lorazepam 2mg–4mg bd is useful to supplement opioid analgesics.

Regional techniques

Regional analgesia including spinal or epidural analgesia, can provide excellent pain relief but because of the prolonged healing of burns and the high risk of infection, these techniques are often contraindicated

Topical analgesia

EMLA® cream for debridement reduces overall pain scores. The use of morphine topically in wounds, using hydrogel as a carrier, has also shown some benefit.

Poorly controlled pain

When pain is not adequately controlled with the agents previously listed, any or all of the following may be necessary:

Ketamine

Ketamine reduces central sensitization by blocking NMDA receptors in the DH. It has been used successfully for over 40 years in the treatment of burn pain.

Dose: 0.1–0.25mcg/kg/h as an IV infusion.

Propofol

Analgesia with morphine IV 15min before the procedure can be supplemented by patient-controlled sedation with propofol using a starting dose of 0.3mg/kg and a lockout of 5min. Respiratory rates, oxygen saturation, and blood pressure should be monitored. Oxygen via nasal insufflation prevents hypoxia.

Lidocaine

Systemic lidocaine has been shown to be effective in the short term at reducing neuropathic pain and secondary hyperalgesia. The administration of lidocaine may lead to a reduction in the procedural and background pain levels of burn patients, leading to lowered opiate requirements and consequently less associated complications.

Dose: IV lidocaine bolus 2mg/kg, then infusion 3mg/kg/h for 1h.

Antidepressants

Amitriptyline at night helps patients to sleep and may reduce neuropathic pain symptoms.

Anticonvulsants

Gabapentin or pregabalin can be titrated to reduce neuropathic pain and may have an opioid-sparing effect. They are also effective for the management of neuropathic itching as the wounds begin to heal.

Management of procedural pain in the healing phase

Principles

Wound debridement and the removal of previous dressings is intensely painful during the procedure and results in an increase in the level of background pain post-procedure.

The type of analgesic used should have a short time to peak effect, be easily titrated to changing requirements, and cause minimal side effects.

- Adequate analgesia following the procedure is essential but oversedation undesirable.
- Healing requires good nutrition and hydration so excessive fasting should be minimized.

Intravenous opioids

- Morphine: 2–5mg. Delayed onset (10min) and prolonged effect make individual titration difficult.
- Alfentanil: 10mcg/kg. Can be titrated to effect and a continuous infusion of 2mcg/kg/min will provide postprocedural pain relief.
- Remifentanil can be titrated to give adequate analgesia during dressing changes but requires continuous tapering infusion postprocedure due to its extremely short duration of action.

Entonox®

Entonox® can be used during the procedure to provide additional analgesia but its efficacy is limited (see ☐ Entonox p84).

Oral medications for mild pain

Morphine is often used preprocedure but needs to be given at least an hour prior to the dressing change. It is commonly used in both adults and children. The recommended dose is 0.3–1.0mcg/kg. The main drawbacks are:

- It has reduced and uncertain bioavailability (15–50%)—oxycodone has more reliable absorption.
- Severe pain during the procedure is difficult to treat.
- Long lasting postprocedural sedation.

Fentanyl lozenges

The fentanyl is absorbed via the oral mucosa and GI tract giving a rapid onset (minutes) and prolonged effect. They work well for dressing changes and physiotherapy. The starting dose is 200mcg and a second lozenge can be administered after 15min. No more than 2 should be used for each episode.

Intranasal drugs

Diamorphine, 0.1mg/kg in 0.2mL saline, works well for some children who undergo short but painful procedures. The potency is 50% of the IM dose and it lasts 15min.

Midazolam nasal spray 0.2–0.4g/kg will last 10–15min and can be used to supplement analgesia.

Non-pharmacological therapies

Anticipation of pain can increase pain intensity and discomfort, therefore distraction may produce a significant analgesic effect. The same is true for hypnosis, which is used by some burn teams. Cognitive behavioural strategies such as relaxation, imagery, and hypnosis have been described by burn survivors as very helpful. These interventions are intended to supplement, not replace, pharmacological interventions.

Recovery phase

This commences as soon as the burned surfaces have been covered or have healed. The primary target is functional rehabilitation. During this phase the patient may experience local discomfort and paraesthesia and itching. These symptoms can be as unbearable as the initial burn pain and may require long-term treatment. Most patients manage with paracetamol with the addition of codeine in some cases. However, a significant proportion will continue to need antidepressants and anticonvulsants for many months.

Rheumatological pain

The common rheumatic conditions are classified by the WHO under four headings:
- Osteoarthritis (OA)
- Inflammatory arthropathies:
  - Symmetrical, e.g. rheumatoid arthritis (RA)
  - Monoarthropathy
- Regional 'soft tissue' disorders, e.g. tendonitis, capsulitis, bursitis
- Back pain (see 📖 Chronic low back pain p.272).

Osteoarthritis

OA is asymptomatic in the majority of cases. Pain is usually related to activity and is the primary presenting symptom and the chief cause of functional loss.

OA pain can be bony, chondrophyte and osteophyte growth under damaged cartilage cause stretching of the highly innervated periosteum, or soft tissue in origin, e.g. ligamentous, capsular, synovial, or muscular. Oedema and effusion can alter the normal mechanical sensitivity of nociceptors, as can inflammatory mediators released from the damaged tissue.

Epidemiology
- ♀*:♂ ratio of OA in the knee is 3:1.
- OA is found in >80% of those aged >75 years.
- Knee OA functionally affects 10% of the population aged >50 years.
- Ethnic variation of site (hip OA rare in black and Asian populations).
- Risk factors:
  - Aging.
  - Obesity*—increased weight precedes the disease not vice versa.
  - Injury.
  - Inflammation—preceding infection or inflammatory arthropathy.
  - Others: acromegaly, haemochromatosis, ochronosis, dysplasias.

Clinical features
- Joint pain, usually hip or knee pain.
- Morning stiffness* and stiffness upon resuming activity.
- On examination there may be crepitus*, bony enlargement, joint instability, effusion, and joint locking due to loose bodies.

(*Patients with these features are more likely to report pain.)

Investigations
Radiological features include joint space narrowing, osteophyte formation at the joint peripherary, subchondral bone sclerosis, and pseudocyst formation. There is a poor correlation between pain and structural damage seen on X-ray films.

Treatment
Guidelines were published in 2000 by the American College of Rheumatology and in 2008 by NICE. The major points are shown in Table 3.2.

Table 3.2 Therapies for OA

Non-pharmacological therapies	Pharmacological therapies
Social support	Topical—NSAID, capsaicin
Patient education and self-management programmes	Oral—paracetamol, NSAIDs, COX-2 specific inhibitors
Exercise—aerobic, physical therapy, or muscle strengthening	Intra-articular injections—corticosteroid
Weight loss (if overweight)	Other analgesics—tramadol, opioids
Splints, insoles, patellar taping	
Surgery—arthroscopic washout, cartilage debridement, osteotomy, or joint replacement	

Rheumatoid arthritis

RA is a systemic, chronic, inflammatory disease which primarily affects peripheral synovial joints in a symmetrical fashion. Its aetiology is unclear, though it is thought that both inherited and environmental factors are involved.

Inflammatory synovitis leads to synovial hyperplasia which is accompanied by T- and B-cell infiltration. Pannus (mononuclear cells, fibroblasts, and proteolytic enzymes which penetrate the cartilage) formation also typifies RA. Lymphocytes, TNF-α, and interleukin-1 are prevalent in synovial fluid in RA.

Epidemiology
- 0.5–1.5% prevalence in adults in Western countries.
- $\female$:$\male$ ratio is 2.5:1.
- Peak incidence is in the 4th and 5th decades of life.
- HLA-DR4 and DR1 are associated (it is unclear as to whether they increase susceptibility to, or severity of, the disease).
- Variation exists between ethnic groups.
- 25% concordance is present between monozygotic twins.
- 90% of RA sufferers will develop cervical spine involvement
  - risk of radiculopathies.
- 20–40% have extraarticular features.

Clinical features
- Onset is usually insidious (5–10% experience an acute onset) which can be systemic (malaise, decreased weight, pyrexia)or articular in nature.
- Articular presentation is usually a symmetrical polyarthritis of the hands and/or feet. Wrist, ankle, C-spine (atlantoaxial subluxation), knee, or temporomandibular joints may be involved.
- Joints are erythematous, swollen, tender, stiff, and pain is more tenacious than in OA; occurring at rest as well as with activity.

- Characteristic hand deformities that develop later are Boutonnière and swan neck of the fingers and 'Z deformity' of the thumb.
- Extra-articular complications:
  - Cardiac—pericarditis.
  - Pulmonary—fibrosing alveolitis.
  - Neurological—entrapped nerves, cervical myelopathy, vasculitis of the vasa nervosum leads to glove stocking sensory loss, mononeuritis multiplex is more severe with loss of sensation and power.

Investigations

High rheumatoid factor (RF) titres indicate a poor prognosis (only 80% of RA patients are RF positive). Erythrocyte sedimentation rate (ESR) and C-reactive protein (CRP) are useful for monitoring disease progression. Early radiographic changes comprise soft tissue swelling, periarticular osteoporosis, and bony erosions. Late signs are loss of joint space and synovial cyst formation. Disease progression on X-rays is an indicator that more aggressive therapy is needed.

Treatment

Pharmacological treatments

- Disease-modifying antirheumatic drugs DMARDs: trials show that these drugs improve symptoms (including pain), global well-being, functional status, and retard radiological disease progression. Some studies have shown better outcome (symptoms and joint inflammation) measures if the DMARDs are introduced as soon as possible after diagnosis. There are a number of different drugs used to modify the course of RA including methotrexate, sulfasalazine, parenteral gold, and TNF-α blockers.
- NSAIDs: given topically or orally they reduce morning stiffness, pain, and swelling.
- Corticosteroids: used often as a 'bridge' in severe inflammation until DMARDS kick in. They can be given orally as, IV/IM injections, or directly into joints.
- Other analgesics/agents: paracetamol, codeine, tramadol, and antidepressants (amitriptyline).

Non-pharmacological treatments

Joint splintage to prevent deformities developing may help in the short term. There is little proof to support resting during periods of active inflammation and exercise does not appear to exacerbate joint symptoms. Podiatry, occupational and physical therapy, TENS, cold and warm packs, and cognitive therapy all have a role. Surgery may be indicated for pain relief and improvement of function.

Acute monoarthropathy

An isolated inflamed joint should usually be aspirated for confirmation of inflammation and to look for the presence of bacteria or crystals.

- Bacterial infection of a joint presents as acute inflammation of the joint and systemic features may occur especially in children. Onset can be more insidious with infection of a prosthetic joint. Bacterial arthritis is a rheumatological emergency as there is a 25–50% chance of developing irreversible loss of joint function. Treatment should be early and aggressive with the relevant antibiotic. Open surgical drainage may be needed and prosthetic joints are usually removed.

- Crystal arthritis such as gout and pseudogout are diagnosed by the presence of uric acid crystals and calcium pyrophosphate crystals respectively in the synovial fluid along with a neutrophil leucocytosis. Treatment of gout and pseudogout includes relief of the acute episode with oral NSAID (except aspirin), oral prednisolone, or intra-articular corticosteroid. Oral colchicine may be used but is often poorly tolerated, causing diarrhoea and vomiting. Drugs which alter plasma urate (aspirin, allopurinol) should not be used in the acute phase. Preventative treatment should be started once the acute phase has subsided, such as allopurinol (xanthine oxidase inhibitor) or probenecid (uricosuric agent).

Regional 'soft tissue' disorders

Upper limb

A classification has been published for the diagnosis of upper limb disorders depending upon the findings in the history and examination:

- Rotator cuff tendonitis
- Bicipital tendonitis
- Shoulder capsulitis
- Lateral or medial epicondylitis
- De Quervain's disease—pain at base of thumb
- Wrist tenosynovitis
- Carpal tunnel
- Non-specific forearm pain.

Controversy surrounds whether there is an association between elbow, forearm, and hand conditions with repetitive, strenuous jobs. Equally controversial is the association of psychosocial, cognitive, and behavioural traits as risk factors for upper limb disorders.

Treatment comprises paracetamol, NSAIDs (both topical and oral), and rest. Subacromial and intra-articular steroid injections for the shoulder may be of short-term benefit where mobility is severely impaired. Injections for forearm/hand disorders are beneficial but relapse is common.

Lower limb

The hip has a large number of bursae which if inflamed (may be associated to OA, RA, or spondylosis of the hip) can lead to soft tissue pain. Trochanteric bursitis is the most common and presents as lateral upper thigh pain exacerbated by lying on that side or activity.

Knee pain in adolescents may be chondromalacia patella. If there is a history of repetitive trauma and a fluctuant swelling over the patella there may be a prepatellar bursitis. Further conditions include iliotibial band syndrome (lateral thigh and knee), meniscal tears, and synovial plicae.

The Achilles tendon or the plantar fascia may become inflamed due to excessive sporting pursuit. Obesity and poor footwear also contribute to plantar fasciitis.

Simple analgesia, NSAIDs, and rest are the most useful treatments. Injections of steroids or LA along with physiotherapy are of unproven benefit.

Acute back pain •

Definition
Low back pain (LBP) of <6 weeks' duration. It is mostly managed in the community by GPs.

Epidemiology
Lifetime prevalence in adults is up to 80% and around 80% of episodes are self-limiting, resolving within 2 weeks. The total economic burden of back pain resulting from incapacity to work has been estimated in the UK as being twelve billion pounds.[1]

Causes
The majority of cases will have non-specific 'mechanical' back pain (around 85%) and the remainder are likely to be due to nerve root compromise/ irritation (e.g. intervertebral disc prolapse). It is important to exclude the small number of serious pathological conditions which can give rise to back pain:
- Underlying systemic disease presenting with back pain
- Infection
- Malignancy
- Unrecognized trauma
- Neurological compromise, nerve root damage, spinal stenosis, cauda equina syndrome.

Risk factors
Premorbid psychosocial factors (low social support, low job satisfaction) cigarette smoking, and obesity are all associated with LBP.

History and examination
This should be conducted as described on 🕮 Acute pain assessment p.5. It is important to question the patient for features suggesting serious spinal pathology, termed 'red flags' (see Table 3.3). Search for symptoms of neurological compromise (e.g. pain in legs on walking suggests neurogenic claudication in spinal stenosis). Also assess for factors which are likely to present barriers to recovery—so called 'yellow flags' (see box).

Examination should include observation of the patient's behaviour, inspection of the back for deformity (e.g. scoliosis), and palpation for spinal or paraspinal tenderness, muscular spasm, and trigger points. Assess the mobility of the lumbar spine and perform a straight leg raise. Neurological examination of the lower limbs for reflexes, power, and sensory disturbance should be performed and documented carefully.

Investigations
In the absence of factors suggesting a 'red flag' condition, imaging can be deferred unless the pain persists beyond 6 weeks. MRI and plain X-ray should be reserved for people in whom malignancy or infection is suspected. Blood tests should be ordered if 'red flag' symptoms are present and choice of test will depend on the condition that is suspected.

Table 3.3 Red flags: features which suggest serious spinal pathology

Pathology	Accompanying clinical features
Cauda equina syndrome	Urinary retention
	Faecal incontinence
	Perineal anaesthesia
	Leg weakness/abnormal gait
Malignancy (<1% of LBP)	Age >50 or <20 years
	Previous history of malignancy
	Unexplained weight loss
	Progressive symptoms despite treatment
	Pain not relieved by bed rest
Infection	Systemically unwell e.g. fever
	History of IV drug use, HIV, TB
Fracture	History of trauma
	Long-term steroid therapy
	OA—common in patients over 70 years
Inflammatory conditions e.g. ankylosing spondylitis	Morning stiffness, improvement with exercise, slow onset <40 years
	Family history
	Peripheral joint involvement
	Associated phenomena (iritis, rashes, colitis, urethritis)

Yellow flags: psychosocial predictors of chronicity
- A negative attitude that back pain is harmful or potentially severely disabling
- Fear avoidance behaviour and reduced activity levels
- An expectation that passive rather than active treatment will be beneficial
- A tendency to depression, low mood and social withdrawal
- Social or financial problems

Management

Pain is usually managed by the patient with advice from the GP. The mainstays of management are simple oral analgesics and encouragement to mobilize. Short information booklets can be helpful, e.g. *The Back Book*.[2]
- **Medication:** regularly for the first few days rather than PRN. First-line drugs are paracetamol +/− NSAIDs. Due consideration should be given to use of NSAIDs and COX-2 inhibitors in elderly people with regard to side effects and a proton pump inhibitor (PPI) may need to be co-prescribed to patients over the age of 45, if they are likely to remain on the NSAID beyond the first few weeks. Weak opioid preparations (e.g. codeine and dihydrocodeine) may be necessary as a second-line for more severe pain. These also have side effects (e.g. constipation, nausea).

- *Exercise:* bed rest encourages immobility and leads to stiffness. Patients should be encouraged to keep as mobile as possible. Active exercise should be encouraged (e.g. walking and swimming). Patients will need advice on pacing and must understand that they will not harm themselves by being active.
- *Other treatments:* manual therapy including simple manipulation can be helpful. Acupuncture and a structured exercise programme should be considered if the pain persists beyond 6 weeks.

Surgery is rarely indicted for acute LBP apart from emergency decompression for cauda equina syndrome.

References

1 http://www.dh.gov.uk/en/Publications and statistics/Publications/AnnualReports/DH_096206
2 Royal College of General Practitioners and NHS Executive (2002). *The Back Book: the Best Way to Deal with Back Pain; Get Back Active*. Stationery Office Books, London.

Pain in childbirth: introduction

Pain and the development of pain relief in childbirth have been and remain heavily influenced by social and cultural beliefs. Traditionally pain has been regarded as an integral and even necessary part of childbirth. In the 1400s in England, labouring women and caregivers were burnt at the stake for seeking pain-relief techniques in labour. It was not until the late 1800s and early 1900s that, against the resistance of the medical establishment, analgesic techniques started to gain acceptance culminating in the land-mark administration of chloroform to Queen Victoria by John Snow for the birth of her 8th child, Leopold.

Pain pathways in labour (Fig. 3.2)
- First stage of labour: body of uterus-11th and 12th thoracic roots.
- Second stage of labour: cervix, vagina, and perineum-2nd, 3rd, and 4th sacral roots.
- Dystonic labour: duration and intensity of pain may be increased and there may be greater sacral representation of pain—particularly when the fetal head occupies an occipitoposterior position in the pelvis.

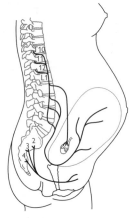

Fig. 3.2 Pain pathways in labour. Normal first stage accompany sympathetic afferents to T10–L1, second stage from perineum (and occipitoposterior position in first stage) accompany pudendal nerve to S2–S4.

Pain in childbirth: non-pharmacological analgesia

Attendance at antenatal classes

- Psychoprophylactic preparation (e.g. Grantly Dick Read in *Natural Childbirth (1938)* and Ferdnand Lamaze in *Painless Childbirth, 1984*).

Although reportedly effective in the hands of the original enthusiasts, these complex psychoprophylactic techniques have been less successful for other educators. Modern antenatal classes draw on many of the ideas of Read and Lamaze but generally present a more balanced view. Ultimately, mothers benefit from antenatal classes although attendees may represent a self-selecting group. Antenatal preparation must be delivered in such a way so as not to engender feelings of 'failure' in individuals who choose pharmacological methods of pain control once in labour.

Intrapartum support

This may be provided simply by a midwife or doula, or by more complex strategies such as hypnosis or hypnotherapy. Constant attendance of a trained attendant improves the outcome of labour; more complex strategies confer little further benefit.

Physical techniques

A wide range of physical analgesic techniques have been described to relieve labour pain. Randomized controlled trials have failed to demonstrate efficacy. Nonetheless, these techniques are invariably harmless and help many women cope with the pain of labour.
- Breathing exercises, touch, and massage
- Labouring in water (not to be confused with delivering in water)
- Mobilizing (birthing balls or rocking bars)
- Acupressure and acupuncture

Transcutaneous electrical nerve stimulation

TENS has received a lot of attention over the years and has been perceived as an effective analgesic technique in labour.
- Electrodes placed over posterior rami T10–L1, S2–4.
- Pulses of 0.1–0.5ms, 50–200Hz.
- 5–10mA to maximum 50mA boosts during contraction.
- May act via Aβ fibre stimulation.
- May cause neuronal release of endorphins.
- Early, unrandomized studies suggest TENS may be helpful in 75–90%.
- Randomized studies comparing with 'dummy' TENS show little benefit.

Summary

Intrapartum guidelines[1] state that there is little evidence to recommend the use of any non-pharmacological techniques but women who wish to use them should be supported in their choice.

Reference

1 NICE (2007). Intrapartum Care. Available at: ☞ http://www.nice.org.uk/nicemedia/pdf/IntrapartumCareSeptember2007mainguideline.pdf

Pain in childbirth: pharmacological therapy

Systemic pharmacological techniques

Inhalational analgesia

Entonox®(See Entonox section p84)

- 50:50 mixture of O_2 and N_2O.
- Most commonly used form of inhalational analgesia used in labour.
- Technique: start to inhale Entonox® as soon as a contraction begins and stop as it peaks. Systemic levels are highest with the peak of the contraction and the Entonox® is breathed out as the contraction wanes.
- The discipline of breathing may act as a distraction from the pain in itself.
- Stronger concentrations of N_2O have been used—including 100% N_2O—'the black gas'. Though effective, the side effects of such hypoxic mixtures are obvious—hence the 50:50 mixture is all that is available in the UK today.

A number of studies have tried improving the efficacy of Entonox® by either adding a constant background flow of Entonox® to the patient or by adding small quantities of other volatile agents—isoflurane, sevoflurane, or desflurane.

- Addition of background Entonox® appears to aggravate the side effects—nausea and dysphoria—without improving analgesia.
- Addition of volatile agents increases sedation and amnesia without analgesic benefit.

In summary, Entonox® appears to provide analgesic benefit to many women. It is unlikely to be harmful to mother or fetus. The principal side effects are nausea and lightheadedness in the labouring woman and these are shortlived (minutes) once she stops using it.

Parenteral analgesics

Parenteral medicines, opioids in particular, have been used to attempt to provide pain relief in childbirth for hundreds of years making it all the more remarkable that in all that time caregivers have failed to accept that they are not only ineffective but, unlike the techniques mentioned earlier, may actually cause harm to both mother and baby. Greek and Roman texts report the use of opium, sometimes mixed with mandragora, an extract from the Mandragon plant containing hyoscine. However, up until the development of the hollow needle in the late 1800s, these potions were taken orally or topically.

Pethidine

Introduced in the 1930s as an alternative to morphine, said to produce 'effective analgesia with reduced side-effects'—an ill-founded claim that has been repeated with the development of every subsequent opioid agonist or partial agonist but never substantiated by proper trials. The popularity of pethidine was and remains cemented in widespread availability due to its licensing rather than any evidence of its efficacy.

Randomized trials suggest that pethidine given either IM, IV, or by PCA does not produce pain relief in labour although reports suggest that it may make some women 'care less about their pain'. At the same time numerous studies show that pethidine causes unpleasant side effects for the mother and the baby (Table 3.4).

Table 3.4 Side effects of pethidine

Mother	Fetus	Neonate
Dysphoria	CTG: ↓variability*	Respiratory depression
Sedation	↓fetal scalp oxygen tension*	↓Apgar scores
Hypoxia (between contractions)	↓fetal activity*	↓breastfeeding
↓gastric emptying		Impaired thermoregulation
Nausea/vomiting		

CTG, cardiotocography. *May result in obstetric intervention

Other parenteral opioid agonists and partial agonists
- Morphine
- Diamorphine
- Meptazinol
- Nalbuphine
- Tramadol.

All appear equally ineffective although side-effect profiles vary.
- Fentanyl given via PCA may have fewer long-term effects on the neonate and is often used as an alternative to regional analgesia when the latter is contraindicated.
- Remifentanil has proved the most promising alternative but remains less effective than regional analgesia; it must be carefully titrated to avoid maternal sedation and respiratory depression, and has yet to be investigated as exhaustively as traditional opioids such as pethidine.

In summary, systemic opioids in general are ineffective at providing pain relief in labour while causing unpleasant side effects in both mother and baby. Disappointingly, the NICE intrapartum guidelines[1] continue to recommend the availability of pethidine and diamorphine—perpetuating this aspect of substandard care that has been provided to women in labour for over 200 years.

Reference

1 NICE (2007). Intrapartum Care. Available at: ℘ http://www.nice.org.uk/nicemedia/pdf/IntrapartumCareSeptember2007mainguideline.pdf

Pain in childbirth: regional analgesia

Regional analgesia (epidural, spinal, or combined spinal epidural (CSE)) is the most effective form of pain relief for labour. However, there remains concern with regard to the possible detrimental effects regional techniques may have on the progress or outcome of labour.

Local anaesthetics

Epidural analgesia in labour has gained popularity since it became widely available in the 1980s. Bupivacaine has been the LA of choice since it has a longer duration of action and exhibits less tachyphylaxis than its predecessor, lidocaine. Early epidurals were administered as bupivacaine alone in relatively high concentrations (0.25%)—either as intermittent boluses or infusions. In the early 1990s there was concern that 'immobility' was detrimental to the progress and outcome of labour and this resulted in the development of 'low-dose' techniques, in combination with neuraxial opioids, that allowed more movement and even ambulation (see 📖 Mobile epidural p.109).

Concerns over the risk of bupivicaine toxicity led to the introduction of single isomer LAs:

- Ropivacaine (S-propivacaine) was marketed with the alleged added benefit of a relative reduction in motor block. Subsequently, however, most studies suggest that it is simply a slightly 'weaker' LA.
- Levobupivacaine (l-bupivacaine) has a very similar profile to racaemic bupivacaine.

LA toxicity is now less of a concern as most units use very low doses. It may be a risk when using large volumes to top-up an epidural for Caesarean section. However, a number of deaths have occurred when bags containing large volumes of low-dose LA were mistaken for IV crystalloid and infused intravenously. Most units have now adopted a protocol for treating accidental LA toxicity that includes IV lipid infusion (see box).

Treatment of cardiac arrest with lipid emulsion

- Basic Life Support/Advanced Life Support.
- Bolus Intralipid® 20% 1.5mL/kg over 1 min[*].
- Start infusion Intralipid® 20% at 0.25mL/kg/min[*].
- Repeat bolus x2 at 5min intervals[*].
- Increase infusion to 0.5mL/kg/min[*].

([*]If adequate circulation has not been restored.)

Adapted from AAGBI guidelines (🖰 http://www.aagbi.org)

Epidural opioids and other adjuncts

A number of strategies have been adopted for increasing mobility in labour. Such strategies have improved maternal satisfaction and probably reduced the increased instrumental delivery rate associated with regional analgesia in labour (evidence suggests that regional analgesia does not increase the Caesarean delivery rate). These strategies include the addition of opioid to the LA. Opioids have a direct effect on the spinal cord rather than simply working centrally (following systemic absorption from the epidural or subarachnoid space). This has a dose-sparing effect on the LA resulting in reduction in the incidence of hypotension and motor block. In larger doses (e.g. >100mcg fentanyl) opioids may still result in detrimental effects on mother and baby.

'Mobile epidural'

CSE: a spinal 'starter' of 2.5mg bupivacaine and 25mcg fentanyl followed by intermittent epidural boluses of 0.1% bupivacaine containing 2mcg/mL fentanyl.

- Rapid effective analgesia
- Minimal motor blockade ± ambulation.

There is debate as to whether performing a CSE in all cases is either necessary or safe. The 'starter spinal' is an extra procedure that breaches the protective barrier of the dura mater and a number of case reports of meningitis emerged. Although the 'starter spinal' is now accepted as safe, most units limit CSEs to specific situations (e.g. rapidly progressing labour, occiptoposterior position).

The majority of units have adopted 'low-dose' regimens employing dilute LA/opioid combinations, allowing the most of women to mobilize if not ambulate. This change has reduced the rate of instrumental vaginal deliveries associated with regional analgesia in labour and improved maternal satisfaction (COMET trial).[1]

Other adjuncts:

- Clonidine, an α-2 agonist has been perhaps the most promising although it can cause sedation and hypotension.
- Adrenaline has also been widely investigated but seems to be associated with an increase in motor block.

Several other adjuncts have been investigated but add little benefit while frequently increasing side effects: neostigmine, for example, increases nausea and vomiting particularly when used via the intrathecal route.

Most additives complicate the procedure and add little benefit because investigators fail to reduce the dose of the principal agents (i.e. LA) to allow the dose-sparing benefits of the adjuncts to become apparent.

Infusions, boluses, or PCEA

Intermittent boluses

- Delivered by the midwifery staff.
- Reduced total dose.
- Concerns that doses may be withheld in the second stage of labour[*].
- Increased workload for staff.

([*]Epidural analgesia should not be withheld in the second stage.)

Infusions

- Maintained throughout labour.
- Decreased workload: need for intermittent top-ups is reduced.
- Total dose is likely to be increased.
- Incidence of motor block increases.

PCEA

- Intermittent bolus top-ups ± low-dose background infusion.
- Gives the labouring woman control of her pain.
- Decreased workload for staff.

Side effects of regional analgesia

In January 2008, the Obstetric Anaesthetists Association published a summary information card detailing incidence of problems and side effects of regional analgesia:

- Failure (1:8)
- Hypotension (1:50)
- Severe headache (1:100)
- Temporary minor nerve damage (1:1,000)
- Severe permanent nerve injury (1:250,000).

Regional analgesia is not believed to increase the risk of Caesarean section. It may be associated with a doubling of the risk of instrumental vaginal delivery.

All labour wards offering regional analgesia should have an obstetric anaesthetist available 24/7. Epidurals should be followed-up during labour and checked for efficacy. Inadequate epidurals should be adjusted and re-sited if necessary. The anaesthetist should evaluate whether an epidural is effective enough to be topped-up for Caesarean section.

Accidental dural tap and/or intrathecal catheter placement should be identified either at the time of Tuohy needle placement, aspiration of the catheter, or by the onset of unexpected significant motor block. If identified at the time of Tuohy needle placement, the catheter can be threaded into the CSF to give predictable analgesia or anaesthesia. All boluses must be given by an anaesthetist due to an increased risk of high block.

All women having regional analgesia in labour must be followed-up. If not catheterized all women should pass urine within 6h of delivery. Any patient with postdural puncture headache (PDPH) should be followed up and offered therapeutic blood patch if necessary. Nerve injury most commonly results from obstetric causes, but central neuraxial complications must always be excluded.

Summary

Pain relief in labour remains a complex sociological issue both in developed and undeveloped regions of the world. Regional analgesia remains the only effective form of pain relief, though is not without significant side effects. There are numerous strategies that help women cope with the birth experience and all, with the exception of parenteral opioid techniques, should be supported by care providers.

Further reading

Chamberlain G et al. (1993). *Pain and its relief in childbirth: the results of a national survey conducted by the National Birthday Trust.* Churchill Livingstone, Edinburgh, pp.1–9.

Collis RE et al. (1995). Randomised comparison of combined spinal-epidural and standard epidural analgesia in labour. *Lancet* **345**:1413–16.

NICE (2007). *Intrapartum Care.* Available at: ℛ http://www.nice.org.uk/nicemedia/pdf/IntrapartumCareSeptember2007mainguideline.pdf

Reference

1 Comparative Obstetric Mobile Epidural Trial (COMET) Study Group UK (2001). Effect of low-dose mobile versus traditional epidural techniques on mode of delivery: a randomized controlled trial. *Lancet* **358**:19–23.

Neonatal pain: introduction

Neonates and small infants respond to painful stimuli in a largely similar manner to older children and adults. They exhibit characteristic behavioural, physiological, and hormonal responses to painful stimuli. However, these responses can be inconsistent, making attempts at quantifying pain very difficult.

Traditional definitions of pain, such as '*an unpleasant sensory and emotional experience usually associated with tissue damage...*' are difficult to apply as they require the ability to communicate and are inappropriate when considering the pain experience of neonates. Consideration of nociception is more appropriate and embodies the anatomical pathways, structures, and physiological responses to a nociceptive stimuli.

All neonates have iatrogenic pain, at the least, the stimulus of a heel lance for metabolic screening. 1 in 12 neonates will have repeated painful procedures (e.g. venepuncture), tissue trauma from surgery, and the continuous stimulation from an endotracheal tube, mechanical ventilation, and repeated suctioning. The very premature neonate, receiving prolonged intensive care, can have hundreds of invasive procedures.

- There are various classifications of painful stimuli in older children and adults that are equally applicable to the neonatal population such as:
  - Acute/chronic
  - Physiological/inflammatory/neuropathic/visceral
  - Mild/moderate/severe
- It is more useful, in the clinical environment, to consider the 3 common scenarios in which the neonate is subjected to painful stimuli:
  - Invasive procedures
  - Mechanical ventilation
  - Surgery.

Fetal development of nociceptive pathways

- At 6 weeks' gestation the sensory neurons form synapses with the DH.
- The sensory neurons grow peripherally to reach skin of limbs by 11 weeks, the trunk by 15 weeks, and mucosal surfaces by 20 weeks. Nociceptor receptor density at term is equal to the adult.
- From 13–30 weeks' gestation there is increased organization of the laminar structure of DH.
- By 24 weeks, the thalamocortical tracts have developed with myelination being completed by 30 weeks.
- C-fibres become functionally mature in the 3rd trimester; however, A β fibres can transmit nociceptive signals at a much earlier gestation.
- Descending inhibitory tracts are not fully developed until post term. There is increased afferent nociceptive transmission in the spinal cord.
- Somatosensory evoked responses are present from 28 weeks suggesting intact, functioning afferent pathways from periphery to brain.
- The preterm neonate consequently has an underdamped, poorly discriminative afferent nervous system which can result in exaggerated responses to noxious stimuli.

Effects of nociception

There are various consequences of not treating pain:

- Changes in pain sensitivity/pain processing: preterm infants have short-term hypersensitivity and hyperalgesia after heel lancing. This can cause hyperinnervation and allodynia.
- Neurodevelopmental/behavioural/cognitive changes in later childhood:
  - Longer-term responses to repeated noxious stimuli as a neonate include a persistence of immature pain responses at 18 months and an increase in somatization at 4–5 years.
  - Even single painful events such as an awake circumcision leads to an exaggerated pain response at 3–6 months.
- Increased incidence of intra- and postoperative complications:
  - A noxious stimulus results in a rise in blood pressure and intracranial pressure from 18 weeks' gestation. In the preterm infant in particular this can lead to neurological complications (intraventricular haemorrhage and periventricular leukomalacia).
  - Neonatal stress response to surgery is greater but shorter lived than older infants. Inadequate treatment results in poor outcomes.

Measurement of pain

Numerous pain assessment tools have been validated for very specific clinical situations. Most require some degree of training and are unwieldy in a clinical setting.

Unidimensional pain scales

Make assessment of behavioural responses to pain (obviously these have no utility in paralysed neonates):

- Neonatal Facial Coding System (NFCS). Uses a variety of facial actions in both preterm and term infants to identify procedural pain.
- EDIN scale (Échelle Douleur Inconfort Nouveau-Né, neonatal pain and discomfort scale) is validated for prolonged pain in preterm infants using 5 behavioural indicators (facial activity, body movement, sleep, contact quality with carers, and consolability).
- Clinical Scoring System (CSS).
- Infant Body Coding System (IBCS).
- Liverpool Infant Distress Score (LIDS). Uses 8 behavioural characteristics to score postoperative pain.

Multidimensional pain scales

Using a combination of behavioural, physiological, and contextual indicators:

- COMFORT scale assesses anxiety as well as pain in ventilated patients on PICU aged from newborn to adolescent.
- Premature Infant Pain Profile (PIPP) is a complex tool that uses brow bulge, eye squeezing, nasolabial furrowing, heart rate, oxygen saturations, gestational age, and behaviour state.
- Neonatal Infant Pain Profile (NIPS).
- CRIES (Crying, Requires increased oxygen administration, Increased vital signs, Expression, Sleeplessness), developed for assessment of postoperative pain.

Neonatal pain: treatment

Opioids

Pharmacological considerations

- Neonates have a higher percentage of body water and less fat than older infants. They have immature hepatic and renal function. Water-soluble drugs (e.g. morphine) will need to be given in relatively large loading doses followed by lower infusion rates than used in older infants as the drug clearance is prolonged.
- Highly lipid soluble opioids (e.g. fentanyl) have a more rapid onset, a greater potency, and a longer duration of action than predicted. This is due to selective redistribution of the drug to the neonatal brain with reduced peripheral uptake.
- Morphine effect site concentrations may also be enhanced due to immaturity of the blood–brain barrier.

Tolerance and withdrawal

- Opioid tolerance can occur over several days due to a combination of true pharmacodynamic tolerance and increased elimination.
- Sudden cessation of morphine administration can lead to opioid withdrawal symptoms, this occurs after between 2–5 days.
- Treatment of opioid withdrawal includes a reducing opioid regimen (using morphine or methadone) or α_2 agonists (clonidine 3–5mcg/kg, PO 8–12-hourly).

Clinical use

- Morphine remains the gold standard analgesic for sedation and analgesia in neonates. Following a bolus it has a slower onset and longer action than fentanyl. However, it has a shorter terminal $t_{\frac{1}{2}}$ than fentanyl, and after a prolonged infusion will have a quicker offset time.
- Nurse-controlled analgesia (NCA) is a useful technique that combines a morphine infusion with additional 'top-up' doses as indicated by the appropriate pain scale.
- Fentanyl is relatively cardiovascularly stable and can be used at very high doses (50–100mcg/kg) to control pulmonary hypertension.
- Opioids should be used with caution in spontaneously ventilating neonates. All infants under 6 months should be monitored, ideally in a high dependency area with a minimal monitoring standard of direct observation, pulse oximetry and ventilatory monitoring.

Paracetamol

- Primarily metabolized by sulphation in neonates (rather than glucuronidation in older children). Once this pathway is saturated, paracetamol is oxidized to a reactive compound that is bound to glutathione with any unbound fraction causing hepatocyte damage. Neonates are relatively protected from the toxic side effects of paracetamol by having slow oxidative metabolism and greater glutathione stores.
- Up to 48h administration of paracetamol in term and preterm neonates is safe, efficacious, and has opioid-sparing effects. After 48h paracetamol may accumulate.
- The dose and interval must be tailored to the gestational age of the neonate.

NSAIDs

- Analgesic, antipyretic, and anti-inflammatory properties.
- NSAID use is limited in neonates due to their side effects:
  - Decreased renal perfusion.
  - Decreased splanchnic perfusion increasing the risk of necrotizing enterocolitis.
  - Reduced platelet function.
  - Reduced cerebral blood flow.
- Indometacin and ibuprofen are used for the medical closure of patent ductus arteriosus. Note some congenital cyanotic cardiac malformations rely on a patent ductus for the delivery of oxygenated blood so avoid NSAIDs in these neonates.
- Ibuprofen has fewer side effects than indometacin and can be used with term neonates. It may displace bilirubin from albumin so caution is needed with jaundiced patients.

Other drugs

- Ketamine is an anaesthetic/analgesic agent that provides reasonable CV stability with bronchodilation. It increases airway secretions and is usually given with an anticholinergic agent (e.g. atropine). It can be given intravenously, intramuscularly, and via the neuraxial route. When used for procedural sedation it is often coadministered with IV midazolam (25mcg/kg).
- Clonidine has analgesic properties and is commonly used via the caudal route (1–2mcg/kg) in combination with LAs.
- Both ketamine and clonidine have the advantage of less respiratory depression than opioids but should be used with caution, as they are associated with apnoea in the preterm neonate.
- Pure sedative drugs have an important role in the management of neonatal pain by reducing anxiety and stress and promoting sleep (e.g. lorazepam, chloral hydrate, promethazine, and triclofos).

Local anaesthesia
- Various modes of administration: topical, local infiltration, local and regional nerve blocks, and neuroaxial (via the caudal, epidural, and subarachnoid routes).
- Provides very effective blocking of nociceptive impulses but techniques are largely in the specialist domain of the paediatric anaesthetist.
- Lower α-1-glycoprotein levels and reduced clearance of amide LAs will result in higher plasma concentrations of LAs and lead to a higher risk of toxicity that will be exacerbated by acidosis, hypoxia, hyponatraemia, and hyperkalaemia.
- Maximum safe bolus dose is 3mg/kg for lidocaine and 2mg/kg for bupivacaine, similar to older children.
- Epidural infusions of bupivacaine (0.2mg/kg/h, 0.125%) can be used safely for up to 48h after which bupivacaine may accumulate in the plasma.
- Topical anaesthesia with amethocaine and EMLA® (2.5% lidocaine and 2.5% prilocaine) reduce the physiological response to certain painful procedures such as venepuncture or circumcision.
- Prilocaine is associated with methaemoglobinaemia—this concern has previously limited EMLA® use in neonates. However, if used infrequently, EMLA® in small quantities is not associated with significant methaemoglobinaemia.

Non-pharmacological
There are various behavioural and non-pharmacological interventions that can both reduce the physiological responses to painful procedures and lead to lower morbidity and earlier discharge from hospital:
- Minimizing painful interventions and clustering them together to reduce the frequency of noxious stimuli.
- Decreasing handling, reducing ambient noise and light, and establishing a circadian day/night cycle.
- Oral sucrose or glucose in concentrations up to 50%.
- A process of 'sensorial saturation' that includes gentle stimulation of the visual, tactile, auditory, and taste senses through the use of sucrose, lights, rocking, and ambient music.

Table 3.5 Suggested analgesic dosing. Neonates receiving opioids must be observed in a high dependency area.

	Dose	Notes
Morphine (ventilated patient)	50–150mcg/kg IV	Loading dose
	5–20mcg/kg/h IV	Infusion
	2.5–10mcg/kg IV	NCA (bolus, max every 30min)
	2.5–10mcg/kg/h IV	NCA (background infusion)
Morphine (unventilated patient)	10–50mcg/kg IV	Slow loading dose
Fentanyl	0.5–10mcg/kg IV	For ventilated neonates only
Codeine	1mg/kg PO/PR	
Paracetamol: maximum daily doses	25mg/kg PO, 35mg/kg PR	Loading dose, all ages
	25mg/kg PO, 30mg/kg PR	30 weeks PC
	45mg/kg PO, 60mg/kg PR	34 weeks PC
	60mg/kg PO, 80mg/kg PR	40 weeks PC
	90mg/kg PO, 120mg/kg PR	60 weeks PC
Ibuprofen	5–10mg/kg PO	Every 12–24h
Ketamine	0.5–1mg/kg IV 3–8mg/kg PR	Coadministration with an anticholinergic advised due to increased respiratory secretions
Clonidine	2–4mcg/kg PO	For opioid withdrawal
Lorazepam	20–100mcg/kg IV	
Chloral hydrate/ triclofos sodium	30–50mg/kg PO/PR	
Promethazine	0.5mg/kg IV/PO	

NCA, nurse-controlled analgesia, PC, post conception.

Table 3.6 Suggested strategies for pain treatment in 3 common scenarios in the neonatal period

1. Procedural analgesia	
E.g. venepuncture or chest drain insertion	Use LA where possible, first establish appropriate safe dose for patient then consider: • Local infiltration • EMLA® (allow skin contact of at least 60min) • Ametop® (allow skin contact of 45min) • Non-pharmacological strategies • Consider single IV opioid bolus

2. Sedation for a ventilated neonate	
	Opioid infusion
	Critically ill baby use fentanyl 2.5–10mcg/kg/h IV
	Otherwise morphine 0–20mcg/kg/h
	Optimize opioid infusion using pain/anxiety scale
	Limit dose to reduce tolerance
	Consider adjuvant drugs to reduce opioid requirements (triclofos or lorazepam)
	Clonidine
	Non-pharmacological strategies

3. Post surgical analgesia	
Non-ventilated baby	Determine opioid history, e.g. loading dose in theatre or long-term administration
	Inadequate analgesia:
	10–50mcg/kg IV morphine bolus over 15min with formal pain scoring at 5min intervals until analgesia is optimal
	Analgesia maintenance:
	0–10mcg/kg/h IV morphine
	Regular paracetamol (caution after 48h—see text) Transfer to enteral analgesics, e.g. codeine, as soon as possible
Ventilated baby	Inadequate analgesia: 50–150mcg/kg IV morphine bolus as required
	Analgesia maintenance: 0–40mcg/kg/h IV morphine
	Regular paracetamol (caution after 48h—see text)
	Fentanyl with critically ill babies (conveys haemodynamic stability)
	0.5–10mcg/kg IV bolus if analgesia inadequate
	2.5–10mcg/kg/h for IV maintenance

Acute pain management in children

Introduction

Historically, pain has been undertreated in children. Young children were thought to feel less pain than adults and assessment of pain was inconsistent and difficult. Less opioid was prescribed due to concerns about excessive sedation, respiratory depression, and a potential for narcotic addiction. In the last 20 years these misconceptions have been dismantled and attitudes have changed. Pain assessment and management is an integral part of the care needed by all children.

Children undergo huge changes, in size, physiology, and psychology which affect acute pain therapy. This chapter will consider pain, assessment, and management in children from 44 weeks post conception age (for neonatal pain management see 📖 p.112). The pharmacodynamics and pharmacokinetics of drugs vary with age. In addition, most children are dependent on their parents with significant psychosocial elements to consider during their management.

Causes of acute pain

- Postoperative
- Procedural (iatrogenic)
- Trauma:
  - Soft-tissue
  - Fractures
- Medical:
  - Inflammatory; arthropathies, tonsillitis, otitis media
  - Cancer-related: tumour, secondary to chemotherapy, i.e. mucositis
  - Sickle cell disease
  - Perthes disease.

Assessment

Regular assessment coupled with appropriate intervention is fundamental to successful treatment of pain. Dependent on age, maturity, and neurodevelopment. Note: children's behaviour may regress when distressed or in pain.

Physiological

Not practical for clinical practice but useful for research projects in neonates and small infants. Neuroendocrine or physiological responses can be measured.

Observational/behavioural

Normally used for preverbal or children with neurodevelopment delay. A multitude of different pain assessment tools described, which indicate there is not a 'gold standard' unlike visual analogue score used in adult practice. Examples are: CHEOPS, OPS, and FLACC, see Fig. 3.3.

Self-rating scores

Well-validated, reproducible, and practical for acute pain management. Children from 4–5 years can use Oucher or Wong–Baker faces (Fig. 1.3). Older children and adolescents can use verbal analogue score or visual analogue scores (see 📖 p.7).

The FLACC Behavioural Pain Assessment Scale

0 No particular expression or smile.	1 Occasional grimace or frown, withdrawn, disinterested.	2 Frequent to constant frown, clenched jaw, quivering chin.
0 Mormal position or relaxed.	1 Uneasy, restless, tense.	2 Kicking or legs drawn up.
0 Lying quietly, normal position, moves easily.	1 Squirming, shifting back and forth, tense.	2 Arched, rigid or jerking.
0 No cry Awake or asleep	1 Moans or whimpers, occasional complaints.	2 Crying steadily, screams or sobs, frequent complaints.
0 Content, relaxed	1 Reassured by occasional touching, hugging or 'talking to'. Distractable.	2 Difficult to console or comfort.

To be used for any child who is unable to report their level of pain.

Fig. 3.3 The FLACC behavioural pain assessment scale.

Consequences of poor pain control

Behavioural

Poor pain control is associated with anxiety, phobic behaviour, and sleep disturbance. These can be ameliorated by good pain control.

Cardiovascular

Tachycardia and hypertension, both systemic and pulmonary, lead to increased myocardial workload and potential for shunt reversal especially in the neonate. In older children and adolescents, immobility, venostasis, and increased clotting may cause venous thrombosis with potential pulmonary embolism

Respiratory

Chest and abdominal pain lead to reduced lung volumes, poor cough with atelectasis, sputum retention, chest infections, and hypoxaemia.

Gastrointestinal

Delayed gastric emptying and reduced intestinal motility. This may also be secondary to opioid use.

Genitourinary

Urinary retention. Exacerbated by immobility but also by opioids and epidural analgesia.

Endocrine/metabolic

Increased release of catecholamines, glucocorticoids, renin/angiotensin, aldosterone, vasopressin, growth hormone, and glucagon with reduced insulin secretion results in increased oxygen consumption, sodium and fluid retention, protein breakdown, raised blood glucose, poor wound healing, and a hypercoaguable state.

Multimodal treatment

Good pain management will usually involve the implementation of a multimodal treatment regimen for children whatever the cause of their admission to hospital but especially following surgery. The aim is to use different modalities, including combinations of analgesic drugs, to reduce pain and distress, improve recovery and mobility whilst minimizing side effects from treatment. On the whole, simple therapies produce the most benefit for least potential harm.

Psychosocial interventions

May focus on the environment, parents, comforters, massage/swaddling, distraction, hypnosis and guided imagery, play and music therapy, and teachers.

Non-pharmacological

Splints, ethyl chloride spray, heat, or cold, TENS and acupuncture. Breast feeding or oral 30% glucose for procedural pain.

Drugs

Prescribe according to age and weight. Many are used 'off label'. Availability of a palatable oral preparation that a child will take influences what is prescribed. IM route of administration must be avoided.

Acute pain management in children: systemic pharmacological treatment

Simple analgesia

Paracetamol

Ubiquitous 'over-the-counter' analgesic and antipyretic. It has no anti-inflammatory effect and its analgesic mechanism is not fully understood (see 📖 Paracetamol p. 24).

Dose (Table 3.7)

Age and route dependant. The oral route is the route of choice and is reliable outside infancy. Rectal absorption is good but there is delayed onset and a higher dose is required when initially loading. Higher doses should be time-limited because of the risk of accumulation and toxicity especially if there is a coexisting fever.

IV paracetamol is useful when the child is vomiting or nil by mouth (NBM) (not recommended for infants <10kg).

Table 3.7 Paracetamol doses

New born (term) infants <10kg	Infants/children 10–50kg	Adolescents >50kg
7.5mg/kg 4–6-hourly	15mg/kg 4–6-hourly	15mg/kg 4–6-hourly
Maximum recommended dose 30mg/kg daily	**Maximum** recommended dose 60mg/kg/day	**Maximum** recommended dose not exceeding 4 g/day

NSAIDs

Ibuprofen is frequently used by parents in the community as an antipyretic and analgesic. It is used for mild to moderate pain or in combination with morphine for severe pain with an associated 30–40% reduction in morphine consumption. It is readily absorbed orally.

Other NSAIDs

Diclofenac and naproxen are useful alternatives, especially if a different route, preparation, or flavour required. Specific COX-2 inhibitors are not licensed for use in children, though controversial issues regarding their use in adults such as increased CV events are less relevant in children.

See Table 3.8 for doses and side effects.

Antispasmodics

Diazepam 0.1mg/kg/8h, is frequently used for children with cerebral palsy who have painful spasms postoperatively, especially following orthopaedic surgery. Baclofen is an alternative. Any children on chronic maintenance treatment must not have it stopped abruptly as this may precipitate severe spasticity and even hyperpyrexia secondary to malignant neuroleptic syndrome.

Table 3.8 Doses of NSAIDs:

Ibuprofen	
Tablets 200mg	5–10mg/kg 6–8-hourly
Elixir 100mg/5mL	**Maximum** recommended dose: 30mg/kg/day not exceeding 2400mg
Diclofenac	
Suppositories: 12.5mg, 25mg, 50mg, 100mg	1–1.5mg/kg 8-hourly
Enteric coated tablets: 25mg, 50mg Dispersible tablets: 50mg	**Maximum** recommended dose: 3mg/kg/day by any route up to 150mg/day
IV diclofenac	
Not recommended in patients <6 months old	
25mg/mL (3mL ampoule)	0.3–1mg/kg 8-hourly
	Maximum recommended dose: 150mg/day for a maximum of 2 days
Naproxen	
Tablets 250mg, 500mg	5–10mg/kg 12-hourly
	Maximum recommended dose: 1000mg/day

Inhalational analgesia

N_2O is an extremely useful short-acting analgesic with a rapid onset (approximately 2min). The simplest way to administer N_2O is as a 50:50 mix with O_2 known as Entonox® via a simple demand valve (see section Entonox p84). Children as young as 3 years of age can trigger the valve and self-administer using a face-mask or a mouthpiece. It causes some transient sedation, excitation/euphoria ('laughing gas'), and occasionally nausea and vomiting.

Indication

Procedural pain control, e.g. drain removal, suturing, bone marrow aspiration, dressing changes, venepuncture.

Contraindications

An insoluble gas that rapidly diffuses into gas-containing spaces, it may change a simple pneumothorax to a tension pneumothorax. Also caution in bowel obstruction, airway abnormality, head injury, and uncorrected congenital heart disease. Care must be taken if other depressive drugs have been used, e.g. benzodiazepines, opioids, and antihistamines, as it may cause excessive sedation and respiratory depression.

It must not be used repeatedly over a prolonged period of time as it affects vitamin B12 metabolism and may cause a macrocytic anaemia and subacute combined degeneration of the spinal cord.

Opioids

Morphine
Gold standard with most paediatric experience, poor lipid solubility results in a relatively slow onset. Principal use is intravenously as an infusion, in NCA or PCA.

Diamorphine
Needs to be deacylated to active component morphine. Lipid soluble with much faster onset than morphine. Mainly used in paediatrics by intranasal administration. 100mcg/kg in 0.2mL normal saline provides rapid analgesia particularly useful in Emergency Department (see 📖 p.88).

Codeine
Commonly used but low potency, dependent on conversion to morphine. As 10% of the population lacks the enzyme then it is variably effective. Must never be used intravenously-causes CV collapse.

Fentanyl
Mainly used intraoperatively by anaesthetists but also provides rapid analgesia in the recovery room. Occasionally used in SC infusion or as the transcutaneous patches for palliative care.

Pethidine
Low potency with some LA and smooth muscle relaxant properties. Has an active metabolite norpethidine that is renally excreted and can accumulate causing excitatory phenomena including seizures.

Tramadol
Weak synthetic opioid agonist but additionally blocks noradrenaline and serotonin reuptake. Used to treat moderate pain.

Side effects
All opioids have a similar range of side effects if given at equianalgesic doses, but there is marked interpatient variability. Side effects include respiratory depression, sedation, dysphoria, miosis, nausea and vomiting, constipation, urinary retention, and pruritus. Small infants occasionally become 'twitchy/jerky' on morphine infusions; this may be a sign of excessive dosing and usually respond to stopping the infusion for an hour and restarting at a lower rate.

Naloxone
Is a specific opioid antagonist at the mu receptor. This can be used to reverse the opioid side effects, especially respiratory depression or excessive sedation. The dose should be titrated to effect to avoid rebound pain, hypertension, cardiac dysrhythmias, and, rarely, pulmonary oedema. Smaller doses can be used to treat urinary retention and pruritus. An infusion reduces recurrent pruritus and resistant nausea without completely reversing the analgesia.

Antiemetics
IV agents e.g. 5HT$_3$ antagonists, ondansetron, antihistamines, cyclizine, or dexamethasone, may be required when opioids are prescribed, especially in adolescent girls and poststrabismus or middle ear surgery.

Antipruritics
Pruritus is often treated with the antihistamine chlorphenamine.

Delivery systems

IV infusion

Use a simple infusion system for young infants and children unable to use a PCA. Titrate to level of analgesia required with a loading dose, maintain above minimum effective analgesic concentration (MEAC), aiming to keep side effects to a minimum i.e. below minimum toxic concentration (MTC). Beware of increasing sedation. It avoids IM injections and recurrent peaks and troughs seen with intermittent IM doses of morphine. Lower doses required in young infants due to pharmacodynamic and kinetic differences.

Table 3.9 IV Infusion of Morphine in infants

Age	Loading doses	Maximum infusion
1–3 months	50mcg/kg	10mcg/kg/h
>3 months	100–150mcg/kg	40mcg/kg/h

Morphine 1mg/kg in 50mL normal saline gives a concentration of 20mcg/kg/mL.

Patient-controlled anaesthesia

PCA is frequently used in paediatric practice both for postoperative pain control and acute painful medical episodes such as sickle cell crisis and mucositis associated with neutropenia induced by chemotherapy. It enables the child to control their pain by keeping the analgesic above the MEAC, without waiting for a nurse to administer the analgesic. Needs careful explanation and reinforcement to child and family and encourage pre-emptive use. Most pumps can limit the total amount given in a fixed 4h period, as a background infusion is usually required in children. There is good evidence that the use of background infusions improves efficacy without the increase in side effects seen in adult practice. The inherent safety of the system is that the child would become sedated and therefore not press the button if they use it too frequently. When initiating treatment, adequate analgesia must be established with IV morphine. The child must be able to understand the concept and be able to physically press the button, so normally applicable to ages of 5 and above. The concentration of the solution used is usually 20mcg/kg/mL up to a maximum of 1mg/mL, i.e. all children over 50kg have a 1mg/mL solution. See Table 3.10.

Complications associated with PCA are usually due to either programming/drug errors or the side effects of opioids. Pump malfunction is now extremely rare.

Table 3.10 PCA

Dose	1mL (i.e. 20mcg/kg) over 1min
Lockout interval	5min
Background infusion	6mcg/kg/h (i.e. 0.3mL/r) on 1st–2nd postoperative day
4h maximum	400mcg/kg/4h

Morphine 1mg/kg in 50mL normal saline gives a concentration of 20mcg/kg/mL.

Nurse-controlled analgesia

NCA is basically a morphine infusion using a PCA pump; it allows the nursing staff to give recorded bolus doses quickly and simply. Used in babies and young children. See Table 3.11.

Table 3.11 NCA

	Over 3 months
Background	10–20mcg/kg/h
Bolus	10–20mcg/kg
Lockout	30min
4h maximum	250mcg/kg/4h

Morphine 1mg/kg in 50mL normal saline gives a concentration of 20mcg/kg/mL.

Other analgesics

Ketamine

NMDA antagonist, a GA, but provides excellent analgesia at lower doses. Racemic mixture or S-enantiomer. S-ketamine has twice the analgesic potency of racemic mixture, with less psychomotor disturbance, less salivation, and shorter recovery. Mainly used as an adjuvant to caudal bupivacaine where 0.5mg/kg prolongs the duration of analgesia up to 12h. Also used intravenously in complex acute pain problems, e.g. mucositis, as an infusion 25–100mcg/kg/h or combined with morphine in a PCA as 50:50 mixture, 20mcg/kg/mL of each. This will often improve analgesia, reduce total morphine consumption, and paradoxically result in less sedation.

Clonidine

An α2-adrenoceptor agonist that is used both for sedative and analgesic properties, especially on PICU. Acts to modulate nociceptive transmission in the spinal cord and brain. Effective orally 1–3mcg/kg, 2–3 times per day. Particularly useful in an epidural infusion combined with bupivacaine for complex multilevel orthopaedic surgery, appears to reduce painful muscle spasms. Side effects—excessive sedation, hypotension, and bradycardia.

Acute pain management in children: local anaesthesia

LA techniques are extensively used in paediatric practice, e.g. to prevent needle phobia by pre-emptive use of topical LA prior to IV cannulation and intraoperatively to provide excellent postoperative pain relief.

Local nerve blocks

Specific nerve blocks performed during anaesthesia, e.g. penile, ilio-inguinal/ilio-hypogastric, sciatic, axillary for postoperative analgesia lasting 4–24h or sometimes in accident department, e.g. femoral, digital to give analgesia for fracture reduction, or suturing. A variety of techniques used to locate nerves including anatomical landmarks, nerve stimulators, or US imaging. Peripheral blocks are associated with less morbidity and possibly mortality compared with neuraxial blocks.

Regional blocks

Spinal

As a sole technique for high-risk ex-premature babies undergoing herniotomy or muscle biopsy. Supplement to GA for high-risk neonatal cardiac surgery where it reduces the stress response to surgery better than high-dose opioids. Becoming increasingly popular with recent concerns about GA and neurodevelopmental delay.

Epidural

Caudal route is a common single-shot access point for postoperative analgesia during sub-umbilical surgery in children. Dose: 0.5–1.0mL/kg 0.25% bupivacaine depending on the height of the block required. The duration of the block can be increased by adding preservative-free clonidine 1–2mcg/kg, ketamine 0.5mg/kg, or morphine 50mcg/kg. See Table 3.12.

Postoperative epidural infusions of LA usually with an adjuvant provides prolonged analgesia 3–4 days after major surgery. An epidural catheter is inserted after induction of general anaesthesia, the level of insertion governed by the site of the surgery, though in young infants some units prefer to always use the caudal route.

Technically, insertion of a catheter into the epidural space of a child needs a skilled, experienced operator. The distance from the skin to the epidural space in the newborn is less than a centimetre; as a general rule, 1mm per kg weight is a useful guide. An 18G Touhy needle is most frequently used though a 19G is required for infants <5kg. This smaller needle comes with a thin-walled single end-holed catheter that is liable to kink and leak. The space is identified with a loss of resistance (LOR) to saline technique (LOR with air has been associated with significant morbidity and deaths). The catheter is usually inserted at the dermatomal level needed to be blocked. The spinal cord is more caudal extending to L3 in the infant, so most epidurals other than caudals are inserted at a level where there is a potential for spinal cord damage.

Table 3.12 Epidural infusions of bupivacaine—loading dose 0.5mL/kg of 0.25% plain bupivacaine

	Epidural solution	Infusion rate	Maximum bupivacaine infusion rate
Child/adolescent	0.1% bupivacaine	0.1–0.5mL/kg/h	0.5mg/kg/h or 15ml/h
	0.1% bupivacaine with 2mcg/mL fentanyl	0.1–0.5mL/kg/h	
	0.1% bupivacaine with 2mcg/ml clonidine	0.1–0.5mL/kg/h	

Advantages of regional analgesia
- Superior postoperative analgesia for major surgery compared to opioids.
- Improved respiratory function.
  - Less atelectasis, better cough, with a reduction in the requirement for postoperative ventilation.
- Earlier discharge from hospital, particularly for high-risk children undergoing open fundoplication.
- Reduced stress response seen during surgery, spinal >epidural >opioid.
- Reduction in postoperative ileus and gastric stasis by blocking sympathetic supply to GI tract and avoidance of systemic opioids therefore earlier enteral feeding and less PONV.

Contraindications
- Lack of patient or parental consent
- Local infection or untreated systemic sepsis
- Bleeding or clotting abnormalities
- Raised intracranial pressure and spinal abnormalities.

Complications
- *Technical:* bloody tap—potential for epidural haematoma; dural tap ± PDPH; accidental total spinal anaesthesia; direct damage to the spinal cord or nerve roots; infection including meningitis and epidural abscess; catheter problems, premature loss, kinking, blockage, leaks (this is very common especially in small infants) and delivery system problems including drug errors and mis-programming of pumps.
- *Physiological:* profound motor block with analgesia has led to pressure ulcers; intense analgesia may cause delay in diagnosis of compartment syndrome; retention of urine in approximately 20% of children so pre-emptive catheterization is usually performed intraoperatively. Hypotension is unusual in children <8 years because of reduced peripheral venous volume, reduced sympathetic innervation to legs, and less cardiac deceleration compared to adolescents and adults. A reversible Horner's block is not infrequent in a high thoracic epidural but rarely associated with significant respiratory embarrassment.

- *Toxic effects of LAs:* seizures and CV collapse have been described especially in infants given excessive initial doses, prolonged infusions, or who received an accidental IV injection of LA.
- *Pharmacological effects of adjuvant drugs:* epidural opioids, clonidine, and ketamine may all cause systemic side effects, though the principal reason for using the epidural route is to use much lower total dose of drug and thereby reduce the incident of this problem.

Paediatric Acute Pain Service (APS)

The use of complex analgesic techniques including epidural infusions, morphine infusions, and PCAs cannot be achieved safely without the investment of a significant amount of professional time and some capital expense (see also 📖 adult APS, p.12). The development of a multiprofessional acute pain team to support these innovations is fundamental to their success. Guidelines on the indication, the prescription of simple analgesic and infusions, the equipment used, and especially the level of monitoring should be developed for each institutions needs and facilities. See Fig. 3.4 for the pain observation chart used in Bristol Royal Hospital for Children. The APS provides ongoing education for nursing and medical staff and sees children and their families on a daily basis to review and audit efficacy. This provides a safe environment for patients.

Further reading

Association of Paediatric Anaesthetists of Great Britain and Ireland. Good Practice in Postoperative and Procedural Pain. Available at: 🔗 www.apagbi.org.uk/docs/APA_Guidelines_on_Pain_Management.pdf

UNITED BRISTOL HEALTHCARE NHS TRUST

BRISTOL ROYAL HOSPITAL FOR CHILDREN

PAEDIATRIC OBSERVATION CHART

ADDRESSOGRAPH LABEL	
Name:	
Date of Birth:	
Hospital No:	
Ward/Hospital:	

Ward Area: .... Date:	
Patient's Weight: .... in kilograms (kg)	
Patient's Height: .... in centimetres (cm)	

PAIN ASSESSMENT TOOLS USED (Please tick)
- ☐ FLACC (Face, Legs, Activity, Cry, Consolability)
- ☐ Wong and Baker (Faces)
- ☐ Visual Analogue Scale (0–10)

NORMAL RESPIRATORY / BP / PULSE RATES **IF RECEIVING O₂ OBSERVATIONS SHOULD BE RECORDED A MINIMUM OF 1 HRLY
UNLESS EXCEPTIONAL CIRCUMSTANCES AND RATIONALE DOCUMENTED IN CARE PLAN / PATIENT NOTES**

Age (yrs)	Respiratory rate	Heart rate	Systolic Blood Pressure
<1	30 – 40	110 – 160	70 – 90
1–2	25 – 35	100 – 150	80 – 95
2–5	25 – 30	95 – 140	80 – 100
5–12	20 – 25	80 – 120	90 – 110
>12	15 – 20	60 – 100	100 – 120

Method of Oxygen administration	
M	Mask
NC	Nasal Cannulae
HB	Head Box
CPAP	Continuous Positive Airway Pressure

Neurology Assessment = AVPU	
A	Alert
V	Responds to Voice
P	Responds to Pain
U	Unresponsive

ANALGESIA

Consider the following:

Increasing pain ⬆

Slight pain

Severe = Paracetamol + NSAID + Morphine (PCA/NCA or epidural)

Moderate = Paracetamol + NSAID + Codeine

Mild = Paracetamol + NSAID

No Pain

In cases of increasing or severe pain, please contact any of the Pain Service Team through switchboard:

- Clinical Nurse Specialist – Paediatric Pain – Bleep No. ....
- Consultant Paediatric Anaesthetist – Paediatric Pain – Bleep No. ....
- SpR Paediatric Anaesthesia – Bleep No. ....

Support Information/Guidelines
Pain Service Website, BRHC Intranet.

Remember
to reassess pain regularly:

Has the severity of pain changed?

What action is needed?

Document findings, actions
and re-evaluate

MONITORING

Whilst on Patient Controlled Analgesia (PCA), IV Morphine or an epidural, monitor BP, pulse, respiratory rate, sedation and pain scores:
- _hourly for first hour
- _hourly for second hour
- then hourly for 24 hours - following this please refer to the 'paediatric acute pain service guidelines'

PAIN SCORE	SEDATION	NAUSEA / VOMITING	PRURITUS	MOTOR BLOCK
0 = No Pain	0 = Wide awake	0 = None	0 = None	1 = Free movement hips, legs & feet
1–3 = Mild Pain	1 = Drowsy	1 = Nausea	1 = Mild	2 = Able to flex hip, knees with free movement of feet
4–7 = Moderate Pain	2 = Asleep but easy to arouse	2 = Vomiting	2 = Moderate	3 = Weakness in hips, knees, unable to lift heels, moves toes
8–10 = Severe Pain	3 = Somnolent and difficult to rouse	3 = Severe nausea or vomiting	3 = Severe	4 = Unable to move legs or feet
	S = Normal sleep			

Fig. 3.4 Paediatric observation chart.

DATE																								

TIME																								

Capillary refill time secs																									
O₂ saturation %																									
Administered O₂ Litres/min or %																									
Method of Administration																									
Blood Glucose																									
PEW Triggered																									

Pain Monitor

Infusion Rate Change																									
Sedation																									
Pruritis																									
Nausea / Vomiting																									
Pain Score Rest 0 - 10																									
Movement 0 - 10																									
Motor Block																									

Fig. 3.4 *(Cont.)*

Acute pain in the elderly

Conditions that commonly lead to acute pain in the elderly include:
- Acute exacerbations of joint conditions.
- Osteoporotic fractures of spine.
- Trauma from falls.
- Cancer.
- Pain from acute medical conditions including ischaemic heart disease, herpes zoster, and peripheral vascular disease.

Advances in anaesthetic and surgical techniques also mean that increasingly elderly patients are undergoing more major surgery.

Barriers to effective pain control in the elderly
- Difficulties with assessment of pain, including problems related to cognitive impairment.
- Higher incidence of co-existent diseases and concurrent medications—increased risk of drug interactions.
- Fear of side effects.
- Fear of prescribing drugs to the elderly.
- False belief that elderly tolerate pain better—pain threshold increases with age but elderly have a reduced ability to endure or tolerate severe pain.

Assessment of pain
The most reliable indicator of the existence and intensity of pain is the patient's self-report. Elderly may use words such as 'ache' or 'sore' rather than 'pain'. Under-reporting of pain is well known in the elderly and it is important to look for behavioural indicators of pain.

Cognitive impairment is common in the elderly and these patients are unable to report pain effectively. Delirium (confusion) is a form of acute cognitive impairment occurring commonly in the elderly during acute illnesses and postoperative setting. Risk factors include old age, infection, pre-existing dementia, hypoxaemia, anaemia, electrolyte imbalance, drugs (e.g. opioids, benzodiazepines, anticholinergics), and unrelieved pain.

Pain assessment scales
Commonly used tools for pain assessment include the numeric rating scale, visual analogue scale, and verbal descriptor scale. For patients with cognitive impairment or those who have difficulty with abstract thinking, simple verbal descriptor scale is preferred, such as one with words 'none', 'mild', 'moderate', and 'severe'.[1]

Pharmacokinetic and pharmacodynamic changes:
Pharmacokinetic and pharmacodynamic changes in the elderly require alterations in drug dosages, as summarized in Table 3.13.

Table 3.13 Pharmacokinetic and pharmacodynamic changes

Physiological changes in the elderly	Pharmacokinetic result	Adjustments needed in drug regimens
CVS		
Cardiac output ↓ 0–20%	↑ peak concentration after bolus dose	Smaller initial dose and slower rate of injection
Hepatic		
Reduced liver mass	↓ clearance of flow limited drugs	↓ maintenance dose
Absolute reduction in liver blood flow by 20–40%		
Hepatocellular enzyme function largely preserved		
Renal		
Renal mass, mainly cortical, ↓ about 30% by the 8th decade	↓ clearance of drugs excreted by kidneys	↓ maintenance dose of renally cleared drugs and drugs with active metabolites cleared by kidneys
Blood flow and plasma flow ↓ 10% per decade	↓ clearance of some drugs and metabolites	
Glomerular filtration rate ↓ 30–50%		
Creatinine clearance ↓ 50–70%		
↓ tubular function		
↓ plasma renin and aldosterone levels		Risk of hyperkalaemia
CNS		
Brain mass ↓ 20% by the 8th decade, CSF volume ↑ 10%	↓ distribution to CNS	No change in dose
Cerebral blood flow ↓ 20%, autoregulation preserved		
Concentration response	↑ response to opioids	Careful titration to effect
Body fluid composition	↓ volume of distribution for water soluble drugs	↓ dose
Total body water ↓ 10%		
Body fat ↑ 10–50%	↑ volume of distribution for lipid soluble drugs	
Plasma albumin ↓ 20%	↑ free fraction of protein-bound drugs	

Management of acute pain in the elderly

Multimodal approach: this is critical to achieve maximal pain relief in the elderly, while minimizing side effects from the drugs. A combination of analgesic drugs, regional techniques, and non-pharmacological treatment techniques should be used. Pain management strategies previously used by the patient should be incorporated into the treatment plan when feasible.

Drug treatment

Paracetamol

Regular paracetamol should be used for treating mild to moderate pain in all elderly patients unless there are contraindications. 1g 4 times a day is suitable for most patients and should be prescribed regularly.

NSAIDs

Elderly patients are more likely to suffer adverse gastric and renal side effects following administration of NSAIDs. Renal failure is of particular concern in the elderly, as they are more likely to have pre-existing renal impairment, cirrhosis, cardiac failure, or be using diuretics or antihypertensive medications. Interaction with drugs such as warfarin, heparin, and potentially nephrotoxic drugs (e.g. aminoglycosides) is more likely in the elderly. For these reasons, NSAIDs should be either completely avoided or used with extreme caution in the elderly population. If prescribed, their use should be limited to a short duration and be combined with PPIs for gastric protection.

Selective COX-2 inhibitors have been suggested to reduce GI side effects. However, the incidence of adverse effects including renal, are similar to non-selective NSAIDs. COX-2 inhibitors are contraindicated in patients with history of CV disease or those with known CV risk factors.

Opioids

Elderly patients are more sensitive to the effect of opioids, however, there is a large interpatient variability and doses must be titrated to effect in all patients. Reduced renal function can lead to rapid accumulation of active opioid metabolites. The active metabolite of pethidine, norpethidine, can accumulate in the elderly and cause CNS excitement and seizures, and hence pethidine should be avoided. The elimination $t_{1/2}$ of tramadol is slightly prolonged in the elderly; therefore lower daily doses should be used.

Elderly patients are more sensitive to side effects such as respiratory depression and appropriate monitoring should be used. Constipation can be a persistent problem and coadministration of laxatives is advisable. Side effects such as nausea and pruritus reduce with age.

Tricyclic antidepressants and other anticonvulsants

These drugs are particularly effective in managing neuropathic pain. However, elderly patients are more prone to side effects such as sedation and confusion. These drugs should be started at low doses and titrated upwards slowly.

Patient controlled analgesia

PCA is an effective method of pain relief in the elderly. However, it cannot be used in those with cognitive impairment or dementia. Factors such as ability to press the button in conditions such as severe arthritis should be taken in to consideration. There is evidence (level II)[2] that PCA results in significantly lower pain scores compared with intermittent SC or IM opioid injections.

Regional anaesthesia

Neuraxial blockade with spinal or epidural administration of LAs as well as the use of selective nerve blocks can be an effective way of managing acute pain in the elderly, especially during the perioperative period. LAs have a low incidence of side effects and can reduce the opioid requirements considerably. Caution is required in patients on antiplatelet drugs and anticoagulants. The recommended safe dose of LAs should not be exceeded under any circumstance.

Non-pharmacological therapy

Physical therapy techniques (e.g. exercise, heat and cold therapy) can be successfully employed in managing acute musculoskeletal pain. TENS can also be a useful adjunct in managing acute pain in the elderly.

Summary of approach to acute pain in the elderly

- Assessment of patient for comorbidities and drug interactions (coronary disease, renal failure, liver dysfunction).
- Cognitive assessment: Is PCA or PRN medication suitable?
- Assessment of pain: use the most appropriate tool on an individual basis.
- Multimodal approach: oral analgesia ± regional techniques.
- Avoid NSAIDs and COX-2 inhibitors if possible.
- Consider PCA.
- Adjuvant drugs: tricyclic antidepressants and anticonvulsants, especially for neuropathic pain.
- Non-pharmacological therapies such as TENS.

Rreferences

1 Closs SJ *et al.* (2004). A comparison of five pain assessment scales for nursing home residents with varying degrees of cognitive impairment. *J Pain Symptom Manage* **27**:196–205.

2 Keïta H *et al.* (2003). Comparison between patient-controlled analgesia and subcutaneous morphine in elderly patients after total hip replacement. *Br J Anaesth* **90**:53–7.

Chronic pain

chronic pain

Basic principles of chronic pain

History

A carefully and sensitively elicited history helps to formulate a diagnosis and gain insight into the patient's hopes, beliefs, and attitudes to therapeutic goals.

Useful information and cues can be gathered in a structured questionnaire completed by the patient in advance of the consultation. A minimum of 45min uninterrupted time is required for a new patient consultation.

▶Use a non-judgemental open style of questioning and allow the patient adequate time to give a full account.

Referral

Record the source of referral; GP, secondary care specialist, physiotherapist, other specialist service, e.g. back pain service, stroke service, or self-referral.

Take time to read the referral letter, other notes, and investigations.

▶Ascertain previous attendance at this or other pain service. Obtain case records to determine findings, treatments, and outcome. Is the patient attending other specialties with this condition? Are other treatment plans in progress or being considered, e.g. physiotherapy, surgery?

Pain history

▶Patients frequently present with more than one complaint. Document each problem and any relationships between them.
- Onset: how and when it started, causative/precipitating factors.
- Pattern: duration, variation over time, remission/quiescent phases.
- Exacerbating/relieving factors.
- Associated symptoms may suggest treatable underlying organic pathology: visual disturbance, skin changes, uveitis, dry eyes, dry mouth, ulcer, rash, photosensitivity, joint stiffness, neurological deficit, swelling.

Pain characteristics

- Quality: sensory/affective/evaluative descriptors.
- Temporal features: fleeting/sustained/paroxysmal.
- Intensity: extremes, periodicity.
- Topography: location, spread, radiation/referral to distant sites, trigger points.

Effects

- On mood, social interactions, work/colleagues, hobbies/interests, finance, family/friends, relationships, life goals.
- Of past and current pain treatments on pain, well-being, and function; side effects and complications.

Strategies

Employed by the patient:
- Medication: pain-contingent or time-contingent dosing (is medication taken in response to, or in anticipation of, the pain, or taken independently of the pain).

- Mechanical/thermal stimulation: rubbing, heat, cold.
- Avoidance of trigger factors/situations.
- Activity/distraction.
- Other agencies sought privately, e.g. osteopathy, acupuncture.

Medical history
- Past and concurrent disease, especially chronic illnesses, e.g. diabetes.
- Surgery/procedure, e.g. spinal surgery.

Drug history
- Comprehensive drug history including medication being taken for other conditions and non-prescription drugs.
- Effects of medication on pain, sleep.
- Significant adverse reactions, e.g. sedation, dry mouth, nausea, epigastric discomfort, constipation, memory impairment, allergies.

Psychological history
- Past and concurrent psychiatric illness: depression, anxiety, psychosis.
- Social phobia, symptoms of post-traumatic stress.
- Physical/emotional/sexual abuse.
- Substance dependence: alcohol, tobacco, non-prescription drugs, opioids, benzodiazepines.

Social and family history
- Marital status, family, pets.
- Family history of illness/pain conditions.
- Occupational history, reasons for changing work.
- Housing: alone, with others, sheltered, residential care.
- Physical ability to manage stairs, access to local amenities.
- Finance: benefits, social finance, charity, dependency on others.
- Legal, e.g. plaintiff in unsettled litigation, work-related compensation claim.
- Travel: to work, family, holidays.
- Care: home help, family carers, professional carers.

Activity
- Typical day: outline how time is spent.
- Sports/exercise: premorbid fitness, previous activities, limitations.
- Sleep: what time retires to bed, falls asleep, wakes up. Waking because of pain or other factors? Daytime somnolence, napping.
- Mobility:
  - Normal.
  - Impaired—no aids/sticks/crutches/walking frame/wheelchair.
- Ability to walk, cycle, use public transport, drive.

Expectations
- Hopes and fears for the future.
- Expectations about pain relief: partial/complete? Are they realistic and achievable?
- Meaning of the pain to the patient: effects on prospects, finance, family, relationships, concern about underlying disease.
- Expectations of others: relatives, friends, employer, referrer.

Examination

General

Observe how the patient enters the room, movements, body symmetry, attire, eye contact, speech, and interactions. Record the use of walking aids, cervical collar, slings, or braces. Remember that on the first visit, the patient is likely to be anxious and this may affect behaviour. Be thoughtful in your physical examination and explain what you are doing—avoid adding to the patient's pain burden. Patients with allodynia may be reluctant to let you approach the painful part. Remember to compare affected sites with normal areas.

The examination can be divided into 2 logical parts: a targeted examination of the painful area and a wider systematic examination.

Examine the pain site

- **Location:** body region, shape, boundaries, adjoining structures.
- **Appearance:** deformity, asymmetry, swelling, oedema, colour, skin changes, hair—absence or excess, muscle bulk.
- **Palpation:** swelling, temperature, tenderness, allodynia, range of movement, pain on movement, pulses, skin perfusion.
- **Percussion and auscultation:** in a patient presenting with chest or abdominal pain, for bruits in suspected vascular disease.
- **Sensation:** test for light touch and pinprick sensation looking for areas of hypoaesthesia/anaesthesia, allodynia, hyperalgesia. Von Frey hairs can help in outlining areas of allodynia. QST remains largely a research tool and is infrequently used in routine clinical examination.

Map and record the boundaries of any abnormality (including the virtual extremity in phantom pain).

Perform a systematic examination

Depending on the pain history and specific pain site examination, a more general examination may be indicated including some or all of:

Musculoskeletal system

- *Spine*: examine for normal cervical and lumbar lordoses, structural abnormalities, scoliosis, reduced height from vertebral collapse, scars from previous surgery, paraspinal muscle wasting and tenderness, range of movement.
- *Lumbar nerve root irritation*: test by performing straight leg raising, crossover or femoral stretch test. A positive test is reproduction of the symptomatic root pain in the affected leg.[1]
- *Joints*: deformity, colour, temperature, stability, range of movement, crepitus, effusion, swelling, bursitis, synovitis, tenderness.
- If *systemic inflammatory arthritis* is a possibility, examine eyes (scleritis, iritis, keratoconjunctivitis, xerophthalmia), parotid glands, mouth (xerostomia, ulcers), lymph nodes, skin (rash, vasculitis, ulcers), nails, chest (pericardial/pleural effusion), abdomen (splenomegaly).
- *Muscles*: size and conformation, symmetry, power, tenderness (diffuse, tender, or trigger points).

Neurological system

- Perform a full neurological examination, including cranial nerves, if a generalized or specific neurological disorder is suspected.
- Examine gait, perform Romberg test, assess mental state (orientation, memory, calculation, neurolinguistic ability, mood).[2]
- Test for motor and sensory function, deep tendon reflexes, coordination.
- Significant deficits may warrant referral to a neurologist, neurophysiologist or neuropsychologist for more detailed assessment.

⚠ In patients with suspected cauda equina syndrome from central disc prolapse, pay attention to sacral nerve roots—check for saddle anaesthesia, progressive lower limb weakness and reduced sphincter tone.

If any of these signs are present the patient should be referred immediately to a neurosurgeon.

Abdomen and pelvis

- Inspection (distension, masses, scars)
- Palpation (masses, organs, deep/superficial/scar tenderness)
- Auscultation (bowel sounds, bruits).

Formulation

After completing the history and examination:

- Document findings.
- Formulate a working diagnosis and problem list.
- Identify psychosocial issues and potential barriers to progress ('yellow flags'). see 🕮 p.101.
- In cases of possible serious pathology, initiate urgent investigation/referral/action.
- Discuss your formulation with the patient.
- Agree and initiate a management plan (this might include further multiprofessional assessment or specific investigations e.g. MRI, electrophysiological tests).
- Communicate your findings and plan with the patient's GP and the referrer.
- Give a written summary to the patient to help them remember the main points discussed and to aid compliance.

References

1 Waldman SD (2006). *Physical Diagnosis of Pain: An Atlas of Signs and Symptoms.* WB Saunders, Philadelphia, PA.
2 Masur H and Papke K (2004). *Scales and Scores in Neurology: Quantification of Neurological Deficits in Research and Practice.* Thieme, Stuttgart.

Measurement of chronic pain

Measurement of chronic pain is essential for the study of pain treatments. It is important to be able to evaluate and quantify the outcomes of various pain therapies and interventions.

Persistent pain is a complex personal experience which makes it difficult to define or measure. It includes both a sensory dimension and dimensions affected by physiological, psychological, and environmental factors. There is no objective measure of chronic pain (e.g. a blood test); evaluation relies on the patient's ability to communicate their pain both verbally and behaviourally.

The widespread impact of chronic pain on physical, emotional and social dimensions needs assessment using quality of life and broad ranging qualitative measures. All assessment should take into account other factors such as cognitive impairment or cultural background.

Pain can be assessed in the following areas:
- Pain intensity
- Measures of physical functioning
- Pain behaviours and experience.

Commonly used pain assessment tools

Unidimensional pain scales
Visual analogue scales (VAS) and numerical rating scales (NRS) (see Measurement of acute pain p.6).

Multidimensional pain scales
Brief Pain Inventory (BPI)
Measures intensity, disability, and affect. Assesses pain and the subjective impact of pain on activity and functional capability. Includes a body outline so that patients can provide a topographical representation of their pain. Short version widely used in pain clinics. See Fig. 4.1.

McGill Pain Questionnaire
Contains 3 major classes of word descriptors: sensory, affective, and evaluative which are used to specify a patient's subjective pain experience. Also contains an intensity scale and other items to determine the properties of pain experience

Pain experience (mood, social functioning)
Hospital Anxiety and Depression Scale (HAD)
Comorbid mental health status can be important. This tool gives an overall impression although tends to measure lack of positive affect rather than depression. Used commonly in pain clinics but not specific for pain.

Short Form-36 (SF-36)
Generic measure of health status, measures impact on functioning, well-being, and overall evaluation of health.

General approach to use of chronic pain assessment tools
- Prior to initial consultation use a multidimensional tool (e.g. BPI) to gain a comprehensive picture of the pain experience.
- Continue to use a multidimensional tool with subsequent follow-up consultations.
- Use specific tools (e.g. neuropathic pain scale) when appropriate.
- Avoid the use of unidimensional pain scales (e.g. VAS) unless for rating intensity of specific episodes.
- Appreciate the need for specific pain scales for particular patient groups (e.g. children, patients with learning or cognitive difficulties).

Assessment of neuropathic pain

Neuropathic pain is caused by a lesion or disease affecting the nervous system, either peripheral or central. This generates the pain rather than the more usual physiological nociceptive pain signalled by peripheral nociceptors. Neuropathic pain is qualitatively different from other types of pain, and the diagnosis often rests on characteristic pain symptoms which usually coexist with signs of altered sensory function.

In peripheral neuropathic pain, symptoms will be localized to the area innervated by the damaged or diseased nerves; in central nerve damage such as poststroke pain or spinal injury, the pain may be more widespread.

Neuropathic pain is associated with large number of diverse aetiologies although there are many shared symptoms and signs.

Common causes of neuropathic pain

- Diabetic peripheral neuropathy
- Postherpetic neuralgia
- Radicular leg pain
- Phantom limb pain
- Trigeminal neuralgia
- Postsurgical scar pain
- Poststroke pain
- Multiple sclerosis
- Cancer pain
- Spinal cord injury pain.

Many of these aetiologies will be covered in separate chapters.

Symptoms

Pain can be spontaneous or evoked. Spontaneous pain is often episodic, coming in sudden paroxysms, but may be continuous. Evoked pain can be initiated by innocuous stimuli such as clothing, breeze or temperature changes. These sensations can be extremely unpleasant and neuropathic pain tends to be rated as more distressing than nociceptive pain of the same intensity.

Characteristic verbal descriptors of neuropathic pain
- 'Burning pain'
- 'Electric shocks'
- 'Shooting pain'
- 'Numbness'
- 'Pins and needles'
- 'Itching'.

Examination

In any patient suspected of having neuropathic pain a full neurological examination is appropriate.

In patients with evoked pain or sensory loss, responses to different sensory stimuli (soft touch, sharp and dull pressure, thermal, and vibration) should be carefully assessed using an unaffected part of the body as a control. Findings may be positive (abnormal or exaggerated evoked sensations) or negative (sensory loss). In patients with episodic spontaneous pain there may be very little to find on examination. It is useful to map out the area of pain and examination findings on a body diagram for future reference as neuropathic pain is not necessarily static.

Positive and negative signs in neuropathic pain
Positive signs
- *Allodynia*: a painful response to a non-painful stimulus (soft touch with cotton wool or brush, gentle pressure, or temperature changes, e.g. cold metal or warm hand—it is usually modality specific).
- *Hyperalgesia*: an exaggerated painful response to a painful stimulus (usually pinprick) in comparison to an unaffected part of the body.
- *Hyperpathia*: repeated innocuous stimulation triggers pain.
- *Autonomic signs*: less commonly, there may be local changes in skin colour, quality, temperature, swelling, and sweating.

Negative signs
- *Hypoaesthesia*: loss of normal sensation to non-painful stimulus (soft touch, pressure, thermal, or vibration).
- *Hypoalgesia*: there may be loss of painful sensation to pinprick. This is very common in peripheral neuropathies and often coexists with intense spontaneous burning pain.
- *Motor deficits*: occasionally weakness, paralysis and loss of reflexes may be found, e.g. poststroke pain or acute demyelination.

Investigations

Neuropathic pain is a clinical diagnosis based on the patient's subjective report of pain plus a simple bedside examination, and there are no investigations which can conclusively prove or disprove the diagnosis. However, investigations which confirm an underlying neurological disorder lend weight to the clinical diagnosis and may be useful to guide management of the underlying problem. There are a number of laboratory-based investigations used in the research setting (QST, nerve and skin biopsy, laser evoked potentials) but none are routinely used in clinical practice.

Diagnostic screening tools

There are a number of validated screening tools available which can aid the diagnosis of neuropathic pain, particularly in primary care or non-specialist settings. These tend to be short questionnaires which rely on the presence of verbal pain descriptors ('burning', 'numbness', and 'pins and needles' are used frequently) to calculate the likelihood of neuropathic pain being present. Diagnosis should not be made solely on the result of a questionnaire, but if a patient scores highly, then a specialist referral to a pain clinic is warranted.

Management

Neuropathic pain tends to be chronic, distressing, and is often unresponsive to conventional analgesics. Pharmacological management includes antidepressant and anticonvulsant medication along with topical treatments, although oral opioids are increasingly used (see 📖 p. 162, 168, 170). Neurostimulation therapy (TENS, spinal cord stimulation) can offer excellent relief in some refractory patients. Full rehabilitation may require physiotherapy and psychology input, and a comprehensive multidisciplinary assessment from a specialist pain clinic is often required.

Epidemiology of chronic pain

Epidemiology has been defined as the study of distribution and determinants of disease in the population and the application of this study to the control of health problems.

Studies reporting the prevalence of chronic pain often give widely differing estimates as to the size of the problem. In his annual report in 2008, Sir Liam Donaldson, the Chief Medical Officer for the UK, presented a variety of commonly accepted prevalence statistics:[1]

- 7.8 million people in the UK suffer with moderate to severe pain persisting for >6 months.
- An estimated 11% of adults and 8% of children experience severe pain.
- One-third of households have someone in pain at any given time.
- Prevalence of chronic pain is 2–3× what it was 40 years ago.
- ♀ report chronic pain more frequently than ♂.
- People from socially or financially disadvantaged groups suffer more chronic pain.
- Some ethnic minority groups have an increased incidence of chronic pain.
- Each year 5 million people in the UK develop chronic pain and only two-thirds will recover.
- Chronic pain becomes more common with age—the probability of suffering chronic pain at age 50 is double that at age 30.
- Most residents of the UK in nursing homes experience constant or frequent moderate to severe pain.
- Chronic pain affects a quarter of school age children with pain lasting on average >3 years.

Specific pain conditions

There are some reports in the epidemiology literature relating to specific chronic pain conditions.

Low back pain

Prevalence

- 58–84% of the population will suffer with LBP at some point in their life.
- 18–50% 1-year point prevalence.
- Commoner in ♀.
- Increases with age until about 60 then declines slightly.
- 1 in 20 adults will consult primary care with LBP in any year.
- 20% children aged 2–15 will get back pain but will not seek medical attention.

Risk factors

- Mechanical risk factors include: moving heavy loads, working at or above shoulder level, and kneeling or squatting.
- Increased risk reported in miners, firefighters, and nurses (10–30%).
- Psychosocial risk factors include: high levels of stress, anxiety, and depression; catastrophizing; and pain behaviours. Dissatisfaction with work doubles the risk of developing back pain.

Headache

Migraine (1-year prevalence)
- 7% ♂:21% ♀ (Western Societies).
- 1.7% ♂: 4.2% ♀ (Ethiopia).
- 2.4 % ♂: 7.8% ♀ (rural Peru).
- Initially there is an increased prevalence with age followed by a decrease in later life.

Non-migraine headache (1-year prevalence)
- Up to 95%.
- Higher in ♀ than ♂ (less pronounced difference than migraine).
- Significant association between depression and anxiety disorders and both migraine and non-migraine headaches.
- Strength of association increases with increasing frequency of symptoms.
- Lack of education and low socioeconomic status double risk of developing symptoms.
- Children with problems at school and a fear of failure are more likely to report weekly headaches. These children are also more likely to have moderate or severe depression or to have a family member with a psychiatric disorder.
- Chronic headache (both migraine and non-migraine) patients have an increase risk of stroke (haemorrhagic and ischaemic).

Upper limb pain
- Shoulder pain reported in 7–61% adults aged 18–65 (1-year period prevalence).
- Excess prevalence in ♀.
- Prevalence increases with age.
- Forearm/wrist pain reported in 9–12% (1-month period prevalence).
- Aetiology multifactorial with mechanical, psychological, and psychosocial factors playing a part.
- Lifting, carrying on one shoulder, pushing or pulling, and working above shoulder level seem to increase risk of developing shoulder pain.
- Low job satisfaction, monotonous work, low social support, and 'high mental load' increase risk.

Forearm pain
- Few studies have been done specifically on forearm pain despite the huge media and public interest in 'repetitive strain injury'.
- Risk factors include: work involving repetitive movements, dissatisfaction with work, high levels of psychological distress, previous somatic symptoms, and illness behaviour.

Lower limb pain
- Prevalence of hip pain 9–14%.
- Only 1.5% will require surgery for hip disease.
- Risk factors: anatomical abnormality (e.g. acetabular dysplasia) in young people, OA, obesity, previous surgery.

- Prevalence of knee pain 25–50% in adults aged 50 or over.
- Risk factors: OA, ♀ gender, obesity, low social class, low educational achievement, anxiety and depression.

Abdominal pain

- Most common symptom in patients with functional GI disorder.
- Prevalence of 5–22% reported.
- Risk factors: high levels of psychological distress, illness anxiety, fatigue, back pain, a relative with abdominal pain.

Orofacial pain

- Prevalence reported at 1–48%. Most report prevalence of about 25%.
- Risk factors: young age, ♀ gender.

Non-cardiac chest pain

Most of the literature on chest pain is concerned with chest pain of cardiac origin and little is known about the prevalence of non-cardiac chest pain. One study reported prevalence of 23%.

Fybromyalgia

- Prevalence 7–14% using American College of Rheumatology (ACR) criteria.
- Peaks at age 60–69.
- Twice as common in ♀ compared to ♂.
- 50% will have persisting symptoms at 1 year and 25% will have persisting symptoms at 7 years.

Further reading

McMahon S and Koltzenburg M (eds) (2005). Epidemiology of pain. In *Wall and Melzack's Textbook of Pain*, 5th edn. Churchill Livingstone.

Reference

1 Annual Report of the Chief Medical Officer (2008). *Pain: Breaking Through The Barrier*. DH, London. Available at: ℗ http://www.dh.gov.uk/dr_consum_dh/groups/dh_digitalassets/documents/digitalasset/dh_096233.pdf

Chronic pain services

The first multidisciplinary Pain Clinic was commissioned at the University of Washington, Seattle in 1960. It is now generally accepted that the effective relief of pain should be a fundamental objective of any healthcare provision.

Establishment

Specialist pain services should ideally be provided regionally (all district general hospitals and most specialist hospitals with provision for care closer to the patient wherever possible and practicable). Pain services vary in the treatments offered which range from outpatient-based pain management services to residential pain management units. All services need adequate resourcing. This should include premises fit for purpose and a staff team that is appropriately skilled. Attention should be paid to ensuring adequate access, allocation of designated beds, and ring-fenced operating theatre and radiology time for both diagnostic and therapeutic procedures, and adequate tools should be provided for all professional groups within the multidisciplinary team.

Not all hospitals have a specific pain clinic, but may have a consultant who has a special interest in pain and can offer pain control interventions such as medication or injection. Staffing should comprise fixed sessions for consultant specialists and their job plans should reflect the difference between this work and other anaesthetic roles. Other healthcare professionals are equally important, including specialist psychologists, nurses, physiotherapists, occupational therapists (OTs), and others. These teams should be supported with adequate secretarial and administrative cover and up-to-date IT and technical facilities for all staff.

Approach

A comprehensive, individualized, multidisciplinary approach is essential to address the impact of chronic pain on an individual's quality of life and functioning. Good communication is vital between pain management services and other healthcare groups including primary care, palliative care, and also with relevant external resources such as vocational advisors, drug and alcohol services.

Arrangements should be made to accommodate all patient groups across the lifespan at all levels of functioning and understanding, including those who are disabled, intellectually handicapped, and speakers of other languages. It must be a priority to ensure equitable provision for all patients, taking their social, economical, and cultural needs into account. Clear written information should be available to patients to ensure they are in a position to make informed decisions about their care.

Pain management specialists should provide an active programme of education in chronic pain for other professionals engaged in the care of this population, and undertake continuing evaluation and audit of their services.

Referral

Patients are generally accepted by referral from a GP and will have had pain for >3 months which is not resolved by the usual medical interventions.

Treatment

Medical interventions may include comprehensive assessment, education, TENS, medication, acupuncture, nerve blocks, and neuromodulation.

Patients may often be referred on for individual or group-based interventions including advice, education, pacing and goal setting, and exercise. These may be covered by multidisciplinary Pain Management Programmes, run by specialist psychologists, physiotherapists, and nurses or OTs often with the support/leadership of a pain consultant. Pain Management Programmes aim to teach patients about pain, coping strategies, and how to live a more active and fulfilled life. Such programmes promote a return to normal physical and psychological functioning and thereby a shift from unhelpful reliance on healthcare resources (see ⬚ Pain Management Programmes, p.262).

Further reading

The Royal College of Anaesthetists and The Pain Society (2003). *Pain Management Services: Good Practice*. Available at: ℘ http://www.rcoa.ac.uk/docs/painservices.pdf

Pharmacological therapies

Introduction

Although some of the analgesics commonly used for acute pain also have a role in the management of chronic pain, there are often cautions about their use over the long term. There is a more limited evidence base upon which to base prescribing decisions for patients with chronic pain. Several classes of drugs are employed in the treatment of chronic pain (e.g. anti-convulsants or antidepressants) that have little or no analgesic efficacy in the treatment of acute pain. These are particularly employed in the treatment of neuropathic pain but their use has expanded into other settings. All of these pharmacological treatments need to be employed in tandem with physical, psychological, and alternative therapies if significant improvements in outcome are to be realized.

Opioids for chronic non-cancer pain

Opioid drugs have been used effectively for many years for the management of acute pain and cancer pain. Two decades ago, their use in persistent non-cancer pain was rare and the literature suggested that the drugs had poor efficacy in the management of chronic pain. Since then, there has been a steady flow of clinical trial data and some systematic reviews which suggest that opioids may be useful for a number of chronic pain conditions including neuropathic pain[1] although some important questions remain unanswered, including:

- Can data from short-term clinical trials answer questions about safety and efficacy of long-term opioid use?
- Do opioids improve quality of life as well as reducing pain intensity?
- What is the risk of developing a substance misuse problem from prescribed opioids?

Scrutiny of clinicians' opioid prescribing habits, well established in the USA, is now more common in the UK and might be expected to impose a disincentive to prescribe. However, the prescription of strong opioid drugs continues to increase. Guidance on opioid prescribing has been developed (see British Pain Society recommendations[2]) to provide information regarding the appropriate context in which opioids should be used and to highlight where problems might arise.

Weak and strong opioid drugs

Opioids are traditionally categorized as weak or strong (see 📖 Fig. 2.1, p.34).

- Weak opioids include: codeine, dihydrocodeine, and tramadol.
- Commonly used strong opioid drugs include: morphine, oxycodone, fentanyl, buprenorphine, and methadone. Note the use of pethidine is not recommended for chronic pain (issues with metabolites and dependency).

This division is somewhat arbitrary as the inappropriate use of weak opioids should prompt equivalent prescriber concern to that invoked by worrisome use of stronger preparations.

Opioids used for chronic pain are usually prescribed in sustained release formulations (oral or transdermal). Immediate release preparations, although probably equally effective, may predispose to tolerance and problem drug use, but they do have a role in the treatment of recurrent intermittent pain. There is rarely (if ever) any indication for the use of injectable opioids to manage long-term pain.

Are opioids effective in treating chronic pain?

There is published clinical experience reporting efficacy of opioids for a variety of pain conditions. Evidence from randomized controlled trials (over the short term) suggests that these drugs are effective in OA (including back pain), postherpetic neuralgia (PHN), diabetic neuropathy, and central pain. Doses of opioids used in practice often exceed those in clinical trials. Few trials draw firm conclusions about whether opioids bring about improvement in other important domains including sleep, mood, and physical function.

Starting opioid therapy

Opioids should only be prescribed for chronic pain as part of a wider pain management plan supported by use of other drugs where indicated, physical interventions, and advice regarding activity and rehabilitation. The primary goal of therapy is pain relief but improvement in other domains, such as sleep, is desirable and should be evaluated. Complete pain relief is rarely achievable: a reduction in pain intensity allowing improved function should be the goal.

- The patient should be assessed comprehensively making note of known influences on the experience of pain.
- Desired outcomes of treatment should be discussed and documented.
- Where possible, the decision to start opioids should be agreed by all health-care professionals contributing to the patient's management.
- The patient should know what side effects to expect and how these might be managed. The time over which a trial of opioid therapy should be conducted can be agreed (2–3 months typically).
- Follow-up should occur within 1 month after dose adjustments.
- The clinician initiating the opioid trial should, where possible, carry out the evaluation and provide the prescriptions during this period.
- If, after reasonable dose manipulation, the patient experiences intolerable adverse effects or does not achieve substantial relief with attainment of agreed goals, the opioid trial has been unsuccessful— consider opioid rotation.
- The patient must take responsibility for deciding whether they are fit to drive. They should discuss treatment with their insurance company and the Driving and Vehicle Licensing Agency. Patients should be advised that it is unwise to drive when first starting opioids and after dose escalations.
- Sudden reductions or cessation of opioid dose can result in withdrawal symptoms. These can be very unpleasant and recognition of withdrawal symptoms forms an important part of the discussion needed to support safe and tolerable opioid treatment.
- Patients should be reminded that the supply and use of opioid preparations is controlled by law and that it is an offence for these drugs to be used by anyone other than the intended recipient.

If the opioid trial is successful it is usual for the patient's primary care practitioner to take over prescribing and follow-up but specialist pain teams must be willing to review patients if concerns regarding continued effectiveness or tolerability arise.

Side effects of opioids

Adverse effects occur in up to 80% of people taking opioids. Side effects should be actively managed where possible. Tolerance to some side effects may occur within the first few days of dosing although some problems, particularly constipation, tend to persist.

Common adverse effects of opioids include:

- Nausea, vomiting, and constipation—constipation often prevents the patient continuing with therapy.
- Drowsiness, sedation, and impaired concentration.

- Respiratory depression: commoner when using parenteral opioids for the treatment of acute pain but caution should be exercised when co-prescribing with other CNS depressants.
- Pruritus.
- Possible immune and hormonal suppression (can lead to subfertility and loss of libido).

Problem drug use

Concerns are frequently expressed, by both prescribers and patients, regarding the propensity of opioids to cause problems of tolerance, addiction, and dependence. These terms are often misunderstood in the context of prescribing opioids for pain relief. Useful definitions have been derived by the American Pain Society and the American Academy of Pain Medicine (2009).[3]

Physical dependence

Physical dependence is a state of adaptation that is manifested by a drug class-specific withdrawal syndrome that can be produced by abrupt cessation, rapid dose reduction, decreasing blood level of the drug, and/or administration of an antagonist.

Tolerance

Tolerance is a state of adaptation in which exposure to a drug induces changes that result in a diminution of one or more of the drug's effects over time.

Addiction

Is characterized by behaviours that include one or more of the following: impaired control over drug use, compulsive use, continued use despite harm, and craving. Addiction is a primary, chronic, neurobiological disease, with genetic, psychosocial, and environmental factors influencing its development and manifestations.

It should be noted that tolerance and dependence are expected pharmacological consequences of long-term opioid use and do not per se constitute problem drug use.

The likelihood of chronic pain patients developing an addiction syndrome to prescribed opioids has proved difficult to quantify. Patients with the following factors are more at risk of running into problems:

- A past history of substance misuse.
- A family member who has a drug problem.
- Psychiatric comorbidity.

Careful assessment of a patient before starting opioid therapy should always include a sensitive discussion of substance misuse issues. A current history of substance misuse does not preclude the use of opioids for chronic pain therapy but such cases need to be managed by a multidisciplinary team with experience in both addiction and pain problems.

If a patient is at risk of developing a substance misuse problem it may be helpful to detail the types of behaviours which are likely to prompt concern. If opioids are to be prescribed in these circumstances the patient should agree to comply with regular review, which may need to be frequent. When concerns regarding problem drug use arise, prescriptions should be issued from a single prescriber and, if necessary, dispensed from an identified pharmacy. It may be necessary to provide prescriptions for small quantities of drug on each occasion.

Conclusion

Opioids are an effective and important tool in chronic pain management but relatively little is known about the benefits and adverse effects of these drugs in the long term. Side effects are common and should be actively managed where possible. Concerns regarding addiction remain prominent for prescribers and patients alike and highlight the importance of comprehensive assessment and ongoing surveillance of opioid therapy.

References

1 Kalso E et al. (2004). Opioids in chronic non-cancer pain: systematic review of efficacy and safety. Pain **112:**372–80.
2 British Pain Society website: ℘ http://www.britishpainsociety.org/
3 American Pain Society and the American Academy of Pain Medicine (2009). ℘ http://www.jpain.org/article/P11S 1526590008008316/fulltext

NSAIDs for chronic pain

NSAIDs, including traditional non-selective NSAIDs and the newer COX-2 selective inhibitors (coxibs), are amongst the most frequently prescribed medication worldwide because of their anti-inflammatory and analgesic properties. Their efficacy has been demonstrated in a wide range of acute and chronic pain conditions. However, in chronic pain conditions, a major limitation on their use is their potential for adverse effects, namely GI, renal, and more the more recently identified CV toxicity.

Mechanism of action

NSAIDs act by blocking the enzyme COX which is a key component of the prostaglandin synthetic pathway. Two isoforms have been identified: COX-1 and COX-2. COX-1 is constitutively active in most cells and is associated with the homeostatic regulation of the GI and renal tracts, platelet function, and macrophage differentiation. COX-2 has less of a constitutive role in homeostasis; however it can be strongly induced by peripheral as well as central inflammation. It was proposed that blockade of COX-1 was responsible for the adverse effects of NSAIDs, thus the selective blockade of COX-2 should produce anti-inflammatory and analgesic effects with fewer side effects.

Clinical efficacy

NSAIDs are the standard treatment for inflammation and pain due to inflammatory arthropathies. Although there are fewer RCTs of efficacy for chronic LBP or OA, NSAIDs have been tested in chronic LBP showing moderate efficacy and similar findings were reported for OA of the hip and of the knees. As might be expected, there is minimal evidence of effectiveness in neuropathic pain conditions. In the management of chronic pain there is little evidence to guide selection of particular NSAIDs or COX-2 selective inhibitors in term of efficacy. However, there are data relating to the risk of GI and CV side effects (see following section).

Adverse effects

Gastrointestinal

These side effects are very common, with up to 60% of NSAID users experiencing dyspepsia and heartburn and 20–30% developing ulcers. The annual incidence of NSAID-related complicated and symptomatic ulcers is 2.5–4.5% and the annual incidence of serious complications (perforation, haemorrhage) is 1–1.5%. Risk factors for GI toxicity are:

- Type, dose, and duration of NSAIDs.
- Use of concomitant medications such aspirin, corticosteroids, and anticoagulants.
- Patient history of dyspepsia, peptic ulcers, *Helicobacter pylori* status.
- Age.

The mechanism of GI damage is linked to COX-1 inhibition or dual inhibition of COX-1 and COX-2. Thus COX-2 selective inhibitors carry less risk of symptomatic peptic ulcers than non-selective NSAIDs and probably less risk of serious GI complications. However, caution in prescribing is still required if patients have risk factors for GI complications. To decrease NSAID GI toxicity in at-risk patients it is appropriate to co-prescribe a PPI.

Cardiovascular

NSAIDs increase both systolic and diastolic blood pressure, in a dose related fashion, and can precipitate congestive heart failure. Thus they are relatively contraindicated in patients with hypertension or heart failure. In addition, coxibs may interfere with the endothelial function promoting platelet aggregation.

Most NSAIDs tend to increase CV risk, and a recent analysis of 9218 cases of first MI suggested an increased risk of MI with use of rofecoxib, diclofenac, and ibuprofen, but not with naproxen (perhaps related to the degree of COX2:COX1 inhibition). This association with the coxibs saw rofecoxib withdrawn from the market and prescribing restrictions placed on the use of coxibs in patients at high risk of CV events.

Renal

NSAIDs can produce a spectrum of renal diseases including functional renal insufficiency, nephritic syndrome with or without interstitial nephritis, renal papillary necrosis and chronic interstitial nephritis, renal acute tubular necrosis, vasculitis, glomerulonephritis, and obstructive nephropathy. Moreover, NSAIDs can interfere with fluid and electrolyte homeostasis. The prevalence of nephrotoxicity in NSAID users is low, but risk factors include:

- Age.
- Comorbidity, such as hypertension or diabetes.
- Co-medication reducing renal perfusion, such as ACE inhibitors or diuretics.

In the clinical setting of reduced renal perfusion, the kidneys are protected through the action of prostaglandins and the use of NSAIDs is contraindicated because of the risk of precipitating renal failure.

Conclusion

For long-term use as in chronic pain, the therapeutic index of NSAIDs is narrow and they are better employed in short courses for pain 'flare-ups' rather than on continuous repeat prescription. Regular monitoring of blood pressure and of renal function is warranted in at-risk patients.

Further reading

Aronson JK (ed) (2006). *Meyler's Side Effects of Drugs*, 15th edn. Elsevier.

Hardman JG and Limbird LL (eds) (2001). *Goodmann and Gilman's. The Pharmacological Basis of Therapeutics*, 10th edn. Mc Graw Hill.

Jones R et al. (2008). Gastrointestinal and cardiovascular risks of non-steroidal anti-inflammatory drugs. *Am J Med* **121**:464–74.

Onk CKS et al. (2007). An evidence-based update on non-steroidal anti-inflammatory drugs. *Clin Med Res* **1**:19–34.

Roelofs PDDM et al. (2008). Non-steroidal anti-inflammatory drugs for low back pain. *Cochrane Database Syst Rev* **1**:CD000396.

Antidepressants

Antidepressants are widely prescribed for the management of chronic pains, such as neuropathic pain, headaches, fibromyalgia, or rheumatological conditions such as LBP.

Importantly, several studies have shown that their effect on pain is independent of the mood-enhancing properties of these drugs and they are effective in patients without mood disorders.

Multiple mechanisms of action have been suggested but they are believed to act mainly by reinforcing descending monoaminergic inhibitory pathways by blocking reuptake.

Tricyclic antidepressants (TCAs) are more effective than selective serotonin reuptake inhibitors (SSRIs) but their use is somewhat limited by adverse effects. In that respect new 'balanced' serotonin and noradrenaline reuptake inhibitors (SNRIs) are of interest because of better tolerability.

Tricyclic antidepressants

Amitriptyline is the prototypic TCA but 2nd- and 3rd-generation agents are also used in treatment of chronic pain (e.g. nortriptyline). TCAs inhibit the reuptake of noradrenaline (NA) and serotonin (5-HT) but they are relatively promiscuous compounds with actions at a number of other receptors (cholinergic and histaminergic) and ion channels (e.g. Na^+ channels) that are responsible for many of their adverse effects.

The efficacy of the TCAs has been robustly demonstrated and they are recommended as a first choice in the treatment of peripheral and central neuropathic pain, as well as in the prevention of tension headaches and migraines or as coanalgesics in LBP and fibromyalgia. The analgesic effect exhibits a delayed onset of action (typically taking 3–6 weeks) and they are often used at lower doses than that required for antidepressant action.

Dizziness, sedation, orthostatic hypotension, dry mouth, and constipation are common side effects of TCAs which may be intolerable. These effects tend to decrease with continued treatment and can be minimized by gradual dose escalation. Moreover TCAs are contraindicated in patients with glaucoma, prostatic hypertrophy, or cardiac conduction disturbances.

▶ TCAs are particularly toxic in overdose and they should not be prescribed to patients at risk of self-harm.

Serotonin and noradrenaline reuptake inhibitors

This group includes venlafaxine, duloxetine, and milnacipran and they are dual inhibitors of 5-HT and NA reuptake. They have a good selectivity profile with low affinity for cholinergic and histaminergic receptors.

There are, however, considerable differences in their selectivity for monoamine reuptake. Venlafaxine has a high affinity for the 5-HT transporter but not the NA transporter and at low doses probably acts as an SSRI. Duloxetine has a more balanced affinity but is still more selective for the 5-HT transporter and milnacipran may be slightly more noradrenergic than serotonergic.

Venlafaxine has been shown to be effective in a number of chronic pain conditions, including fibromyalgia. In neuropathic pain its efficacy was demonstrated in a randomized controlled study on diabetic polyneuropathy, painful neuropathy, and neuropathic pain due to breast cancer.

Milnacipran has been tested with positive results in a RCT on fibromyalgia.

The efficacy of duloxetine has been demonstrated in 3 RCTs in patients with diabetic polyneuropathy and in those with fibromyalgia. The onset of pain relieving action is quicker than with the TCAs at about 2 weeks.

Adverse events of SNRIs typically occur early in treatment with a mild to moderate severity and with a tendency to decrease with continued treatment. The most frequent adverse effect is nausea. At high doses, venlafaxine can increase blood pressure, and can have a proarrhythmic effect so it should not be used in patients who are severely hypertensive or with a history of cardiac failure, coronary artery disease, or electrocardiogram abnormalities. The cardiotoxicity of milnacipran or duloxetine seems minor.

Conclusion

Antidepressants and TCAs in particular are first choice agents for the treatment of chronic pain. However, the new balanced SNRIs, although less studied so far, seem to have an advantageous risk/benefit profile.

Further reading

Attal N et al. (2006). EFNS guidelines on pharmacological treatment of neuropathic pain. *Eur J Neurol* **13**:1153–69.

Dworkin RH et al. (2007). Pharmacologic management of neuropathic pain: evidence-based recommendations. *Pain* **132**:237–51.

Saarto T and Wiffen PJ (2007). Antidepressants for neuropathic pain. *Cochrane Database Syst Rev* **4**:CD005454.

Anticonvulsants

Anticonvulsants are front-line treatments for neuropathic pain, having been found initially to be effective in empirical clinical trials. They act by blocking voltage-gated ion channels on sensory neurons, which are key elements in the state of hyperexcitability seen in neuropathic pain. Among them, gabapentin and pregabalin are most widely prescribed, and following large RCTs they were licensed in neuropathic pain.

Gabapentin/pregabalin

Gabapentin and its sibling compound pregabalin preferentially act on the $\alpha2\delta$ subunit of presynaptic Ca^{2+} channels which causes a reduction in neurotransmission in abnormally active sensory neurons.

The efficacy of gabapentin has been recently reviewed in a meta-analysis and its NNT for a significant improvement in chronic neuropathic pain, was 4.3 (95% CI: 3.5–5.7). The magnitude of effect of pregabalin is similar with a NNT of 3.7 (for 50% pain relief). Gabapentin and pregabalin are considered as first choice treatments of all types of peripheral neuropathic pain and have also shown some degree of efficacy in central neuropathic pain. Recently beneficial effects of pregabalin have been reported in fibromyalgia.

The main differences between gabapentin and pregabalin lie with the pharmacokinetic profile of these compounds. Gabapentin has a non-linear and dose-dependent profile of absorption that brings a high intersubject variability to the absolute bioavailability. In practice, gabapentin needs individual dose titration, which increases the time needed to establish whether a patient is a responder. In contrast, pregabalin has a linear pharmacokinetic profile, with a bioavailability of 90%, which makes its effect far more predictable. Furthermore, the onset of the pain-relieving action of pregabalin is quicker, often taking <1 week.

The main adverse effects of gabapentin and pregabalin are sedation and dizziness.

Carbamazepine

Carbamazepine blocks voltage gated Na+ channels but has a number of actions at other targets. Carbamazepine is effective in diabetic neuropathy but its principal indication remains trigeminal neuralgia (TN). Carbamazepine is the treatment of choice for TN with a NNT of 1.8 (95% CI: 1.3–2.2) with an effect on both the frequency and intensity of paroxysms.

However, the use of carbamazepine is complicated by pharmacokinetic issues. It induces hepatic microsomal enzyme system and may influence the metabolism of several drugs. Besides common side effects including dizziness and sedation, are more severe issues such as anaplastic effects, hepatitis, skin toxicity, and hyponatraemia. As a consequence, patient compliance is a significant limiting factor. Oxcarbazepine (a sister compound) seems to have a similar efficacy to carbamazepine in TN with a better tolerability. It is recommended as a first choice in TN but with a lower strength of evidence.

Others

Several other anticonvulsants, such as lamotrigine and topiramate, have been tested in neuropathic pain but the results to date are not especially compelling. Given the risk of potentially serious cutaneous reaction and the availability of more effective treatments, lamotrigine does not have a significant place in therapy at present. Despite its interesting action on AMPA/kainate glutamate receptors, topiramate has yet to find a niche in the treatment of neuropathic pain.

Conclusion

Anticonvulsants are amongst the first choice for the treatment of chronic neuropathic pain. Gabapentin and pregabalin have the best risk:benefit profile and are extensively prescribed.

Further reading

Attal N et al. (2006). EFNS guidelines on pharmacological treatment of neuropathic pain. *Eur J Neurol* **13**:1153–69.

Gidal BE et al. (2000). Inter- and intra-subject variability in gabapentin absorption and absolute bioavailability. *Epilepsy Res* **40**:123–7.

Van Seventer R et al. (2006). Efficacy and tolerability of twice-daily pregabalin for treating pain and related sleep interference in postherpetic neuralgia: a 13-week, randomized trial. *Curr Med Res Opin* **22**:375–84.

Wiffen PJ et al. (2005). Gabapentin for acute and chronic pain. *Cochrane Database Syst Rev* **3**:CD005452.

Antiarrhythmics

The antiarrhythmic drugs that can relieve pain are those with LA properties that, by blocking ion channels, can slow action potential propagation in heart or nerve. LAs were developed originally for blockade of peripheral nerves, a practice that continues to be employed in the treatment of both acute and chronic pain. However, it was subsequently noted that systemic administration of low doses of lidocaine could effectively (if transiently) treat neuralgias.

Mechanism

The antiarrhythmics are thought to exert their beneficial effects through a dampening of ectopic firing in sensitized circuits. This is thought to be achieved via blockade of Na^+ channels. In patients with neuropathic pain this occurs at low dose, consistent with the idea that there is an upregulation of Na^+ channel activity. There has been much recent interest in the possible use of subtype-specific Na^+ channel blockers. These may discriminate between the channels in peripheral nociceptors and those on the heart, thereby minimizing side effects. However, to date none of these agents has made it through clinical trials.

Lidocaine

Systemic administration has been shown to be effective (5mg/kg infused over 30min) for neuropathic pain but the duration of effect is short and the requirement for IV administration makes long-term therapy impractical. In contrast, lidocaine patches have been shown to be efficacious in the longer-term treatment of postherpetic neuralgia and diabetic neuropathy (see 📖 Topical analgesics, p.174). Some clinicians employ a trial of IV lidocaine as a mechanistic test to indicate whether a patient is likely to respond to oral mexiletine. Although this is an enticing concept it appears to have a poor predictive value.

Mexiletine

This orally administered antiarrhythmic drug (like lidocaine it belongs to class Ib) has been advocated as a possible treatment for neuralgia. Several studies have examined its efficacy in diabetic peripheral neuropathy as well as in spinal cord injury pain and HIV associated pain. However there is limited evidence of efficacy and its use is limited by prominent GI and neurological side effects. If a trial of mexiletine is to be undertaken it needs to be initiated at low dose, gradually titrated up, and the patient carefully monitored for side effects.

Conclusion

The rationale for the use of Na^+ channel blockers is enticing, particularly in peripheral neuropathic pain, but as yet the clinically available compounds have not proved especially useful and are limited by side effects.

Topical analgesics

Topical analgesics are potentially extremely valuable in chronic pain because they allow a high concentration of drug at the site of pain initiation with low systemic drug levels, thus potentially reducing adverse drug effects.

By definition, topical drugs act locally on damaged or dysfunctional soft tissues or peripheral nerve endings. As chronic pain can involve changes in both peripheral and central elements, topical analgesics are particularly useful when there is a significant peripheral component.

To date, beneficial effects have been demonstrated for topical NSAIDs in chronic OA and lidocaine and capsaicin in peripheral neuropathic pain.

Topical NSAIDs

Topical NSAIDs are superior to placebo in single joint arthritis and rheumatologic disorders, improving pain, stiffness, and function. However, there is a large intersubject variability of responses with the percentage of patients achieving pain relief in active groups being 30–95%. The incidence of side effects was low with mostly local reactions (itching, burning, or rashes). In chronic painful conditions, topical NSAIDs do not appear to be more efficacious than oral preparations. However, this apparent equivalent efficacy is associated with a better side-effect profile leading to the inclusion of topical NSAIDs in treatment guidelines.

Lidocaine

Lidocaine is a LA which prevents generation and conduction of nerve impulse along primary afferent axons by blocking Na^+ channels. Topical lidocaine patches (5%) are used when tactile allodynia is a prominent symptom and their efficacy has been formally studied in postherpetic neuralgia. For this indication, lidocaine was only moderately superior to placebo in relieving pain but its good side-effect profile has led to its inclusion in recent guidelines on the treatment of neuropathic pain.

Capsaicin

Capsaicin, the 'hot' compound in chilli peppers, binds to and activates TRPV1 channels on C-fibre nociceptors in the skin. This causes an initial excitation of the sensory neuronal terminals in the skin and a period of enhanced sensitivity and pain. This is usually perceived as itching, pricking, or burning, with cutaneous vasodilation, and is thought to be due to release of inflammatory mediators including substance P. This is followed by a refractory period with reduced sensitivity and, after repeated applications, persistent desensitization, due to depletion of C-fibres in the skin which produces the analgesic effect.

Capsaicin (0.025–0.075%) has been tested in randomized trials in neuropathic and musculoskeletal pain, outperforming placebo, with a mean response rate of ~60% after 4–8 weeks of treatment Significantly more patients had local adverse events and adverse event related withdrawals with capsaicin than with placebo but no systemic adverse effects were notified. A patch formulation of high dose capsaicin (8%, Qutenza®) has recently been licenced for use in neuropathic pains and has shown some efficacy. Its use is currently restricted to specialist centres.

Although topically applied capsaicin has only moderate efficacy in the treatment of chronic musculoskeletal or neuropathic pain, it may be useful as an adjunct or sole therapy for a small number of patients who can tolerate the initial burning sensation.

Conclusion

In general, topical analgesics have limited efficacy; however, on an individual basis, they can be valuable tools in chronic pain management because of their large therapeutic index.

Further reading

Attal N *et al.* (2006). EFNS guidelines on pharmacological treatment of neuropathic pain. *Eur J Neurol* **13**:1153–69.

Mason *et al.* (2004). Systematic review of topical capsaicin for the treatment of chronic pain. *BMJ* **328**:991.

Moore RA *et al.* (1998). Quantitative systematic review of topically applied non-steroidal anti-inflammatory drugs. *BMJ* **316**:333–8.

Novel and atypical agents

A number of other drugs have been employed in the treatment of chronic pain whose mechanism of action falls outside the classes of drugs described in the preceding chapters.

Ketamine

Is an intravenous anaesthetic agent which can be analgesic at subanaesthetic doses. It has a multitude of actions but its analgesic effect is probably exerted by a non-competitive blockade of NMDA glutamate receptors. These receptors are involved in the synaptic plasticity of nociceptive circuits associated with chronic pain and their blockade has been shown to prevent or reverse such sensitization. Clinical studies have shown that the acute administration of ketamine is analgesic in a number of neuropathic pain syndromes such as phantom limb, PHN, and central pain. However, over the long term, ketamine is poorly tolerated because of psychomimetic side effects (confusion, hallucinations, delirium) and the requirement for parenteral administration. It is also a drug of abuse with clear potential for addiction. Additionally, reports have emerged of long-term users developing chronic lower urinary tract pain. Preclinical studies indicate a pre-emptive role for NMDA receptor antagonism in the prevention of chronic pain but this has been difficult to discern in clinical trials.

Baclofen

Is a GABA$_B$ agonist which acts to depress synaptic transmission and has been used for a number of years as an antispasmodic agent. It was believed that any analgesic effects were secondary to this central muscle relaxant action. However, it has subsequently been shown to be effective in trigeminal neuralgia suggesting that it can act as a direct analgesic. It has also been licensed for intrathecal administration by continuous infusion which can circumvent the sedative side effects.

Clonidine

This relatively selective α2-adrenoceptor agonist can produce a similar analgesic effect to opiates without the respiratory depression and with less abuse potential. It has been licensed for intrathecal use in refractory cancer pain by continuous infusion from an implanted pump. Much of its analgesic effect is achieved at a spinal level; however, actions at brainstem and higher CNS levels cause hypotension and sedation that limit its usefulness as a systemically administered agent. Nonetheless it has been shown to have some beneficial actions in the treatment of PHN and diabetic neuropathy.

Neither clonidine nor baclofen should be stopped abruptly due to the risk of rebound hypertension and delirium (respectively).

Ziconitide

Is a synthetic derivative of a conus toxin (marine snail) that binds avidly (practically irreversibly) to N-type calcium channels. These channels are involved in neurotransmitter release from synapses and intrathecal administration of ziconitide has been licensed for the treatment of severe, intractable pain. It has been shown to be analgesic in such refractory cases and there is no evidence of tolerance developing. However, it has a narrow therapeutic range and is associated with a number of predictable side effects including confusion, dizziness, nausea, memory impairment, and nystagmus. The drug requires careful incremental titration to achieve acceptable benefits.

Calcitonin

Is a peptide hormone involved in the regulation of bone resorption through the inhibition of osteoclasts. It has demonstrated efficacy in the management of osteoporotic vertebral wedge fractures. Some studies have also indicated efficacy in the management of metastatic bone pain and, intriguingly, in phantom limb pain. The latter suggests that its effects are unlikely to all be mediated via actions on osteoclasts and it may have a central analgesic action. It can be administered by nasal spray or IM/SC. The clinically used preparation is derived from salmon calcitonin.

Cannabinoids

There has been considerable interest in a potential role for cannabinoids in the management of chronic pain. To some extent this interest has been triggered and driven by anecdotal patient reports of benefit from cannabis use. Subsequent epidemiological studies showed that a significant proportion of patients suffering from chronic non-cancer pain smoke or ingest cannabis for pain relief.

The recent discovery of the endocannabinoid system with specific CB1 and CB2 receptors and the development of agonist and antagonists as well as encouraging results from preclinical studies point to a role of cannabinoids as a therapeutic option.

However, although animal work continues to suggest that cannabinoids may be useful for neuropathic and inflammatory pains, to date the results in clinical studies have been relatively modest and rather controversial.

Pharmacological considerations

Herbal cannabis contains a variable mixture of cannabinoids, with Δ9-THC, Δ8-THC, cannabidiol, and cannabinol being the major pharmacologically active components. These plant-derived cannabinoids have poor oral bioavailability, their lipophilicity limits GI absorption, which restricts their use in therapeutics. Inhalation of smoked cannabis provides a more predictable and titratable route of administration, but given the risks of combusted cannabinoid inhalation (emphysema, obstructive airways disease, and risk of lung cancer) it cannot constitute an appropriate therapeutic strategy. Some efforts are being made to take advantage of the lipophilicity and employ nasal or buccal administration of drug. Another consequence of the high lipid-solubility of cannabinoids is that they are sequestered into fatty tissue, leading to a long elimination $t_{1/2}$, extending from days to weeks.

Clinical efficacy

Cannabinoids have mostly been studied in cancer pain and in central neuropathic pain (and spasm) associated with multiple sclerosis (MS). A meta-analysis of trials published up to 1999 (5 on cancer pain, 2 on chronic non malignant pain, and 2 on acute pain) examined the effects of either Δ9-THC or levonantradol. The cannabinoids were estimated to be approximately equianalgesic to codeine 50–120mg, but adverse effects were common (see later), being reported in all studies.

More recently, Δ9-THC/cannabidiol (oromucosal spray) or dronabinol (taken by mouth) produced a significant decrease in the mean intensity of pain and reduced sleep disturbance in patients with MS. These results were replicated in an uncontrolled open-label extension study, which confirmed the benefit at 2-year follow-up of the oromucosal spray. Despite these results in MS, cannabinoids cannot yet be considered as a first choice in the treatment guidelines for neuropathic pain.

Adverse effects

The currently employed cannabinoids have both short- and long-term adverse effects that compromise their therapeutic use. The short-term adverse effects are mainly CNS (dizziness) and GI (nausea and vomiting).

More importantly, there are concerns regarding the long-term risk of developing mental illness with regular cannabis use. Cohort studies have demonstrated a dose-dependant increased risk of schizophrenia in regular cannabis users, notably in those with a predisposition to psychosis at baseline and similar findings are reported for depression and anxiety. Moreover there are data indicating cumulative, dose-dependent deficits in cognitive function in regular cannabis users. Finally, driving regulations and legislation limit the use of cannabinoids in some European countries.

Many of these side effects are a consequence of CNS effects of the cannabinoids which may be overcome by peripherally restricted CB2 antagonists which have some analgesic and anti-inflammatory action.

Conclusion

While there are strong laboratory data supporting the analgesic effects of cannabinoids, there is a need for more evidence in man. Despite evidence of a modest efficacy in neuropathic pain associated with MS, cannabinoids should not be currently be considered as a front line option in the treatment of chronic pain, because of the incidence of adverse effects.

Further reading

Attal N et al. (2006). EFNS guidelines on pharmacological treatment of neuropathic pain. Eur J Neurol **13**:1153–69.

Campbell FA et al. (2001). Are cannabinoids an effective and safe treatment option in the management of pain? A qualitative systematic review. BMJ **323**:13–16.

Ware MA et al (2003). Cannabis use for chronic non-cancer pain: results of a prospective survey. Pain **102**:211–16.

Placebo

The term placebo derives from the Latin meaning 'I shall please' and was originally used as a derogatory term denoting ineffective treatments employed to appease patients. However, its meaning has altered greatly and there is now a widespread recognition that both active and sham treatments can produce a useful therapeutic response, independent of their presumed biological efficacy. The placebo effect was defined as 'any effect attributable to a pill, potion, or procedure, but not to its pharmaco-dynamic or specific properties' by Wolf et al. in 1959.[1]

This placebo response is easily demonstrated in pain studies where a patient's belief in the potency of a treatment can produce a 20–30% improvement in their pain symptoms. Therefore, all meaningful trials of analgesics must include an appropriate placebo group to be able to demonstrate the efficacy of a novel treatment or intervention. Conversely nocebo effects are also encountered, where subjects report specific adverse effects from sham treatment. For example, in trials of opiates the placebo group has reported the anticipated opiate side effects of nausea, vomiting, itching, and constipation. Thus the form of the placebo and nocebo effect can be influenced by the patient's expectation of the actions of the active treatment.

Other interesting characteristics of the placebo effect include the findings that it operates in a somatotopic-specific[2] and a dose-dependent manner.[3]

Mechanism

There has been much research into the psychology and neurobiology of the placebo response. It is clear that the placebo effect is best engaged by a powerful medical figure who engenders confidence and trust in the patient. However, even in the absence of such a personal interaction, patients who believe that the treatment is potent and likely to be of benefit gain an additional therapeutic response compared to those who are unaware of its potential up-side. Furthermore, more complex, expensive, invasive, or high-tech interventions evoke greater placebo responses. There is little evidence to support the idea that only susceptible (and by implication weak) individuals are more likely to experience placebo effects.

Recent pharmacological and functional imaging studies have shown that some placebo responses in pain studies are due to the engagement of the endogenous opioid system and can be reversed using the opioid antagonist naloxone. Cholecystokinin exerts an anti-opioid action, and antagonizing this has been shown to increase the placebo effect. Other placebo responses appear to engage reward circuitry involving dopamine release and are less opioid-sensitive. It is possible to demonstrate objective alterations in pain perception associated with placebos emphasizing the potential utility of these responses in treatment.

Ethical considerations

The placebo effect is the basis by which quacks and snake-oil salesman have historically been able to peddle ineffective medications with some evidence of apparent benefit. Much of health-care regulation aims to prevent the abuse of patients by individuals and organizations offering treatments that are actually no better than placebo. This situation is most clearly apparent in the pain field where all treatments must be compared against placebo before they can be claimed beneficial.

It has also been thought that fraudulent and malingering patients could be identified by administering 'placebo' medication. However, an appreciation of the neurobiology of the placebo response reveals why this sort of 'test' is logically flawed and the ethics of such placebo trials are clearly unsound.

However it is considered ethical and legitimate to take advantage of the beneficial placebo effects when administering active treatments and a confident, professional manner and good communication have been shown to add additional therapeutic value to treatments.

Conclusion

The neurobiology underlying placebo effects is beginning to be better understood. Placebo responses are intrinsic to much of medical practice and are present in almost all pain consultations. They can be usefully engaged to enhance treatment efficacy by the skilled physician but must always be suspected in considering the evidence for a particular intervention.

Further reading

Benedetti F et al. (2005). Neurobiological mechanisms of the placebo effect. *J Neurosci* **25**:10390–402.

Petrovic P (2008). Placebo analgesia and nocebo hyperalgesia—two sides of the same coin? *Pain* **136**:5–6.

References

1 Wolf S (1959). The pharmacology of placebos. *Pharmacol Rev* **11**:689–704.

2 Benedetti F et al. (1999). Somatotopic activation of opioid systems by target-directed expectations of analgesia. *J Neurosci* **19**:3639–48.

3 Price DD et al. (1999). An analysis of factors that contribute to the magnitude of placebo analgesia in an experimental paradigm. *Pain* **83**:147–56.

Interventional therapies

Peripheral nerve blocks

Peripheral nerve blockade can be used to treat a wide variety of acute and chronic pain conditions. However, these techniques are not without risk. Good knowledge of anatomy and stringent safety precautions are essential. Modern techniques have been modified to include the use of nerve stimulators and, more recently, U/S to identify the nerves to be blocked. Catheters can be placed near to nerves or nerve plexuses to permit prolonged infusion and thus increase the duration of pain relief.

Types of peripheral nerve block

Diagnostic blocks

These can help to locate the source of pain.

Therapeutic blocks

These are most often used for acute pain after surgery or trauma, but repeated LA blocks are also commonly used in the treatment of chronic pain conditions, e.g. localized cancer pain. Performed with or without corticosteroids, they may provide pain relief for far longer than the duration of action of the LA. This may be due to the prevention of reflex muscle or sympathetic nervous effects, reduced ephaptic transmission or reduced excitability of nociceptive nerve fibres in recurrent spinal circuits. However, the evidence for benefit of repeated blockade from RCTs is not strong. Regional blocks can also be used to improve circulation to ischaemic limbs (see 📖 Sympathetic blocks, p.198), and to facilitate physiotherapy in CRPS.

Neurolytic blocks

These blocks employ chemical, thermal, or cryogenic techniques to destroy nerve tissue thereby preventing nociceptive impulses. They are covered elsewhere in this book (see Neurolytic blocks p 210).

General principles

General indications

- Intraoperative anaesthesia and postoperative analgesia
- Analgesia after trauma
- Treatment of dynamic (movement-induced) pain to aid rehabilitation after trauma or surgery
- CRPS, especially to facilitate physiotherapy
- Diagnostic blocks
- Neuralgia and nerve entrapment
- Cancer pain
- Muscle spasm
- Ischaemia (sympathetic blocks).

Contraindications

Absolute
- Patient refusal
- Local infection
- Lack of resuscitation facilities.

Relative
- Anticoagulation or coagulopathy.

Informed consent

A full discussion with the patient should take place and should include a full medical and anaesthetic history, the indication for the block, and possible complications, allowing patient consent to be obtained.

Preparation

- Secure IV access.
- Full airway and CV resuscitation equipment and expertise should be immediately available.
- Patients should be fully monitored.
- Aseptic technique should be employed, using antiseptic solution, sterile gloves, and sterile disposable needles.

Nerve identification

Landmarks

- Bony prominences or arterial pulses can be used, e.g. in inguinal field and femoral nerve blocks.
- Arteries lying within nerve sheaths (e.g. the axillary artery) can also be transfixed to aid localization.

Measured needle insertion

- The needle is inserted to a predetermined depth based on anatomical knowledge, as in the intercostal block.

Loss of resistance

- Loss of resistance to the injection of air or saline.
- Used in epidural, psoas compartment, and paravertebral blocks.

Eliciting paraesthesia

- Causing a prickling or tingling sensation in the distribution of the nerve to be blocked.

Peripheral nerve stimulators

Still the most commonly used method of nerve identification. Uses electrical impulses delivered via the needle to elicit either paraesthesia or a characteristic pattern of muscle movement. They reduce the potential for nerve damage as the nerve can be identified without the needle coming into contact with neural tissue

- Can be used with the patient awake, sedated, or under GA, although not when muscle relaxants have been used.
- Connect the anode to a large ground electrode at least 20cm from the needle insertion site, and the cathode to a stimulating needle (patient positive, needle negative).
- Set duration of impulse at 100microsec or less and frequency 1–2Hz.
- Initially set delivered current at 1–2mA.
- Look for synchronous muscle movement in the desired distribution.
- Reduce the current. Movement should still be present at 0.5mA but should disappear at 0.2mA; otherwise the needle may be within the nerve.

- Aspirate to check for intravascular placement. Inject 1mL of LA solution. Motor response should disappear due to displacement of the nerve from the needle tip.
- Injection should be painless and without resistance. If not, consider re-positioning.

Inject in divided doses with repeated aspiration for blood to check that needle tip has not migrated into a blood vessel.

Ultrasound
- This technique is gaining popularity with the increased availability of high resolution portable U/S scanners. It enables visualization of the nerve, surrounding anatomical structures and needle in real time.
- The spread of LA around the nerve can also be seen and predicts a successful block.

Needles
- Standard hypodermic, epidural, and spinal needles can be used to perform peripheral nerve and regional blocks.
- Several types of specially designed, insulated and non-insulated needles are available for use with nerve stimulators. Insulated needles are generally preferred as they require half the current of non-insulated needles. They also produce fewer false positives (from nerve stimulation by the needle shaft).
- Long-bevelled needles (angle 10–14°) penetrate tissues more easily and therefore give less feel when passing through tissue planes. They are more likely to cut nerve fibres.
- Short-bevelled needles (angle 18–45°) give more feel to the operator, especially when 'popping' through tissue planes. They have also been shown to produce nerve trauma.
- Pencil-point needles have a side injection port which is designed to prevent intraneural injection. They separate nerve fibres rather than cutting them, which may help to prevent nerve damage.

Local anaesthetic solutions
Lidocaine
- Rapid onset and short duration of action.
- Causes vasodilatation at the site of injection.
- Addition of adrenaline (1:200,000) slows systemic absorption and prolongs duration of block.
- Maximum dose is 3mg/kg or 7mg/kg if adrenaline added.
- In toxicity, cerebral irritation typically occurs before myocardial depression.

Avoid preparations containing preservatives as these may be neurotoxic.

Bupivicaine
- Slower onset and longer duration of action (lasts 2–3× longer than lidocaine).
- Does not cause vasodilation.
- Consequently the addition of adrenaline does not slow systemic absorption or prolong duration of block.

- Maximum dose is 2mg/kg.
- In toxicity, myocardial depression may progress to refractory ventricular fibrillation and cardiac arrest.
- Some preparations contain preservatives which may cause nerve injury.

Levobupivicaine
- S-enantiomer of bupivicaine.
- Maximum dose 2mg/kg.
- Believed to be less cardiotoxic.

Ropivicaine
- Onset of action similar to bupivicaine.
- Causes vasoconstriction which may prolong duration of block.
- Maximum dose 2mg/kg.
- Reduced motor block and cardiotoxicity compared to bupivicaine, may be due to its lower potency.

Prilocaine
- Rapid onset of action and short duration.
- Similar potency to lidocaine.
- Does not cause vasodilation.
- Maximum dose 6mg/kg, or 8mg/kg with addition of adrenaline 1:200,000.
- Rapid metabolism by hydrolysis, reducing risk of systemic toxicity.
- Metabolized to o-toluidine, which may cause methaemoglobinaemia.
- Agent of choice for IV regional anaesthesia (e.g. Bier's block).

Adjuvant drugs
Adrenaline
- Slows absorption of LA solution, thereby increasing duration of action and decreasing potential for toxicity.
- Less effective with longer-acting LA solutions.
- Also has an analgesic property due to α_2 -adrenoceptor agonism.
- Avoid in extremities such as finger and penile blocks—risk of ischaemia.

Corticosteroids
- Enhance the pain relieving effects of LAs by anti-inflammatory and also by direct analgesic effects.
- May also prevent or decrease both peripheral and central neuronal hyperexcitability.

Clonidine
- α_2 adrenergic agonist.
- Prolongs duration of block, including post-block analgesic effect.
- Dose for peripheral nerve blocks 0.3–1.0mcg/kg.

Opiates
- Shown to give synergistic analgesic effect when combined with LAs in neuraxial blocks. Benefit in peripheral blocks less certain.

General complications

- Needle injury to nerves.
- Repeated doses at high concentration can be toxic to nerves, muscles, and tendons.
- Haemorrhage or haematoma.
- Infection.
- Intravascular injection (e.g. into cerebral circulation causing seizure).
- Systemic toxicity (see following section).
- Anaphylaxis.
- Subdural or subarachnoid injection.
- Pneumothorax.

⚠ Local anaesthetic toxicity

- Caused by exceeding recommended maximum dose, prolonged infusions, or direct intravascular injection.
- More likely in more vascular areas, e.g. intercostal, epidural, and brachial plexus blocks.
- Less likely with dilute solutions, slower injection, and the addition of adrenaline to lidocaine.
- Neurological symptoms are initially excitatory, with agitation, tremor, visual disturbance, tinnitus and tingling around the mouth. There is progression to neurological inhibition, with respiratory depression, decreased conscious level, convulsions, and coma.
- Myocardial effects depend on the agent used: lidocaine produces prolongation of the PR interval and QRS duration, while bupivicaine has a negatively inotropic effect and produces more tachydysrhythmias. Both agents eventually cause CV collapse.
- Effects are more pronounced with acidosis, hypercarbia, and hypoxia.

⚠ Treatment

- Immediately stop injection or infusion.
- Assess and manage airway, breathing, and circulation.
- In mild cases, administer midazolam to decrease the chance of seizures.
- If decreased conscious level, convulsions, or CV collapse, intubate trachea and ventilate.
- In CV collapse, start cardiopulmonary resuscitation and consider administration of IV lipid according to local protocol (e.g. 1mL/kg Intralipid® over 1min, repeated up to twice at 3–5min intervals, then infusion of 0.25mL/kg/min).

Specific nerve blocks

It is beyond the scope of this book to describe fully the many peripheral nerve blocks that can be employed in the treatment of pain. What follows is a list of the most commonly employed blocks and their specific indications (besides surgical anaesthesia and analgesia). Plexus blocks are described elsewhere (💭 Plexus blocks, p.192).

Head and neck

Occipital nerve

● Repeated injections of LA and steroids can be used in the diagnosis and treatment of occipital neuralgia.

Trigeminal nerve

● This can be blocked at the level of the Gasserian ganglion or by blocking its peripheral branches (mental, infraorbital, supraorbital, and supratrochlear).
● Neurolytic blocks of the Gasserian ganglion with glycerol or radiofrequency ablation are used in TN as an alternative to microvascular decompression (see Trigeminal Neuralgia p.302).
● Also blocked for atypical facial pain, cluster headaches, and cancer pain.

Upper limb

Suprascapular nerve

● Used in the assessment of shoulder pain and to facilitate physiotherapy in CRPS.

Nerve blocks at the elbow

● The median, ulnar, radial, and cutaneous nerves of the forearm can be blocked for diagnosis, analgesia, and to facilitate physiotherapy.

Nerve blocks at the wrist

● The median, ulnar, and radial nerves can also be blocked at the wrist.

Thorax and abdomen

Thoracic, paravertebral, and intercostal blocks

● Blocks can be performed at any paravertebral or intercostal level for rib fractures, pleuritic pain, thoracic spinal pain, and acute herpes zoster.
● Can be used to distinguish between somatic, visceral, and referred pain of the chest and abdomen.
● With added steroid, used for analgesia after thoracotomy and in PHN.
● Neurolytic techniques are used in thoracic spine, chest wall, and abdominal wall cancer.

Ilioinguinal, iliohypogastric, and genitofemoral nerves

● Used in ilioinguinal–iliohypogastric neuralgia, genitofemoral neuralgia, chronic testicular and neuroma pain.

Lower limb

Femoral nerve

● Analgesia for femoral or patella fracture.

Sciatic nerve
- Analgesia for fractures of the lower limb.
- Also used for ischaemic pain and in CRPS.

Obturator nerve
- Blocked for nerve entrapment.
- Neurolytic block used in adductor muscle spasticity.

Lateral cutaneous nerve of the thigh
- Used in the diagnosis and treatment of meralgia parasthetica (a painful mononeuropathy).

Nerve blocks at the knee
- Used in chronic pain syndromes of the knee and lower leg.
- Techniques include intra-articular block, saphenous nerve block, and popliteal fossa block (tibial and peroneal nerves).

Nerve blocks at the ankle
- 5 nerves can be blocked at the ankle:
  - Sural
  - Saphenous
  - Tibial
  - Deep and superficial peroneal.
- Used for local painful conditions and CRPS of the foot.

Plexus blocks

LA blockade of several nerves at a time can be achieved by the employment of plexus blocks. The plexuses most commonly blocked in the chronic pain setting are brachial, lumbar, and sacral. These blocks are frequently employed for surgical anaesthesia and postoperative analgesia, but can also be used for the management of chronic pain by intermittent bolus or continuous catheter infusion techniques.

The agents used, the general principles, and the safety precautions are largely the same as for peripheral nerve blocks (see 📖 Peripheral nerve blocks p.184). Care should be taken when combining plexus blocks, as the maximum dose of LA is likely to be exceeded. Success rates can be improved with the use of nerve stimulators and/or U/S. The application of digital pressure to ensure proximal spread of LA can also improve success. For catheter techniques, initial distension of the nerve sheath with LA facilitates catheter insertion.

Brachial plexus blocks

Indications
- Anaesthesia and postoperative analgesia
- CRPS (especially useful to facilitate physiotherapy)
- Diagnostic or differential blocks
- Tumour invasion of brachial plexus.

Approach
There are 4 main approaches to the brachial plexus: interscalene, supraclavicular, infraclavicular, and axillary.

Interscalene block
- Best for shoulder analgesia
- Often misses ulnar nerve territory.

Technique
- Position patient supine with head on a pillow turned away from the side of the block.
- Identify the midpoint of the posterior border of sternocleidomastoid (at level of cricoid cartilage).
- Lateral to this point, palpate the interscalene groove between scalenus anterior and medius. The groove runs at approximately 30° to sternocleidomastoid. Palpation can be aided by asking the patient to sniff or lift their head.
- After local skin infiltration, insert a 25–50mm insulated needle, aiming towards the contralateral elbow. Specific motor stimulation should be elicited at 10–20mm.
- Endpoints are deltoid contraction or elbow flexion.
- Aspirate for blood or CSF, then inject 10–40mL of LA in divided doses, depending on indication.

Specific side effects and complications
- Phrenic nerve palsy (100%). Use with caution in patients with respiratory disease.
- Horner's syndrome (stellate ganglion affected in 10–25%).
- Epidural or intrathecal injection (results in a high spinal block).

- Vessel puncture (jugular vessels, carotid and vertebral arteries).
- Pneumothorax.
- Bilateral spread.
- Recurrent laryngeal nerve palsy causing hoarse voice (10%).

Supraclavicular (subclavian perivascular) block

- Gives the best chance of blocking the entire arm.

Technique

- Position patient supine with head on a pillow turned away from the side of the block.
- Identify the interscalene groove as described for interscalene block.
- Standing at the patient's side, follow the interscalene groove down until it meets the clavicle. Place your index finger in the groove at this point. The subclavian artery pulsation can be felt in approximately 50% of patients.
- After local infiltration, insert a 50mm insulated needle behind your index finger, aiming posteriorly to the subclavian artery and in the horizontal plane. Specific motor stimulation should be elicited at 10–40mm.
- Endpoints are flexion and extension of wrist and fingers.
- Aspirate for blood, then inject 10–40mL of LA in divided doses, depending on indication.

Specific side effects and complications

- Pneumothorax (1 in 1,000, can be delayed)
- Subclavian artery puncture (20%, aim more posteriorly)
- Intravascular injection
- Recurrent laryngeal nerve palsy causing hoarse voice
- Horner's syndrome.

Infraclavicular block

- Good for elbow, forearm, and hand, and often used for continuous catheter techniques.

Technique

- Position patient supine with head on a pillow, arm abducted.
- Identify the midpoint, on the underside of the clavicle, between the anterior process of the acromion and the jugular notch.
- Palpation of the subclavian pulse above the clavicle will help you to imagine the course of the artery to the axilla. The needle entry point will be at the midpoint of the clavicle, and lateral to the course of the artery.
- After local infiltration, insert a 50mm insulated needle directed posteriorly at 90° to the skin. Do not deviate medially. Specific motor stimulation should be elicited at 30–50mm.
- Endpoint is flexion or extension of wrist and fingers.
- Aspirate for blood, then inject 10–40mL of LA in divided doses, depending on indication.

Specific side effects and complications

- Pneumothorax (1 in 1000)
- Vessel puncture (subclavian artery or vein, 15%, move laterally)
- Intravascular injection.

Axillary block
- Good for elbow, forearm, and hand; often used for continuous infusion techniques.
- Risk of complications is low.
- Often misses axillary and musculocutaneous nerves.
- Intercostobrachial nerve will require a separate block.

Technique
- Position patient supine with arm abducted at 90° and elbow flexed at 90°.
- Palpate the axillary arterial pulse at the lateral border of pectoralis major.
- Fix the artery with the palpating finger.
- After local infiltration, insert a 25–50mm needle above or below the artery at 45° to the skin. Direct the needle parallel to the artery. Specific motor stimulation should be elicited at 10–15mm.
- The insertion point can be altered depending on which nerves need to be blocked in preference—above the artery for median and musculocutaneous, below the artery for ulnar, and behind the artery for the radial nerve. Alternatively, a multiple injection technique can be used.
- Endpoints are index and middle finger flexion (median nerve), thumb adduction and little finger flexion (ulnar nerve), thumb extension (radial nerve), and elbow flexion (musculocutaneous nerve).
- Aspirate for blood, then inject 10–40mL of LA in divided doses, depending on indication.
- The transarterial technique is an alternative. A non-insulated needle attached to an extension tube is inserted into the artery and beyond (guided by the ability to aspirate blood). Half of the LA solution can be deposited posterior to the artery, and half anteriorly on withdrawal of the needle (position again being guided by the ability to aspirate blood).
- The development of a palpable sausage-shaped distension of the plexus sheath suggests successful injection.

Specific side effects and complications
- Vessel puncture and intravascular injection.

Lumbar plexus blocks

Indications
- Anaesthesia and postoperative analgesia for surgery involving hip, thigh, or upper leg.
- Cancer pain from hip or upper femur.
- With a sacral plexus block, for anaesthesia and analgesia of the leg.

Approach
The lumbar plexus can be blocked with a posterior or inferior approach.

Posterior approach or 'psoas compartment block'

Technique

- Use the lateral position, with the side to be blocked uppermost.
- Mark a line running parallel to the spinous processes at the level of the posterior superior iliac spine, and a line joining the iliac crests. The intersection of these lines marks the insertion point.
- Insert a 100mm insulated needle at 90° to the skin, with a slight caudal angulation. Motor stimulation should be elicited at 70–100mm. If the transverse process of L4 is encountered, realign to pass beneath it.
- Endpoint is quadriceps contraction ('patellar twitch').
- Aspirate for blood, then inject 10–30mL of LA in divided doses, depending on indication.
- An alternative is the loss of resistance technique using a Touhy needle. The needle is 'walked off' the inferior surface of the L4 transverse process, and loss of resistance encountered after a further 0.5–1cm.

Specific side effects and complications

- Inadvertent epidural or intrathecal injection
- Vessel puncture and intravascular injection.

Inferior approach or '3 in 1' block

- Aims to block the femoral nerve, the obturator nerve, and the lateral cutaneous nerve of the thigh.
- Not always reliable as the latter nerve is often missed.

Technique

- Position the patient supine.
- Mark a point 1cm lateral to the femoral arterial pulse and 2cm below the inguinal ligament.
- After local infiltration, insert a 50mm insulated needle at 45° to the skin aiming proximally and parallel to the artery. Specific motor stimulation should be elicited at 30–50mm.
- Endpoint is quadriceps contraction ('patellar twitch').
- Aspirate for blood, then inject 20–30mL of LA, applying distal pressure to encourage cephalad spread.
- The lateral cutaneous nerve of the thigh can be blocked separately by injecting 10mL of LA beneath the fascia lata at a point 2cm medial and 2cm inferior to the anterior superior iliac spine.

Specific side effects and complications

- Nerve damage.

Sacral plexus block

Indications

- In conjunction with a lumbar plexus block, for anaesthesia and analgesia of the hip, thigh, or leg
- Cancer pain in the distribution of the sacral nerve roots
- Temporary relief of sciatica.

Approach
There are 2 approaches to the sacral plexus: parasacral and transforaminal. Only the former is described here.

Parasacral approach
Technique
- Place patient in lateral position, with the block side uppermost.
- Mark a point 6cm caudal to the posterior superior iliac spine on a line connecting it to the ischial tuberosity.
- After local infiltration, insert a 100mm insulated needle at 90° to the skin. Aim to hit bone and then redirect caudally. Specific motor stimulation should be elicited at 60–80mm.
- Endpoint is plantar flexion of the foot.
- Aspirate for blood, then inject 10–20mL of LA in divided doses. It is best to avoid the use of adrenaline near the sciatic nerve as its blood supply may become compromised.

Specific side effects and complications
- Loss of parasympathetic innervation to bladder and bowel
- Perforation of bowel
- Intravascular injection.

Sympathetic blocks

Visceral afferents travel along the sympathetic nerves to reach the DH of the spinal cord. These afferents can be blocked with LA or neurolytic techniques, for example, in the management of pain from gastric or pancreatic cancer. Sympathetic nerves are also responsible for the maintenance of vasomotor tone, meaning that sympathetic blockade is also useful in the treatment of ischaemic limb pain. The sympathetic nervous system also has a role in the generation of pain itself. In certain pain states, there is an abnormal response of the primary nociceptive afferents to sympathetic stimulation. Peripheral sensitization occurs, with reduced excitatory thresholds and the production of ectopic impulses. The afferent fibres also have increased adrenoceptor sensitivity, such that norepinephrine released from sympathetic nerve terminals causes further sensitization. This sympathetically mediated pain is sometimes seen in CRPS.

Sympathetic nerves are often blocked along with somatic nerves, as in epidural and brachial plexus blockade. Where there is anatomical separation, however, the sympathetic components can be targeted alone.

Anatomy

Preganglionic, myelinated (white) fibres originate from the cell bodies located in the lateral horn of the spinal cord. They exit the cord with the ventral nerve roots of the 1st thoracic nerve down to the 2nd to 4th lumbar nerve (the 'thoracolumbar outflow'). These fibres then pass into the sympathetic chain. This chain of ganglia lies on the anterolateral surface of the vertebral bodies in the cervical and lumbar regions, being more laterally placed along the necks of the ribs in the thoracic region.

Once in the sympathetic chain, preganglionic fibres either synapse in ganglia immediately or may travel up or down a variable number of segments. Alternatively, they may exit the chain as a splanchnic nerve and synapse in a prevertebral ganglion, for example, within the coeliac plexus.

The sympathetic chain receives visceral afferent fibres from the extremities, the head and neck and the organs of the thorax, abdomen and pelvis.

General principles

General indications

Acute visceral pain
- Pancreatitis
- Renal colic
- Uterine contractions
- Cardiac ischaemic pain.

Acute ischaemic pain
- Limb embolus
- Vascular and re-implantation surgery
- Frostbite
- Raynaud's disease
- Vasospasm from accidental intra-arterial injection of irritant drugs, e.g. thiopental.

Chronic pain
- Limb ischaemia causing rest pain where surgery not possible
- Phantom limb pain
- Central pain after stroke
- Chronic pancreatitis
- Cancer of upper abdominal or pelvic organs
- CRPS.

General contraindications, informed consent, and preparation
- As for peripheral nerve blocks (see 📖 Peripheral nerve blocks p 184).

Local anaesthetic solutions
- When used for diagnostic and prognostic sympathetic blocks, these are as for peripheral nerve blocks (see 📖 Peripheral nerve blocks p 184).

Neurolytic solutions
- Phenol 5–6%
- Ethanol 50–100%.

Neurolytic blocks are described in detail in Neurolytic blocks 📖 p.210, with particular reference to the coeliac plexus block, which is therefore omitted here.

Stellate ganglion block

Anatomy
- The stellate ganglion consists of a fusion of the lower cervical and upper thoracic sympathetic ganglia.
- It is located between the carotid sheath and the fascia overlying the prevertebral muscles at the level of the seventh cervical vertebra.
- Closely related are the dome of the pleura (below) and the vertebral artery (behind).

Specific indications
- CRPS of the upper limb
- Acute herpes zoster and PHN in the trigeminal nerve distribution
- Phantom limb pain
- Upper limb ischaemia
- Inadvertent intra-arterial injection of substances causing vasospasm, e.g. thiopental
- Cardiac ischaemic pain
- Hyperhydrosis.

Approach
- The aim is to place LA solution at C6 with caudal spread blocking the ganglion, as a direct approach risks entering the dome of the lung or the vertebral artery.

Technique
- Position patient supine, with the neck extended.
- Palpate the carotid pulsation at the level of the cricoid cartilage.
- Move sternocleidomastoid and the carotid artery laterally and palpate the transverse process of C6 ('Chassaignac's tubercle').

- After local infiltration, insert a 25G needle perpendicularly to the skin, and advance towards the tubercle until bone is contacted. Then withdraw by 3–5mm.
- Aspirate for blood, and then inject 0.5mL solution as a test dose. Then inject 15–20mL of low concentration LA solution (e.g. 0.5% lidocaine or 0.125% bupivicaine) in 5mL increments.
- Sit patient up to aid caudal spread toward the stellate ganglion.
- Signs of a good block are those of Horner's syndrome: ptosis, miosis, anhydrosis, and enophthalmos. Patients may also get a unilateral blocked nose due to vasodilatation of the nasal mucosa.

Specific side effects and complications
- Intra-arterial injection, e.g. into the vertebral artery causing seizures
- Intrathecal injection causing a high spinal
- Recurrent laryngeal nerve palsy causing hoarseness
- Haematoma
- Cervical or brachial plexus block
- Pneumothorax
- Phrenic nerve palsy: do not perform bilateral blocks.

Thoracic sympathetic block

Anatomy
- The thoracic sympathetic chain is located along the necks of the ribs, in close approximation to the pleura and the somatic nerve roots and their dural cuffs.

Specific indications
- In conjunction with stellate ganglion block, to achieve sympathetic blockade of entire upper limb.
- Ischaemic cardiac pain.

Approach
- Due to the anatomical position of the thoracic sympathetic chain, there is a high risk of pneumothorax, somatic nerve root damage, and intrathecal injection with needle techniques. For this reason, they have been largely superseded by thoracoscopic techniques, especially if neurolytic agents are to be used.

Specific side effects and complications
- Pneumothorax
- Intrathecal injection
- Intra-arterial injection
- Somatic nerve root injury.

Lumbar sympathetic block

Anatomy
- The lumbar sympathetic chains lie on the anterolateral aspect of the lumbar vertebrae, separated from the somatic nerves by the psoas muscle and fascia.
- Anterior relations are the aorta on the left and the inferior vena cava on the right.

Specific indications

- Lower limb ischaemia
- CRPS of lower limb
- Phantom limb pain
- Renal colic
- Urogenital pain.

Approach

- The aim is to place LA solution around the lumbar sympathetic chain from the 2nd to 4th lumbar vertebrae.
- This can either be achieved by a single injection at L3, or 2 separate injections at L2 and L4.

Technique

- Position patient laterally with side to be blocked uppermost.
- Identify the midpoint of the spinous process of the desired lumbar vertebra.
- Mark a point 8cm laterally.
- After local infiltration, and with image intensifier guidance, insert a 12cm, 22G needle at 45° to the skin, aiming medially towards the body of the vertebra.
- The body lies at a depth of about 8cm. If bone is encountered at 4–5cm, it is likely to be transverse process. Redirect cranially or caudally.
- When the body of the vertebra has been identified, redirect needle to pass just anterolaterally.
- A loss of resistance may be felt as psoas fascia is exited.
- Aspirate for blood or CSF, then inject test dose of LA mixed with radiographic contrast.
- Lateral and anteroposterior images should be obtained to ensure correct needle placement.
- Images should show a band of contrast within the psoas compartment and covering the relevant lumbar vertebral levels. If contrast dissipates quickly, needle may be in a vessel. Other appearances may indicate retroperitoneal spread or injection into the psoas muscle.
- Inject dilute LA depending on indication. For diagnostic block inject 5–10mL lidocaine 0.5% or bupivicaine 0.25%. For therapeutic block use 20–25mL in 5mL increments.
- For neurolysis, inject 5–6% phenol or 50–100% ethanol: 3mL at each level or 6mL at one level.
- Leave patient on side for at least 5min to prevent lateral spread of solution, then supine for 1h.
- Check blood pressure.

Specific side effects and complications

- Inadvertent intravascular injection into aorta or inferior vena cava.
- Intrathecal injection.
- Profound hypotension.
- Ureteric damage.

- Ejaculatory failure (bilateral blockade).
- Postsympathectomy neuropathic pain can occur with neurolytic techniques. Anterolateral thigh pain is common, though usually transient. Genitofemoral neuritis, a state of hyperaesthesia in the L1 dermatome, is more troublesome.

Intravenous regional sympathetic block

Mechanism of action

- This technique aims to block sympathetic nerve fibres by local absorption of guanethidine, a drug which acts by blocking the reuptake of released noradrenaline at sympathetic nerve terminals.

Specific indications

- Acute and chronic ischaemic vascular conditions
- Chronic obliterative arterial disease
- Frostbite
- Inadvertent intra-arterial injection of irritant drugs
- Raynaud's disease
- CRPS.

Approach

- Position patient supine.
- Ensure full monitoring is in place.
- Draw up sedative and analgesic drugs (e.g. midazolam, alfentanil) to treat tourniquet pain and the exacerbation of symptoms caused by released noradrenaline.
- Insert an IV cannula in the affected limb, as close to the site of pain as possible.
- Place a second IV cannula in another limb for emergency use.
- Prepare guanethidine solution. The dose of guanethidine is 10mg for the first block and 20–30mg for subsequent blocks, diluted in normal saline, 25mL (upper limb) to 40mL (lower limb).
- Apply an appropriately sized gas powered tourniquet.
- Exsanguinate limb and inflate tourniquet to 50–100mmHg above patient's systolic blood pressure.
- Slowly inject diluted guanethidine solution into the cannula in the affected limb.
- Leave tourniquet inflated for 20min.
- Deflate tourniquet.
- There will be a rise in heart rate and blood pressure as the noradrenaline not taken up by the sympathetic nerve terminals is released into the systemic circulation.

Specific side effects and complications

- High systemic levels of injected agent due to tourniquet failure, rapid injection, or passage through incompressible blood vessels within bone. This may cause hypotension or CV collapse, especially if LA solution has been used.
- Dysrhythmias
- Bronchoconstriction in asthmatics
- Allergy to guanethidine
- Blocked nares due to vasodilatation in nasal mucosa.

Intrathecal and epidural drug delivery systems

Introduction

These systems can be used in patients whose pain and spasm problems have not responded to less interventional modes of treatment.

This is an invasive mode of pain relief and should only be used in a multidisciplinary context by clinicians familiar with their use. In addition there should be access to neurosurgical expertise.

These modes of treatment are relatively underused due to lack of awareness and limited local availability of expertise.

Scientific rationale

Higher concentrations of drugs can be obtained at spinal cord receptors by local as opposed to systemic delivery. The total dose used is much less which can frequently avoid the systemic side effects.

Indications

There are 3 broad indications for neuraxial drug delivery:
- Painful and non-painful limb spasm
- Cancer pain
- Chronic non-malignant pain (CNMP).

It should be clearly understood that the majority of patients in these groups will respond to less invasive modes of management.

Painful and non-painful limb spasm

Some patients with significant neurological injury will develop profound limb spasm. This can be either due to disease, e.g. MS, or trauma and can be managed in a multidisciplinary context with oral antispasmodics such as baclofen or tizanidine. However, in patients who develop side effects or have a poor response, direct drug delivery should be considered.

Children with cerebral palsy and/or gait problems should be managed in an appropriately resourced and experienced specialist centre.

Pharmacological assessment should involve a test dose of intrathecal baclofen. The usual dose in adults is 40–50mcg and less in children. A one-off test dose is adequate. This should be delivered in an appropriate clinical environment. Ideally there should also be a psychological assessment prior to the procedure to explore the patient's expectations, beliefs, and understanding of the procedure.

Cancer pain

Severe pain which is not responsive to standard methods of management can be significantly improved with neuraxial drug delivery.

Pharmacological trial assessment can be by bolus opiate test dose or by infusion. The usual adult bolus is 0.5–1.0mg morphine. Ideally a psychological assessment should take place prior to the procedure although occasionally clinical need may make this impractical.

Chronic non malignant pain

CNMP is the most difficult to assess. Psychological assessment is most important and without this an implant should not proceed.

Pharmacological assessment should ideally be by infusion of opiates over a number of days. Bolus injections can be used but they will probably need to be repeated several times.

Evidence for effectiveness

- **Spasm**: there is excellent evidence for the treatment of spasm arising from disease and trauma.
- **Cancer pain**: there are numerous case reports describing the effectiveness of the technique and one comparative study. One recent study has also demonstrated prolonged patient survival.
- **CNMP**: although there are several open studies demonstrating that implanted systems can deliver good quality pain relief there are no RCTs.

Types of delivery system

Partially implanted

These can either be an implanted intrathecal or epidural catheter attached to an external pump or alternatively with a SC port through which medication is infused continuously or by bolus.

They have the advantage of being simple but are more prone to infection than totally implanted pumps and catheters. Epidural systems are more appropriate for bolus use but will need greater volumes of drug than intrathecal systems. These systems are most frequently used in the setting of limited life expectancy and will restrict a patient's mobility.

Fully implanted

These systems are for intrathecal use. They can be divided into fixed rate and variable (programmable) rate pumps.

Fixed rate

These pumps rely on a pressurized chamber to deliver a drug through a fixed orifice. They are cheaper than a programmable pump but they are less flexible. The only way that the quantity of medication delivered can be changed is by refilling the pump with a different concentration of drug. They are more appropriate for situations where life expectancy is short or when a pump replacement is indicated when a programmable pump comes to the end of its life and the patient's medication dose has stabilized. These pumps have variable reservoir volumes and flow rates. An appropriate pump is chosen for a patient's clinical condition. In general, malignant disease is best managed with higher flow rates.

Variable (programmable) rate pumps

These pumps are mechanically driven and highly flexible. They are programmed externally and can deliver variable amounts of medication over a 24-h cycle. They are highly sophisticated and more expensive than fixed rate pumps. They are more appropriate for situations where the need for medication is variable or difficult to predict.

Medications used

Only morphine, baclofen, and ziconitide are licensed for intrathecal use (see novel and atypical agents p 176). Other drugs such as LAs, clonidine, and hydromorphone have been used intrathecally. The lack of a licence for either the pumps or medications in combination should not deter experienced clinicians from using this technique when it is in the best interests of the patient. The patient should be fully informed at all times of what is in the pump and any potential side effects. The polyanalgesic consensus guidelines 2007 should be read in these circumstances.

Organizational issues

Patients needing neuraxial drug delivery systems have by definition severe and ongoing problems. An implant is not a one-off event but marks the start of an ongoing relationship. Clinicians, their teams, and patients need to accept this. After an implant frequent visits will be needed to optimize appropriate dosage and the patient will need to attend for refills at variable intervals, usually about every 5–6 weeks.

A 24h on call system is necessary and patients' GPs must be fully involved in their management.

Complications

These are can be divided into general, pump-related, and drug-related.

General

Complications relating to the surgical insertion of the pump. These include pump pocket infection, meningitis, local or spinal haematoma, and CSF leak. They are managed as appropriate with the relevant specialities.

Pump related

Pump problems include catheter displacement, disconnection and pump unit failure.

Drug related

There have been reports of LA toxicity and implanting teams need to be aware of this. A rare complication is the development of catheter tip granuloma. This seems to be related to the medications in the pump, the flow rate, and the position of the catheter tip. The long-term use of diamorphine in pumps is felt to be unwise due to interaction with the pump materials.

Opioids can also cause endocrine side effects including weight gain, oedema, excessive perspiration, loss of libido, hypogonadotrophic hypogonadism, hypocorticism, headache, memory or mood changes, and constipation.

Pump refills should always involve double-checking of the programming and medications to prevent errors.

References

1 ℘ http://www.interscience.wiley.com/journal/118536422/abstract

Facet joint injections

Anatomy

Facet or zygoapophyseal joints are true synovial joints in that they are lined with a synovial membrane, have cartilaginous surfaces, and a fibrous capsule. The joints are formed by the articulation of the superior and inferior facets of adjacent vertebrae. They are richly innervated, each joint receiving fibres from the medial branch of the dorsal ramus at the same level as the vertebra as well as from the vertebra above.

Facet joints develop the same degenerative changes as other peripheral joints and are affected by both RA and OA. They are also susceptible to injury during acceleration/deceleration injuries.

Facet syndrome

Facet syndrome is said to occur when there is a symptom complex consisting of LBP which radiates from the low back into the hips, buttocks, and thigh. The pain is in a non-dermatomal distribution. The pain is associated with a decreased range of movement at the lumbar spine and spasm of the lumbar paraspinous muscles. The pain is continuous and is worsened by rotation and extension. There is often tenderness over the joints and paravertebral muscles.

Investigations

All types of imaging of the lumbar spine including radiographic and MRI scans of the spine will demonstrate degenerative facet joint disease in a large, pain-free, proportion of the population. There is no correlation between the degree of degeneration seen on imaging and the degree of pain experienced by patients.

Facet joint procedures

Pain arising from facet joints can be alleviated by either injecting steroid and LA into the joint itself or by blocking the nerves which supply the joint.

Intra-articular injection

This technique is indicated as a diagnostic test to prove whether or not a specific facet joint is responsible for pain. LA and steroid are injected into the joint under fluoroscopic imaging.

Medial branch block

In this technique the medial branch of the dorsal ramus supplying the joint which is thought to be the pain generator is blocked using either LA and steroid or radiofrequency lesioning. Because each joint receives innervation from the dorsal ramus at the same level of the vertebra and also from the medial branch of the vertebra above, both nerves need to be blocked in order to produce pain relief.

Evidence of efficacy

There are conflicting reports in the literature regarding the efficacy of facet joint procedures. A recent Cochrane review[1] concluded that there is no strong evidence for or against the use of any type of injection therapy for individuals with subacute or chronic LBP. The latest NICE guidelines for non-specific low back pain recommended that doctors should not offer injections of therapeutic substances into the back. They recommended that: 'Robust trials, including health economic evaluations, should be carried out to determine the effectiveness and cost effectiveness of invasive procedures—in particular, facet joint injections and radiofrequency lesioning'.[2]

References

1 Staal JB et al. (2007). Injection therapy for subacute and chronic low-back pain. *Cochrane Database Syst Rev* **1**:CD001824.
2 NICE (2009). *Low Back Pain*. Available at: ℘ http://guidance.nice.org.uk/CG88

Neurolytic blocks

Neurolytic blocks involve placing a toxic chemical in or around a nerve in order to permanently disrupt its function. When successful, neurolytic blocks can significantly reduce the pain and the need for other analgesics such as opioids. However, neurodestructive procedures can have serious side effects and are now rarely performed other than in patients with a limited life expectancy due to malignant disease.

Possible complications are:
• Deafferentation pain can develop in the area supplied by the damaged nerve.
• Damage to adjacent nerves such as motor nerves leading to paralysis.
• Reduced effectiveness over time requiring a repeat procedure.

The most commonly used agents for neurolytic procedures are phenol, ethyl alcohol and glycerol. Only commonly used neurolytic blocks will be described.

Coeliac plexus block

Injection of neurolytic agents into the coeliac plexus blocks the nerve supply to the upper abdominal viscera and can be useful in the treatment of pain due to either carcinoma of the pancreas or proximal small bowel. The quoted success rates for this procedure vary but in some reports up to 80% of patients have a reduction in opioid requirements and an improved quality of life. In 10–24% of patients, pain is abolished altogether.

There are several techniques used for coeliac plexus block. The most common is the 2-needle retrocrural technique. In this technique the patient is placed prone and the coeliac plexus is approached from the L1 level. Other techniques include the 2-needle transcrural technique, the single-needle periaortic technique, the single-needle transaortic technique, and the single-needle anterior technique. Detailed description of these techniques is beyond the scope of this book. Typically 10–12mL of 6% aqueous phenol is injected.

Complications of coeliac plexus blockade include diarrhoea, pneumothorax, kidney and ureter damage, and, most seriously, paraplegia.

Trigeminal ganglion block

Blockade of the trigeminal ganglion is sometimes still used in the treatment of trigeminal neuralgia if surgery is not feasible and drug treatment ineffective (see 📖 Percutaneous ablative treatments p.231).

The trigeminal ganglia lies in the foramen ovale in the middle cranial fossa. Under fluoroscopic guidance, a needle can be inserted near the ganglion and a small amount of neurolytic agent, usually phenol, injected.

There are many possible complications with this procedure including anaesthesia dolorosa, intrathecal injection, retrobulbar haematoma, and cavernous sinus fistula.

Lumbar sympathetic block

Sympathetic denervation by blocking the lumber sympathetic chain is used in the diagnosis and treatment of sympathetically maintained pain originating from the lower part of the body. It is sometimes used in the treatment of CRPS of the lower limbs and also to treat the pain secondary to vascular insufficiency of the lower extremities.

A needle is inserted 8–12cm from the midline at the L3 level from a posterior approach. The needle is directed to lie just anterior to the anterior border of the L3 vertebra. LA or phenol is injected to block sympathetic innovation, either temporarily or permanently.

Complications include epidural or intrathecal injection, intraperitoneal injection, genitofemoral nerve damage, diarrhoea, sexual dysfunction, and postural hypotension.

(See also 📖 Sympathetic blocks p.198.)

Other interventional techniques used in chronic pain

There are many interventional techniques which aim to reduce suffering in people with persistent pain problems. There is very little evidence for most of these techniques and therefore only the most commonly used will be discussed.

Before considering any of these invasive techniques it is important that patients are assessed in a multidisciplinary setting and all non-invasive therapies explored. Invasive techniques should only be considered when other methods of both controlling the pain and of reducing its impact have failed.

Intra-articular injections

Intra-articular injections of LA and steroids, either alone or in combination, are often used in an attempt to alleviate pain secondary to arthritis. Any joint can potentially be injected with therapeutic substances but the most commonly targeted joints are the knees, elbows, and shoulders.

Most published data on intra-articular injections are of poor quality and at best only report on short-term symptomatic relief. There is very little compelling evidence to suggest that intra-articular steroids and/or LAs have any influence over long-term prognosis. However, many patients are grateful for the short-term relief they gain from these techniques.

Botulinum toxin

Botulinum toxin blocks the release of acetylcholine from the neuromuscular junction and reduces spasticity. It is often used by direct injection to affected muscle groups in the treatment of spasticity secondary to cerebral palsy. Some studies show short-term benefit in this group of patients but a recent Cochrane review concluded that there was little evidence to either support or refute its use.

Botulinum toxin is also used in the treatment of muscle spasm secondary to myofacial pain syndrome. There is limited evidence to suggest that this may be useful but further RCTs are needed.

Cervical dystonia has been treated successfully with injection of botulinum toxin. There are several short-term studies which show benefit in this condition and other long-term studies which suggest repeat injections continue to confer benefit. Adverse events include dysphagia and dry mouth.

Botulinum toxin has also been used for the treatment of many different headache disorders. There is some evidence of efficacy in these situations.

Cryoanalgesia

Cryoanalgesia is defined as the relief of pain by the application of cold. This can refer to the application of cold packs to a painful area but more commonly refers to the application of a cryoprobe to a nerve in order to produce nerve injury by freezing the nerve (cryoneurolysis).

Cryoneurolysis results in axonal disruption followed by degeneration of the axon distal to lesion with the preservation of the fibrous architecture of the nerve. This allows regeneration of the axon without neuroma formation and with a very low incidence of neuritis.

Cryoprobes work on the principle of high-pressure gas expansion where a high-pressure gas is allowed to expand rapidly causing a rapid decrease in temperature. These probes can reach temperatures of −60°C to −70°C. N_2O is the most commonly used gas.

Cryoanalgesia is most commonly used to produce neurolysis of peripheral nerves in chronic pain conditions caused either by dysfunction of a particular peripheral nerve or where the nerve innervating a painful area can be readily accessed. It has been used during surgery to block the ilioinguinal nerve during repair of inguinal hernias and also to block intercostal nerves during thoracotomy.

The nerves most commonly targeted by cryoanalgesia are the intercostal nerves, the medial branches of the posterior primary rami of the spinal nerve roots, the greater occipital nerves, and neuromas.

Radiofrequency (RF) lesioning

Radiofrequency lesioning produces heat within tissues by applying a high-frequency current between 2 electrodes, one within the tissue and one on the surface of the body. The high-frequency current results in an electric field which causes ions to vibrate rapidly and thereby generate heat. The heat produced results in thermocoagulation. In pain management, RF is usually applied to nerves but in other situations it can be applied to any tissue, for example, it is used in the destruction of hepatic metastases.

One of the first clinical applications of RF lesioning was percutaneous cervical cordotomy. This is performed for patients with severe unilateral pain secondary to cancer where all other therapies have failed. It is rarely performed now as other treatment options can often give satisfactory results with less potential risk. It is still sometimes used in the treatment of pain secondary to unilateral mesothelioma. An electrode is placed within the spinothalamic tract and a radiofrequency lesion made.

RF lesioning is still used to treat trigeminal neuralgia when surgery is not indicated and other less invasive treatments have failed.

The most common use of RF lesioning is in the treatment of facet joint syndrome (LBP secondary to facet joint disease). If patients respond to a diagnostic block of the medial branch of the dorsal ramus with LA, proponents of RF lesioning would suggest applying this to the nerve. The evidence for long-term benefit is contradictory.

Complications include paralysis, urinary retention, and respiratory depression.

Spinal endoscopy

Spinal endoscopy is a relatively new technique for the treatment of chronic sciatica. The aims of spinal endoscopy are to place LA and steroids directly onto the nerve root responsible for the radicular pain of sciatica and also to divide any adhesions which may be contributing to the irritation of the nerve root.

The technique involves placing a fine endoscope (diameter 0.9mm) within the epidural space via the caudal route and manipulating the scope to the level of the nerve root that is thought to be responsible for the symptoms. This is done under fluoroscopic control. Once the nerve root has been identified any adhesions are divided and LA and steroids are injected.

There is little good quality evidence to support this technique. A comparison between targeted steroid placement using spinal endoscopy and traditional 'blind' caudal injection showed no difference between these approaches.

Further reading

Dashfield AK (2005). Comparison of caudal steroid epidural with targeted steroid placement during spinal endoscopy for chronic sciatica: a prospective, randomized, double-blind trial. *Br J Anaesth* **94**:514–19.

Neuromodulation

Transcutaneous electrical nerve stimulation

TENS has been with us for over 40 years since its first description by Wall and Sweet.[1] TENS units deliver electrical impulses across the skin with the aim of activating sensory nerve afferents, particularly Aβ fibres, which are normally responsible for touch sensation. This stimulation is delivered by a battery-powered generator through self-adhesive electrode pads applied to the painful region. Despite the fact that there are limited controlled studies showing benefit from TENS, it is often empirically tried for a variety of conditions. It is non-invasive, has an excellent safety profile, and is relatively cheap. A significant proportion of patients report it to be beneficial.

Mechanism of action

TENS was developed to exploit the prediction from the gate control theory of Melzac and Wall that activity in Aβ afferents would obtund incoming pain signals at the spinal segmental level. There is now experimental evidence that the beneficial effects of TENS are mediated at both spinal and thalamic levels and may also involve activation of endogenous opioid systems.

Practicalities

Most TENS units allow the user to control the pulse parameters, such as amplitude, frequency, duration, and pulse pattern. There are a number of different stimulation paradigms which can be split into:

- Conventional TENS (50–120Hz) where the aim is to stimulate Aβ fibres with pulses below the pain threshold.
- High intensity TENS where stimulus amplitude is increased above the pain threshold to stimulate Aδ fibres and evoke local muscle twitches.
- A 3rd variant employs bursts of high frequency, high intensity pulses at a low frequency (2Hz) simulating acupuncture (AL TENS).

Although there is no clear rationale for choosing one paradigm over another, the common practice is to start with conventional TENS as it is well tolerated. It should be noted that often patients will have tried a TENS unit (bought over the counter or borrowed) unsuccessfully before presenting to clinic and may need to be encouraged to embark on a medically supervised trial.

Stimulation is applied for periods of at least 30min. The optimal site is usually over the affected dermatome; however, there are a number of reasons to select an alternative area:

- Damaged or fragile skin.
- Hypoaesthetic skin—theoretically TENS should not work and may damage insensate skin.
- Hyperaesthesia or allodynia may make presence of electrodes intolerable.

In these cases electrodes can be applied to paraspinal locations or on adjacent dermatomes.

Indications

TENS is used for both acute and chronic pain although much of this use is unsupported by level 1 evidence. In general, TENS appears best suited to the treatment of continuous rather than phasic pain.

Acute pain

There is evidence for the efficacy of TENS in acute back pain, orofacial and dental pain, fractured ribs, and dysmenorrhoea. TENS can be used to supplement pharmacotherapy for postsurgical analgesia. There is also evidence that TENS can improve angina pain and may act to improve myocardial perfusion. Although commonly used and considered safe there is little evidence of efficacy for pain during labour.

Chronic pain

TENS is often trialled empirically for chronic pain and is commonly used in musculoskeletal pains such as knee OA, hand RA and a variety of mechanical and radicular back pains. There is also some support for the use in neuropathic pains including some patients with postherpetic neuralgia, TN, peripheral neuropathies and CRPS. In these instances the patient will need to be advised that stimulation is likely to be painful initially before any benefit is seen.

Contraindications and cautions

Serious adverse events from TENS are rare. Manufacturers list the following contraindications—pacemakers, implanted defibrillators, epilepsy, and pregnancy—because of legal concerns. In practice, it is possible to use TENS in all of these conditions (with appropriate medical consultation). Caution should be exercised when applying TENS to the anterolateral neck (risk of vagal bradycardia, hypotension, and laryngeal dysfunction), over the anterior chest wall and internally (without designed devices). TENS should probably not be applied immediately before sleep unless the device has a shut off timer.

Reference

1 Wall PD, Sweet WH (1967). Temporary abolition of pain in man. *Science*. **155**:108–9.

Spinal cord stimulation

This technique uses electrodes implanted in the epidural space to deliver electrical impulses which excite fibres and neurons in the spinal cord, with the aim of producing a pleasant paraesthesia over the painful region. Spinal cord stimulation (SCS) has been in use since the late 1960s and the rationale for its development was based on the gate theory of Melzack and Wall, whereby stimulation of non-noxious sensory inputs could block the transmission of noxious information. However, given that it is relatively ineffective for nociceptive pain and it is beneficial in neuropathic pain conditions, it would appear that this is an oversimplification and other mechanisms are engaged.

Indications

SCS has been used for a wide variety of different pain conditions but the strongest evidence (from RCTs) for its benefit is seen in neuropathic pain where dorsal column function is intact.

- Failed back surgery syndrome with radicular pain
- CRPS
- Neuropathic pain secondary to nerve injury
- Chronic critical limb ischaemia
- Refractory angina.

The first 3 indications have been subjected to detailed analysis and meet the NICE cost–benefit criteria and are thus approved indications. NICE concluded that further data was needed to support the use for refractory angina and critical limb ischaemia. The beneficial effects of SCS in these last two indications are to some extent due to alterations in the sympathetic outflow to these territories.

SCS appears to be relatively ineffective for central pain, spinal cord injury pain, and non-ischaemic, nociceptive pain.

Technique

The kit comprises an implantable epidural electrode, programmable pulse generator (analogous to a cardiac pacemaker), and a tunnelled connector lead. The epidural component can have a variety of configurations but most have an array of electrode contacts. It can be inserted either percutaneously under LA or following laminotomy under GA. Each approach has advantages:

- Percutaneous placement allows optimization of electrode position to allow appropriate paraesthesia to be elicited over the affected territory. The procedure can be abandoned if no beneficial paraesthesia is elicited.
- Surgical implantation allows the placement of larger electrodes which are less prone to migration.

After insertion many centres undertake a trial of stimulation with an external stimulator and only implant the permanent system if this is successful. The stimulation parameters can be adjusted to alter the pairs of electrodes used, the frequency, amplitude, and duration of the pulses to best elicit paraesthesia. Patients can be given programmers to tailor their parameters to their own daily activities.

Complications

As well as the complications associated with epidural implantation (infection, nerve injury, dural puncture) and surgery, the most common issues are with lead migration, connector dysfunction, and the predictable issues of battery failure and the requirement for revision. Lead migration is commoner with percutaneous placement and can result in a loss of efficacy. Battery life tends to be 2–4 years depending on the stimulation parameters.

Patient assessment

Implantation of SCS devices represents a long-term and potentially costly therapeutic commitment. Patients should have failed with trials of simpler therapies and been assessed by a multidisciplinary team as being likely to benefit from SCS. An assessment by a pain psychologist is also desirable to assess patients' expectations and beliefs prior to such a major intervention.

Conclusions

SCS has become an accepted and useful therapy for a number of refractory pain conditions. Its use within established centres can produce good results. However, it still represents a considerable investment of resource, has the potential for physical and psychological morbidity, and thus patients need to be carefully selected.

Further reading

British Pain Society and Society of British Neurological Surgeons (2005). *Spinal cord stimulation for the management of pain.* Available at: ℘ http://www.britishpainsociety.org/book_scs_main.pdf

Simpson EL et al. (2008). *Spinal cord stimulation for chronic pain of neuropathic or ischaemic origin. Technology Assessment Report.* Available at: ℘ http://www.nice.org.uk/guidance/index.jsp?action=download&o=40909

Deep brain stimulation

Has a relatively long history in the treatment of pain (>40 years) and involves the long-term implantation of multi-contact stimulating electrodes. This is done with the aim of producing paraesthesia (analogous to SCS) and/or activating an endogenous analgesic mechanism.

Targets

Endogenous analgesic system

- Periaqueductal or periventricular grey (PAG/PVG): believed to be most effective for somatic nociceptive (non-neuropathic) pain, e.g. temporomandibular joint pain or high cervical RA:
  - Descending modulation of spinal nociceptive circuits
  - Warmth in area of stimulation
  - Bilateral analgesia (best on contralateral side).
- Posteroinferior hypothalamus—specifically for cluster headache.

Paraesthesia-producing targets (typically for deafferentation or poststroke pain)

- Ventral posterior (VP) nucleus of thalamus:
  - Activate lemniscal/dorsal column system
  - Aim for somatotopic paraesthesia
- Internal capsule—target if thalamus not intact.

Indications

Although originally thought to be useful only for nociceptive pain there is now increasing interest in the use of DBS for the treatment of refractory neuropathic pain including:

- Post-traumatic brain injury
- Poststroke pain
- Thalamic syndrome
- Cranial nerve pain:
  - Anaesthesia dolorosa
  - Dental pain
  - Postherpetic pain.

Technique

General stereotactic technique

- Target localization with stereotactic imaging performed using one of several imaging modalities: MRI, computed tomography (CT), ventriculography, or a combination.
- Stereotactic coordinates of the target generated either from direct visualization on high-resolution MRI or indirect localization by defining the target in relation to 3rd ventricular landmarks, primarily the anterior and posterior commissures.
- Stereotactic implantation of the electrode through burrhole with accurate localization of the target verified by perioperative imaging or electrophysiological refinement using microelectrode recording and/ or stimulation or macroelectrode stimulation. Electrophysiological methods require the patient to be awake in order to assess optimal effect prior to implantation of the electrode.

- Electrode lead either externalized for trial stimulation prior to internalization with successful effect, or directly internalized and connected via a SC cable to an intermittent pulse generator implanted usually in the infraclavicular region

Complications

- Haemorrhagic stroke (<2% in experienced hands).
- Hardware complications:
  - Lead migration or dislodgement
  - Lead fracture
  - Infection
  - Erosion
  - Electrical short circuit and component malfunction.
- Stimulation side effects as a result of inaccurate electrode placement and or spread of stimulation to surrounding eloquent structures.
- Tolerance with time.

Outcome

- Remains experimental.
- Results so far have been mixed.
- Best results for failed back surgery syndrome, deafferentation pain syndromes, and trigeminal neuropathy.

Motor cortex stimulation

MCS was first reported by Tsubokawa et al. in 1991[1]. It involves the stimulation of motor cortex, using an implanted electrode plate, below the threshold to induce muscle twitching, which can inhibit pain. Although there is a lack of controlled comparative studies, MCS seems to be as efficacious as thalamic DBS (and slightly less invasive) in the treatment of some neuropathic pain syndromes although its use is restricted to a few enthusiastic centres.

Indications

Intractable neuropathic pain syndromes.

Central
- Spinal cord injury
- Thalamic stroke/lesion.

Peripheral
- Trigeminal neuropathic pain
- Peripheral nerve injury
- Phantom pain or plexus avulsion.

Mechanisms of action

The exact mechanism of action is uncertain but there is evidence that MCS may:
- Reinforce action of non-nociceptive sensory inputs on nociceptive systems at level of thalamus, dorsal column nuclei and spinal cord.
- Reduce emotional component of chronic pain by activating anterior cingulated cortex and insula.

Relative preservation of pyramidal tract and somatosensory pathways is essential for good result. Facial pain is most commonly and effectively targeted. This may be explained by the easily accessible and proportionately large area of facial representation on the cortical convexity. Treatment of leg pain is more difficult because of the inter-hemispheric cortical location.

Procedure
- Localization:
  - Preoperative: fMRI, transcranial magnetic stimulation (TMS).
  - Intraoperative: neuronavigation, median nerve somatosensory evoked potential mapping, motor cortex stimulation to evoke twitches in correct area.
- 16–20 plate diagnostic grid to locate target.
- 4-plate electrode secured: anode on sensory and cathode on motor cortex.
- Stimulation cycled (3–12h cycles): onset of pain relief is typically delayed and outlasts period of stimulation.

Outcomes

Figures from case series (% obtaining >50% pain relief):
- Neuropathic facial pain (73%)
- Central poststroke pain (52%).

Response to preoperative transcranial magnetic stimulation may be a useful predictor of response to MCS.

Complications

- Extra/subdural haematoma
- Seizures (0.7%)
- Speech disorders (0.7%)
- Paraesthesia/dysaesthesia (2.2%).

Relative contraindications

- Large cortical stroke with encephalomalacia in region of stimulation
- Significant weakness in painful territory
- Loss of long somatosensory tracts.

Reference

1 Tsubokawa T et al. (1991). Chronic motor cortex stimulation for the treatment of central pain. Acta Neurochir Suppl (Wien) **52**: 137–9.

Surgical techniques

Surgery for back pain: introduction

Non-operative treatment remains the mainstay of the management of back pain.

In general, surgical intervention may be indicated for back pain if it:
- Corrects deformity and instability
- Relieves neural compression
- Eradicates tumour/infection.

There are a number of conditions where surgery is indicated:

Children
- Congenital and developmental disorders, e.g. kyphoscoliosis
- Infection
- Tumours (usually primary).

Younger adults
- Trauma
- Spondylolysis and spondylolisthesis
- Degenerative disc disease.

Older adults
- Degenerative spinal stenosis
- Tumour (usually metastatic)
- Infection.

Infection

Epidemiology
Vertebral osteomyelitis/discitis: 1–3 per 100,000 population per year in developed nations, much higher in developing world. Bimodal distribution with peaks of incidence in mid-childhood and 6th decade.

Aetiology
Origin of infection may be from:
- Haematogenous spread from extraspinal focus
- Direct spread from adjacent focus
- Direct inoculation (e.g. trauma, iatrogenic)
- Unknown.

Causative organisms
- Bacteria (most common):
  - *Staphylococcus aureus*
  - *Escherichia coli*
  - *Pseudomonas aeruginosa*
  - *Klebsiella* (particularly in IV drug users)
  - *Staphylococcus epidermidis*
  - *Streptococcus* (particularly in iatrogenic cases)
- Others (non-pyogenic):
  - *Mycobacterium tuberculosis* (particularly in thoracic vertebral osteomyelitis)
  - *Toxoplasma gondii*.

Clinical features

Back or neck pain is the commonest symptom:
- There is often an insidious onset in adults (resulting in delayed diagnosis).
- More acute onset with fever in children.

The classical triad of neck/back pain, fevers, and neurological deficit is not present in most patients.
  Neurological deficit occurs later and suggests epidural abscess.

Any of the listed features suggestive of infection should prompt urgent referral to a spinal surgeon for assessment and initiation of treatment.

Diagnosis

Bloods
- Elevated CRP and ESR.
- White blood cell (WBC) count may not be elevated, particularly in chronic infection.
- Blood cultures must be taken before antibiotics.

Imaging
- Radiographs usually normal in first 2–4 weeks. Disc space narrowing and endplate changes suggest discitis. Osteomyelitis results in bony destruction (radiolucency), new bone formation (radiodensity), and, later, vertebral body collapse. Paravertebral soft tissue mass may be visible.
- CT shows bony/disc disease and paravertebral mass earlier than X-rays. CT-guided percutaneous biopsy provides tissue for culture.
- MRI shows high signal on T2-weighted scans due to oedema within bone and disc, and provides most detail on associated collections.
- Radionuclide bone scans show increased uptake long before radiographic changes occur. Gallium more useful than technetium for differentiating osteomyelitis from OA/tumour.

Management

Medical
- Broad-spectrum antibiotics initially. Refined if causative organism identified.
- Traditionally, administered parenterally for 6–8 weeks, then orally for variable duration, guided by clinical response and resolution of elevated inflammatory markers.

Surgical
Indicated in:
- Bony destruction resulting in instability.
- Symptomatic neural compression (from kyphosis secondary to vertebral body collapse/instability, abscess, inflammatory mass).
- Systemic sepsis not responding to antibiotics (suggests abscess).

Surgery for back pain: spondylolysis and spondylolisthesis

Definitions

Spondylolysis: defect in the pars intra-articularis (the part of the lamina that connects the superior and inferior articular facets), probably due to stress fractures in genetically susceptible individuals, one of the causes of spondylolisthesis.

Spondylolisthesis: displacement of a vertebral body on the one inferior to it (usually an anterior slip of L5 on S1).

Classification (Wiltse, 1976):
- Type 1: dysplastic (congenital abnormalities of facets).
- Type 2: isthmic (defect in pars intra-articularis including spondylolysis).
- Type 3: degenerative (causing remodelling and instability of facet joints).
- Type 4: traumatic (fractures of posterior elements excluding pars).
- Type 5: pathological (generalized or localized bone weakness).

Incidence

5% prevalence in the general population.

Clinical

Usually asymptomatic in children, back pain may occur during adolescent growth spurt or with high activity levels (competitive sports). Occasionally, leg pain occurs (probably due to L5 root irritation). With increasing slip, children develop deformity (lumbar kyphosis and compensatory lordosis above slip level) and waddling gate; adults more likely to develop radicular signs.

Diagnosis

Imaging: standing lateral radiographs used to estimate severity of slip as a percentage of the width of the vertebral body.

Management

Non-operative: analgesics and NSAIDs, avoidance of aggravating activity, bracing, physiotherapy (core stability). If spondylolysis does not respond, rule out other causes of back pain (infection, tumour, osteoid osteoma).

Operative

Spondylolysis: repair of pars defect with debridement, bone grafting, fixation with wires/screws (only necessary in very small proportion).

Spondylolisthesis

Indications: significant neurological signs, high grade slip (>50%), traumatic and iatrogenic slips, severe persistent symptoms despite non-operative treatment, and postural and gait abnormalities.

Surgical techniques: fusion (posterolateral or lumbar interbody fusion), usually with fixation using instrumentation, decompression for associated radiculopathy, reduction of slip prior to fusion is controversial (improves posture/spinal biomechanics and places less stress on fusion mass but high rates of permanent nerve root injury reported).

Surgery for back pain: degenerative disc disease

Epidemiology
Extremely common with increasing age.

Aetiology and pathogenesis
- Discs consists of concentric rings of fibrocartilage (annulus fibrosus) surrounding the gelatinous nucleus pulposus.
- Disc is avascular in adults—degeneration may be secondary to decreased diffusion through cartilaginous endplate.
  - Stage 1 (age 15–45): tears of annulus, synovitis of facet joints.
  - Stage 2 (age 35–70): progressive disc disruption, facet joint degeneration + subluxation.
  - Stage 3 (age >60): hypertrophic bone formation around discs and facet joints results in ankylosis.

Clinical features
- 'Discogenic' pain (disc itself is poorly innervated, pain probably comes from surrounding structures): aching at level of degeneration.
- Radicular pain/sensory loss/weakness: nerve root compression secondary to disc protrusion or facet joint hypertrophy.
- Neurogenic claudication: pain, loss of sensation and weakness in legs when walking, secondary to spinal stenosis.

Diagnosis
- Radiographs: loss of disc space height, endplate sclerosis, syndesmophytes, facet joint hypertrophy.
- MRI: decreased disc signal on T1 and T2 (decreased water content), disc herniations, nerve root impingement.
- Selective nerve root blocks: useful diagnostic and therapeutic tool.

Management
Non-operative
Analgesics, NSAIDs, muscle relaxants, exercise, physiotherapy, back education, epidural steroid injections.

Operative
Decompressive surgery
Removal of herniated disc or hypertrophic bone/soft tissue that is resulting in radiculopathy or spinal stenosis with pain or significant neurological deficit.
- Discectomy: posterior approach, bulging annulus incised + disc material removed
- Laminectomy ± partial facetectomy: posterior decompression preserving lateral 2/3 of facet joints to prevent iatrogenic instability.

Fusion
For pain secondary to instability. May be posterolateral or lumbar inter-body, with or without instrumentation (pedicle screws/cages provide stability and encourage fusion).

Surgical management of trigeminal neuralgia

When trials of medical therapy have failed there are many different surgical options available for TN (see p302). Many of the procedures available are neuro-destructive and lesion the trigeminal nerve in a variety of ways whereas the 'gold standard' treatment—microvascular decompression—is considered neuroreconstructive. Gamma knife surgery is a non-invasive alternative method of lesioning the trigeminal nerve route. Access to this treatment is limited despite it being a useful, NICE approved, option.

Microvascular decompression

Microvascular decompression (MVD) is the gold standard surgical treatment and procedure of choice for those fit for GA and posterior fossa craniotomy.

Contraindications

Neuralgia secondary to pontine demyelinating plaque or mass lesion.

Advantages
- High initial response rate
- Best long-term cure rates (>80%)
- Low risk of facial/corneal sensory loss (anaesthesia dolorosa).

Disadvantages
- Risk of death (~0.4%).

Factors predicting poor response
- 'Atypical' TN
- Previous ablative procedures
- Venous or unconvincing arterial compression of nerve root on magnetic resonance angiography (MRA).

Procedure
- Microsurgical exploration of trigeminal nerve via a small (2.5cm) posterior fossa craniotomy.
- Cerebellar retraction and arachnoid dissection to visualize the whole extent of the nerve from the root entry zone into the pons to Meckel's cave and identify the possible source of vascular compression along the whole length of the trigeminal nerve. The superior cerebellar artery is the most common culprit.
- Nerve root decompressed by gentle dissection of vessel from the nerve root and either separated by placement of interposing material or by transposition of the vessel with fixation to the tentorium.
- Venous decompression-vessel is either coagulated and divided or mobilized and separated.

Partial sensory rhizotomy (PSR)
- Partial section of trigeminal sensory root is done when there is equivocal or no vascular compression identified or the vessel cannot be mobilized.
- Best for pain in maxillary (V2) and mandibular (V3) divisions.

- Pain fibres in caudal part of sensory root, near brainstem.
- Half section root for V3 pain, 2/3 section for V2 pain.
- These sections aim to produce lower facial analgesia, without anaesthesia and sparing the corneal reflex. However, there is a significant risk of anaesthesia dolorosa, dysaesthesia, and corneal dysfunction.

Complications of MVD and PSR

- Death
- Posterior fossa haematoma/infarction
- Ipsilateral deafness
- Trigeminal sensory loss/dysaesthesia
- Other cranial nerve deficits (IV and VII)
- CSF leak, infective or aseptic meningitis
- Recurrence of pain.

Percutaneous ablative treatments

These percutaneous, injection techniques involve passage of a needle, under brief GA, through the foramen ovale under X-ray control to target the trigeminal ganglion. The ganglion is then lesioned using either radiof-requency thermocoagulation (RTC), glycerol rhizotomy (GR), or balloon compression (BC). Although less likely to be effective over time than the craniotomy-dependent procedures they are often well tolerated and have a negligible mortality rate, thus have a relatively important role in the elderly or frail patient.

Indications

- Medical contraindications to posterior fossa surgery under GA
- Unwilling to have posterior fossa craniotomy
- MS patients or absence of compressing blood vessel
- Recurrence or symptom persistence despite adequate microvascular decompression.

Advantages

- High initial response rate
- Lower risk of major complications/death.

Disadvantages

- Less effective long term with significant recurrence rates
- Increased risk of facial/corneal numbness (which correlates with duration of pain relief)
- Reactivation of HSV.

Stereotactic radiosurgery

SRS is the delivery of a single high dose of radiation to a well-defined target without exceeding the radiation tolerance of surrounding tissues.

Gamma knife

Cobalt-60 is the source of gamma rays in 201 individual capsules arranged around a collimator helmet that targets the radiation to the chosen field. In one of the first uses of the gamma knife, in 1953, Leksell (the pioneer of the gamma knife) targeted the trigeminal ganglion to treat neuralgia.

Mechanism
- SRS induces demyelination and inflammation of trigeminal nerve and selective damage to less myelinated pain fibres.
- The nerve root entry zone is targeted as the oligodendrocytes of the central myelin are more sensitive to SRS than the Schwann cells of peripheral myelin.

Indications
- As for the other ablative percutaneous procedures.
- There are advocates of early treatment with SRS as the risk of facial numbness or dysaesthesia is ~10%.

Advantages
- Non-invasive
- No sedation/anaesthesia required
- Low rates of facial numbness and anaesthesia dolorosa.

Disadvantages
- Very high dose of radiation near brainstem (~90Gy) to small target
- Limited access to gamma knife centres (in UK)
- Delayed effect—latency period of few days–6 months.

Outcome
- Initial rates of effectiveness of >90% are similar to that of other ablative procedures.
- Up to 50% of patients will experience some relapse but in 2/3 of cases the degree of pain relief is nonetheless sufficient to avoid the need for continuing medical treatment.

Physical therapies

Physiotherapy in chronic pain

Definition of physiotherapy

Physiotherapy is a form of treatment which employs physical approaches to promote, maintain, and restore physical, psychological, and social well-being, applicable to a wide range of variations in health status.

Core skills include manual therapy, the application of electrophysical modalities, and therapeutic exercise. Through problem-solving and clinical reasoning the physiotherapist works in partnership with the individual to optimize their functional ability and potential. Physiotherapists work with patients who have neuromuscular and musculoskeletal problems, including pain.

Indications for physiotherapy in the management of chronic pain

Physiotherapy may be indicated in various types of chronic pain, whether of malignant or benign origin. It may be helpful in cancer pain, but this chapter focuses on chronic pain of benign origin, such as mechanical musculoskeletal pain or neuropathic pain. Whatever the origin of pain, physiotherapy may be indicated in the following circumstances when there is:
- Deconditioning.
- Loss of confidence in movement and activity.
- Fear avoidance beliefs and behaviours.
- Activity cycling interfering with effective pain management.

Aims of treatment
- To improve self-management of pain-associated incapacity.
- To reduce the risk of development of pain-associated incapacity.
- To relieve pain.

If pain relief is the main aim, the related incapacity may also be tackled, e.g. stretching within an active exercise programme to avoid/reduce soft tissue contractures. Pain management approaches occasionally result in pain relief but this is not a stated aim.

Principles of treatment
- Assessment including diagnostic triage—to exclude serious pathology and to make clinical diagnosis as a basis for the treatment programme.
- Use of methods to manage or reduce the risk of pain-associated incapacity and improve self-management.
- Use of methods to reduce or relieve pain.

Pain-relieving approaches in physiotherapy

Model of care

Treatment approaches aimed at relieving or reducing pain are underpinned by a tissue-based model of disease, with treatment intended to rectify or reduce the perceived dysfunction in order to relieve the pain. The treatment philosophy is neuromusculoskeletal or biomechanical (i.e. biomedical) and the approach may be manual, electrophysical, or by therapeutic exercise (with or without education). Treatment is on a one-to-one basis except in the latter approach which may also be delivered in a group.

Aims of treatment

At the end of treatment the patient should:

- Report reduced or relieved pain.
- Show practical awareness of the relevance of posture, biomechanics, and movement in the management of pain.
- Implement an exercise programme in order to maintain desirable changes that have been achieved and to increase fitness.

Methods

These fall into 3 categories—manual therapy, electrophysical modalities, and therapeutic exercise.

Manual therapy

This includes:

- Traction
- Massage
- Manipulative therapy.

Traction (no evidence for use in chronic pain)

- This is passive movement applied to spinal joints and is a mobilization technique.

Massage

- Massage is manipulation of soft tissue using various techniques depending on the tissue interface being targeted.
- Therapeutic massage is claimed to have effects on the circulation, muscle, connective tissue, the autonomic nervous system, and on pain and sensation.
- Techniques are effleurage, petrissage, kneading, wringing, rolling, picking-up, shaking, clapping, pounding, vibration, and deep transverse frictions. Techniques are chosen depending on the target tissues. Effleurage, for example, targets superficial tissue whereas deep transverse frictions may target specific, deeper tissues such as ligaments.
- Massage is known to reduce oedema and muscle spasm and may have an effect on pain by breaking into the 'pain–muscle spasm' cycle.

Contraindications

Include: open wounds, inadequate circulation, thrombophlebitis or delicate vessels, haemophilia, psoriasis, haemorrhage, early stages of healing, active bacterial or fungal infection, febrile conditions, acute inflammation, and active bone growth such as at a healing fracture site.

Caution

Malignant disease, fragile skin, collagen weakening such as in long-term steroid use, advanced RA or diabetes, heart problems, the early stages of pregnancy, and over the anterior neck or chest and mid scapular regions where reflex responses may be stimulated.

Evidence for its use in chronic pain supports short-term effects only and it may best be viewed as an active strategy within an overall package of self-management.

Manipulative therapy

There are various theories as to how manipulative therapy acts to reduce pain (although supportive evidence is lacking). These include changing the viscosity of intra-articular synovial fluid, increasing joint accessory range of motion, enhancing endorphin release, and stimulating joint mechanoreceptors so that the inputs from small diameter C-fibres are blocked by closing the pain gate. Physiotherapists may use techniques from different schools of manipulation such as Maitland, Cyriax, or Kaltenborn.

2 types of therapy are applied by physiotherapists:

- Manipulative techniques: small-amplitude, high-velocity thrust applied to spinal or peripheral joints beyond restricted range of motion.
- Mobilization techniques: high-amplitude, low-velocity physiological or accessory passive movement applied to spinal or peripheral joints within or at the limit of range of motion.

Caution should be exercised in the choice between manipulative or mobilizing techniques. Care should be taken but gentle mobilizing techniques may be selected in the following (where manipulative techniques present a risk):

- Some medical conditions such as Paget's disease, RA, osteomyelitis, or ankylosing spondylitis where bone and/or joint structures may be compromised.
- Vertebro-basilar insufficiency.
- Vertigo.
- Generalized joint hypermobility.
- Instability such as spondylolisthesis.

There is evidence for modest effectiveness for manipulative therapy in chronic LBP but no evidence that it is more effective than other treatments such as analgesia or exercise.

Contraindications

Absolute contraindication to manipulative or mobilizing techniques:

- Neurological changes indicating nerve root involvement.
- Cauda equina and cord syndromes.
- Radiological changes such as osteoporosis, bony malignancy, or RA.

Electrophysical modalities

This includes thermal agents such as local superficial heat, deep heat (e.g. electromagnetic energy and US), hydrotherapy and cryotherapy.

Thermal agents

Thermal agents are claimed to produce local metabolic, neuromuscular, haemodynamic, and collagen extensibility changes in tissue. Although it is known that heat elevates the pain threshold, alters nerve conduction velocity, and changes muscle spindle firing rates, the underlying mechanism for pain relief is unclear.

Thermal agents are applied therapeutically to reduce pain and muscle spasm and to increase soft tissue extensibility and may be part of a treatment or self-management package.

Local superficial heat

Can be applied by hot packs or pads (71–82°C), hot baths, paraffin wax (49–54°C), hydrotherapy, or radiant heat.
- Heats tissue up to 3cm from the skin surface.
- Contraindicated by local or systemic inflammatory processes, reduced circulation, decreased skin sensation or integrity, over areas of infection or malignancy and in areas where liniments have recently been applied.

Deep heat
- Delivered with various electrotherapies, mainly electromagnetic energy, US, and laser.
- Heats tissue 3–5cm from the skin surface.
- Contraindicated by local or systemic inflammatory processes, reduced circulation or skin sensation, malignancies, pregnancy, metal implants, or cardiac pacemakers. Should not be applied to areas of high water content such as the eyes or gonads.

Electromagnetic energy

Clinical effects are claimed to be pain relief and improved wound healing as well as other general effects of heat where this is applied. Evidence for pain relief is weak.
- Non-ionizing RF radiation: applies electromagnetic energy to the tissues at a frequency of 27.12MHz.
- Shortwave diathermy: continuous electromagnetic energy is absorbed to produce heat in the tissues.
- Pulsed electromagnetic energy: the waves may be pulsed at regular intervals and may be set to produce heat or not to produce heat.

The intensity, duration, and frequency of the treatment determines how much heat is produced. It is vital that the patient can appreciate and report the sensation of heating in the tissues in order that appropriate adjustments are made.
- Contraindications as listed earlier.

Ultrasound

Acoustic energy converted to mechanical energy which produces heat in tissues. Is non-ionizing.
- Frequency: 1MHz optimum dose for compromise between deep penetration and adequate heating. 3MHz available for superficial tissue effects.
- Continuous waves provide constant intensity whereas pulsed waves provide interrupted intensity (duty cycle of 0.05–0.5).
- Intensity determines the strength of the US beam and gives the rate at which energy is delivered to a unit area. Ranges from 0.5–2 watts per cm^2.
- The greater the intensity, the greater the temperature elevation.
- US is known to reduce the nerve conduction velocity of C-fibres but evidence for pain relief is weak.

- Contraindicated over areas of high fluid content, such as the eyes, malignancies, areas of suspected fracture or reduced bone density.

Hydrotherapy

Movement or exercise in water that uses heat, buoyancy, and turbulence as well as the sedative effects of being in warm water. Therapeutic effects are said to be:
- Reduction in pain and muscle spasm.
- Improved joint motion.
- Re-education and increase of muscle strength.
- Improved circulation and balance.
- Improved confidence and function.

There is a lack of supportive evidence for these effects in chronic pain.

Contraindications
- The presence of open wounds or infections.
- Comorbidities where the application of warmth to the body as a whole may produce harmful effects.

Cryotherapy
- Cold may be applied to reduce pain, muscle spasm, swelling, and as a counterirritant. Can be applied with cold packs (ice or gel at 5–12°C), cold baths, vapocoolant sprays, or local application with ice cubes. Often part of the patient's set of self-management strategies.
- Action is to cool tissue by conduction or evaporation. Has haemodynamic and neuromuscular effects. The greater the temperature gradient between the skin and the cooling source, the greater the tissue temperature change.
- Dose depends on method of application; from 1 min for ice massage to 30min for cold packs.

Contraindications
- Reduced circulation, skin sensation, or integrity.

Therapeutic exercise

The aim of exercise therapy (individual or group), may be to extend joint and soft tissue range of motion, increase muscle strength, improve general, CV, or respiratory function, develop overall mobility and balance, or foster a sense of well-being. Exercise programmes may, therefore, include stretch, muscle strengthening and endurance, and aerobic exercise, as well as exercise aimed at improving balance and coordination. In chronic pain management, the aims are frequently to improve general fitness and function and all these elements may be incorporated into the exercise programme. Some specific exercise approaches claim to relieve pain and this may be reported as a result of general exercise.

Evidence for exercise therapy alone shows it to be slightly effective at reducing pain and improving function in chronic LBP. Evidence for specific (e.g. directional) back exercises rather than general exercises in LBP is unclear. Combined with education (i.e. Back School), exercise does not decrease LBP or work absence, but when delivered in an occupational setting, there is some evidence that it reduces work absence.

Exercise as part of an active rehabilitation programme is effective in improving function, either in a unidisciplinary setting or as part of a multidisciplinary Functional Restoration Programme or an inter-disciplinary Pain Management Programme.

Pain management approaches in physiotherapy

Model of care

Pain management approaches to physiotherapy treatment focus on managing or reducing the development of pain-associated incapacity rather than on the pain itself. They are based on a biopsychosocial rather than a disease model of human behaviour. The biopsychosocial model is the underlying treatment philosophy and a cognitive behavioural approach to physical therapy is used to achieve the aims of treatment. The use of cognitive behavioural approaches is not a physiotherapy core skill and therefore is typically delivered by a specialist pain physiotherapist. Treatment may be individual or in groups.

Aims of treatment

At the end of treatment the patient should be able to:
- Demonstrate and develop principles of pacing with exercise and physical activity.
- Show practical awareness of the relevance of posture, biomechanics, and movement in the management of pain.
- Plan and implement achievable goals using principles learned.
- Reflect on prior physical activity level with a view to developing independence.
- Justify requirement for exercise and explain the effects of disuse and deconditioning.
- Plan continuous development of exercise in order to maintain and improve fitness.
- Show confidence in physical activity and abilities.
- Acknowledge risks and implement plans for setbacks as these occur.
- Employ relaxation and exercise skills as part of an overall stress management strategy.

Methods

Improve fitness, mobility, and posture by exercise; taught using cognitive and behavioural principles. Help the patient return to a range of usual and more satisfying activities by applying improved fitness with goal-setting and a graded increase in chosen activities. Assist the patient in counteracting unhelpful beliefs and improve mood and confidence by:
- Teaching cognitive principles.
- Building steadily on successes.
- Educating about pain and healthy use of the body.
- Identifying and addressing fears relating to movement and activity.

Improve stress management and sleep by:
- Assisting with the identification of stress.
- Teaching strategies to deal with stress including relaxation and exercise.

Choice of whether treatment is with the individual or in a group will be influenced by:

- The existence of comorbidity where specific rather than general messages may be more helpful.
- Ability to communicate in the language used in a group.
- The patient's choice.

Contraindications and cautions

Presence of serious pathology (potentially worsened by physiotherapy) requiring investigation and further medical management.

Evidence

The evidence supporting a cognitive behavioural pain management approach to physiotherapy intervention is growing. Reduced fear-avoidance beliefs and behaviours, negative coping strategies, and disability, and improvements in exercise behaviour have been demonstrated.

Multidisciplinary pain management intervention is more likely to be successful where psychological factors influence adjustment and where these would not be expected to improve with physiotherapy alone.

Conclusion

Physiotherapy in chronic pain may aim for pain management or pain relief. Treatment begins with assessment and diagnostic triage. This leads to clinical diagnosis and an appropriate treatment programme is planned which may be unidisciplinary or multidisciplinary. The aims of treatment are always agreed with the patient. A range of physiotherapy techniques is available and the physiotherapist is best placed to select the most appropriate modality. Many patients with chronic pain develop associated disability and these two factors are only moderately correlated. Treatment emphasis is shifting towards a pain management rather than purely pain-relieving approach, aiming for more effective self-management and improved quality of life. Although the physiotherapist should consider whether patients with complex disability and distress are likely to benefit more from interdisciplinary treatment, many patients benefit from a programme of physiotherapy alone.

Acupuncture

Acupuncture: from the Latin *acus*, 'needle' (noun) and *pungere*, 'to prick' (verb). The treatment modality of piercing the skin with fine needles to elicit a therapeutic effect is one of the best known and most accepted of the complementary therapies. It is practised in primary care and pain centres by a wide variety of health-care practitioners.

Brief history

The development of therapeutic needling has uncertain historical origins. Recent discoveries date the use to 3200BC in Europe with evidence of use in ancient Egyptian, Greek, and Hindu scripts. However, acupuncture is, to the majority, associated with Traditional Chinese Medicine (TCM), the components of which may have originated ~1600BC, and were influenced by the philosophical and cultural framework of Taosim, ~400BC.

In the UK the 2 main schools of acupuncture are:
- Traditional Chinese medical acupuncture
- Western medical acupuncture.

Traditional Chinese acupuncture

This is the use of acupuncture, moxibustion, and Chinese herbal medicine following a detailed assessment (incorporating examination of the tongue and radial pulses) in order to maintain the smooth and balanced flow of Qi (vital energy) through a series of channels (meridians) that exist beneath the skin. The presence of Qi in all living matter is a core belief in Chinese philosophy and Qi moves in equal and opposite qualities (yin/yang). Disease exists when this flow is interrupted. The insertion of fine needles into these channels is believed to stimulate an innate healing response resulting in the restoration of an individual's physical emotional and spiritual equilibrium. The British Acupuncture Council (BAcC ♒ http://www.acupuncture.org.uk) is the main non-statutory registering body for professional acupuncturists in the UK.

Western medical acupuncture

This is a modern scientific approach to acupuncture used in conjunction with orthodox clinical diagnosis, predominantly for the treatment of somatic pain. Specific points are chosen based on neurophysiological principles. The effects of treatment are mediated through stimulation of the peripheral nerves and neuromodulation within the CNS, to provide analgesic and some non-analgesic effects. Points are chosen in order to stimulate localized painful areas (usually myofascial trigger points) or areas which have a spinal segmental innervation corresponding with the painful and dysfunctional area. The British Medical Acupuncture Society (BMAS ♒ http://www.medical-acupuncture.co.uk) represents regulated health-care professionals who use this approach.

Regulation

Presently in the UK, acupuncture is not regulated, although there are moves to address this as appropriate and adequate training can reduce the potential for adverse events.

Acupuncture treatment

Acupuncture is an effective treatment for a range of conditions.

Commonly
- Acute and chronic musculoskeletal problems
- Chronic pain conditions
- Chronic headaches
- PONV.

Also it shows promise in other relevant conditions such as:
- Bladder detrusor instability
- Insomnia
- General well-being, anxiety, and depression.

Mechanism of action for treatment of pain

Traditional Chinese medicine
- By attempting to resolve local or systemic accumulation or deficiencies of Qi. Pain is considered to indicate blockage or stagnation of Qi flow
- TCM treatment attempts to influence interruptions of flow of Qi at specific channels/meridians or in the corresponding yin yang organ (termed *zang fu*) at tender points termed *ah shi* points.

(refer to ☐ Further reading, p.246).

Western medical theory

Stimulation of the peripheral nervous system via Aδ or type II and III afferent nerve fibres induces neuromodulation of the CNS resulting in analgesia and some non-analgesic effects.

There are 4 categories of therapeutic effects:
- Local (immediate vicinity of the needle) release of trophic and vasoactive neuropeptides from the terminals of small-diameter sensory nerves.
- Segmental (within segment of spinal cord where the nerves from needle site enter CNS) at the DH. *Sensory modulation* occurs by inhibition of C-fibre pain transmission to substantia gelantinosa by enkephalinergic interneurons as a result of Aδ afferent stimulation. Most powerful effect.
- Heterosegmentally (all segmental levels of CNS). Projections to sensory cortex via thalamus have brain stem collateral connections to the PAG, where release of β-endorphin results in potentiation of serotoninergic and noradrenergic descending inhibitory pathways. Effect on afferent drive in DH of all spinal segments. Diffuse noxious inhibitory controls contribute in a minor way to the acupuncture effect.
- Generally (on whole body via central and possible humeral release of neuropeptides and hormones into the blood and CSF).

Point selection

The principle of point selection for pain treatment is to stimulate the body as close to the primary site of pain as possible or to a point within the same spinal innervation (segmental acupuncture). Needling occurs at localized tender points, trigger points, or traditional acupuncture points.

Distant points are used to stimulate the required spinal segment, because they are conveniently located and thought to generate strong analgesic effects (heterosegmental and general effects).

Clinical aspects

Technique
- Clinically clean hands (of practitioner).
- Clinically clean needle site (on patient).
- Needles: deposable stainless steel of varying length and diameter with or without attached guide tube.
- Needle is gently inserted to desired depth.
- Duration: 5s to 30min (depending on technique).
- Electroacupuncture (EA): electrical stimulus applied to needles to increase therapeutic effect (especially analgesic).

Strength of stimulus
(Can vary loosely as follows:)
- Depth of needle insertion: from superficial to muscle or fascial level (sensations of *de qi* obtained at this level), or 'pecking' the periosteum.
- Duration of needling: ≤1–30min in chronic cases. Trigger points can be deactivated with very brief needling. No longer than 45min—EA of this duration may result in the release of CCK-8, an endogenous opioid antagonist.
- Amount of needle manipulation: via lift and thrust, and rotation techniques.
- Number of needles: average 4–6 per treatment, initially 1–5, following sessions can be up to 20.
- Frequency of treatments: normally weekly for 6–12 sessions, can be longer and more frequent.

Patient variables
- 10% strong responders—very sensitive and require gentle treatment.
- 10% non-responders.

Needle sensation and treatment responses
Termed *de qi*, describes sensation occurring from needling muscle or some other deep tissue, usually desired effect of acupuncture and occurs with strong responders. Individual variables exist.
- Symptoms: transient sharpness through skin, ache, pressure, swelling, numbness, and pain (caused by type II and III fibre stimulation in muscle).
- Signs: wheal and flare response, localized muscle twitch, and recognition of pain complaint (when needling a trigger point in muscle).

Beneficial therapeutic response
- Relief of pain or reduction in muscle spasm and stiffness (immediately and permanent or gradual over repeated treatments).

Other response
Whole body relaxation, lightheadedness, syncope, catharsis (weeping or giggling), profuse sweating (general or regional), exacerbation of symptoms (usually 24h before improvement, unlikely to be longer than 2–3 days) and general malaise or exhaustion.

Safety aspects

As with any needling therapy there are serious risks associated with transmission of blood-borne infection and direct trauma of vital structures. It is often regarded by the public as being completely safe but clearly piercing the body with sharp metal instruments is not entirely so.

Adverse effects

Pain

- Persistent pain is rare, but commonly a temporary exacerbation of presenting condition may occur for 24–48h.

Syncope and sedation

- Syncope can be reduced by treating patients when they are lying down; however, very rarely profound sinus bradycardia will result in loss of consciousness even when supine.
- Sedation relatively common especially during initial treatments.

Infections

- Very uncommon but nearly always serious. Hepatitis B and C most commonly reported. Others include HIV (unproven claims), bacterial endocarditis (from use of indwelling needles in patients with valvular heart disease), septicaemia, and isolated reports of joint infections.
- Auricular chondritis or perichondritis result exclusively from use of indwelling needles left in the pinna.

It should be noted that the incidence of infections is significantly reduced by the use of sterile disposable needles and the avoidance of indwelling needles or reusable needles requiring sterilization.

Trauma

- Pneumothorax is the most frequently reported serious injury caused by acupuncture with nearly 200 incidents being reported in scientific publications.
- Cardiac tamponade as a result of deep needling through a congenital sternal foramina (10% ♂; 4% ♀) or through precordial rib interspaces.
- Trauma to abdominal viscera, peripheral nervous system, CNS, and blood vessels has also been described.

Contraindications

- Patient refusal.
- Indwelling needles in patients with a prosthetic heart valve or valvular heart disease.
- EA in patients with implanted defibrillators.

Cautions

- Anticoagulant medication
- EA in patients with demand pacemakers
- Hyperaesthetic or anaesthetic areas
- Oedematous tissue
- Tumours or swellings
- Immunosuppression
- Lack of orthodox diagnosis

- Pregnancy (a patient's beliefs are the key concern here rather than any physiological risk).

It should be concluded that acupuncture is a very safe form of therapy in competent hands.

Research

Clinical effectiveness remains controversial. Recently there are an increased number of high quality clinical trials facilitated by development of sham acupuncture needles.

Evidence for effectiveness in:
- LBP, neck pain, and chronic headache
- Osteoarthritis–particularly OA of the knee
- PONV
- Dental and facial pain.

Further reading

British Medical Acupuncture Society (BMAS) website: ⋒ http://www.medical-acupuncture.co.uk
Ernst E and White A (eds) (1999). *Acupuncture-A Scientific Appraisal.* Butterworth Heinemann, Oxford.
Filshie J and White A (eds) (1999). *Medical Acupuncture-A Western Scientific Approach.* Churchill Livingstone, Edinburgh.
Kaptchuk TJ (1983). *Understanding Chinese Medicine: The Web that has no Weaver.* Congdon & Weed, New York.
Maciocia G (1989). *The Foundations of Chinese Medicine: a comprehensive text for acupuncturists and herbalists.* Churchill Livingstone, Edinburgh.
White A, Cummings M, Filshie J (2008). *An Introduction to Western Medical Acupuncture.* Churchill Livingstone, London.

Osteopathy and chiropractic

Osteopathy and chiropractic developed in the late 1800s as alternatives to a conventional medical approach, in which it was believed that if the structural and mechanical integrity of the body could be restored, then function would improve, and health would be restored in a wide variety of conditions. This improvement in integrity was achieved primarily using manual techniques. Since then osteopathy and chiropractic have become primarily recognized in the management of musculoskeletal pain syndromes, and are particularly known for their manipulative approaches. Whilst they developed independently, they have been included together here because of the considerable overlap in approaches used.

What pain syndromes are treated?

A large part of the caseload of most practitioners comprises patients with mechanical spinal and neck pain, headaches, and regional musculoskeletal pain syndromes (e.g. shoulder pain, knee pain, pelvic pain, thoracic spinal/chest/rib pain), often related to work, road traffic collisions, and sports injuries. Both acute and chronic pain syndromes are seen. These services are usually provided on a fee basis within the UK.

Assessment

History and examination

- All practitioners carry out a conventional medical history and examination, with the aim of identifying non-musculoskeletal causes of pain, which will be referred on when necessary. Many chiropractors take X-rays in their own clinics, whereas osteopaths will refer on for imaging (usually to the GP), as well as for any other tests deemed appropriate.
- A detailed pain history is taken, including a psychosocial assessment. Practitioners identify psychosocial yellow flags, such as catastrophizing and fear avoidance, and any other obstacles to recovery.
- Physical examination usually involves a postural and biomechanical assessment, as well as orthopaedic and neurological examination.

Management

Approaches to treatment and management depend on the diagnosis made, on the needs of the patient, and on the training of the practitioner. Relief/reduction of pain and/or restoration of function are the primary aims, using a biopsychosocial model of care. An emphasis is placed on giving patients a positive explanation and encouraging return to work or normal activities as soon as possible.

- Self-management: patients may be given advice on maintaining mobility, work station assessment, posture, and lifting techniques.
- Manual techniques:
  - Mobilization: techniques used include various soft tissue release methods (including massage techniques, stretches, muscle energy technique, trigger point release), joint articulation and mobilization, and harmonic technique.

- Manipulative thrust techniques: this is often the technique for which chiropractors and osteopaths are best known. It involves a high-velocity thrust to a joint taking it beyond its restricted range of motion, but within its normal physiological range of motion. It is frequently accompanied by an audible 'click'. Theories vary as to how it works; however one effect seems to be an increase in joint accessory range of motion, which is essential to normal function.
- Rehabilitation: traditionally regarded more the preserve of physiotherapists, all undergraduate courses now include some training in rehabilitation, including basic exercise prescription. A graded return to activity is encouraged. Many practitioners go on postgraduate courses such as advanced rehabilitation, exercise prescription, or CBT.
- Acupuncture: whilst not taught at an undergraduate level, many practitioners undergo postgraduate training in acupuncture. For most, this is based on a series of weekend courses, learning the fundamentals of 'trigger point' dry needling (though it is acknowledged the evidence in this field is still controversial). Some undergo longer training in traditional Chinese acupuncture.
- Electrotherapy: rarely taught in the undergraduate curriculum, though some practitioners undergo postgraduate training.
- Pharmacology: currently osteopaths and chiropractors are not licensed to prescribe or inject in the majority of countries, with the exception of some states in the USA where osteopaths have full medical practice rights.
- More 'alternative' approaches: both professions have their advocates for more alternative approaches, including release of 'visceral and fascial restrictions', or 'cranial' approaches, which are believed to work on a so-called 'craniorhythmic impulse'. Evidence is currently lacking for any of these approaches.

Evidence

It can be difficult to provide evidence 'for chiropractic' or 'for osteopathy' since most practitioners deliver a package of care using a variety of the aforementioned approaches. Reassuring patients and advice on management are integral parts of a consultation. It is therefore possible to look at whether there is evidence for particular approaches used in particular conditions (e.g. manipulation and acute back pain), or whether there is evidence for an overall package of care (e.g. chiropractic care and neck pain).

With respect to manipulation, for example, most research has been carried out on manipulation and low back pain, with >40 RCTs and numerous systematic reviews. Most trials have not differentiated between manipulative thrust techniques and mobilization, and many trials are of a more pragmatic nature involving a package of care, making it difficult to determine the exact contribution which each manipulation had made. Most national guidelines include recommendations on the use of manipulation/mobilization in the management of acute and chronic low back pain. Because of the overlap between the professions, no national guidelines distinguish between approaches used by physiotherapists, osteopaths, or chiropractors in the management of LBP. A recent Medical

Research Council[1]-funded trial on back pain looked at an overall package of care agreed by chiropractors, physiotherapists, and osteopaths.[1]

Less research has been carried out on osteopathic and chiropractic approaches to limb musculoskeletal pain, pelvic pain, or musculoskeletal chest pain, though many practitioners claim efficacy.

It is hoped that with the increase in research, practitioners will be prepared to adopt approaches for which there is evidence, and reject approaches where there is clear evidence of lack of efficacy or harm.

Differences

With the increase in research and evidence-based medicine, the traditional boundaries between the 3 professions have become more blurred. Traditionally physiotherapy has had a greater emphasis on exercise rehabilitation and electrotherapy, and chiropractic and osteopathy have had a greater emphasis on manipulative approaches. Most osteopaths and chiropractors graduate with extensive skills in musculoskeletal assessment and manipulative approaches. Physiotherapists work in a range of areas including CV, respiratory, and surgical rehabilitation, and musculoskeletal/pain medicine is seen as a postgraduate specialization (see 📖 Physiotherapy in chronic pain p.234). The difference in emphasis is gradually changing, and these days many practitioners will go on postgraduate courses provided by one of the other professions; a chiropractor might have an MSc in core stability, an osteopath in pain management, or a physiotherapist an MSc in manipulation. However, the historical differences are still reflected in current practice. Physiotherapists, for example, may work in pain clinics with a completely hands-off approach, whereas chiropractors and osteopaths will invariably use 'hands-on' approaches.

Training and status in the UK

Both professions have achieved statutory regulation, with the General Osteopathic Council and the General Chiropractic Council performing similar regulatory functions to the General Medical Council. All chiropractors and osteopaths must complete a minimum 4-year full-time degree in chiropractic or osteopathy to achieve registration, with compulsory continuing professional development in order to maintain registration. All courses include training in the basic medical sciences, together with advanced training in musculoskeletal examination and treatment approaches. Many will achieve postgraduate qualifications, including training in acupuncture, ergonomics, or pain management. All undergraduate courses will include training in evidence-based medicine.

The vast majority of practitioners work in private practice. A limited number provide services funded by the NHS, such as Primary Care Trust-funded joint physiotherapy and osteopathy back pain services. Most patients will contact their practitioner directly, though increasingly more are referred by their GP.

Further reading

1 UK BEAM Trial (2004). United Kingdom back pain exercise and manipulation (UK BEAM) randomised trial: effectiveness of physical treatments for back pain in primary care. *BMJ* **329**:1377–81.

2 General Chiropractic Council 🔗 http://www.gcc-uk.org

3 General Osteopathic Council 🔗 http://www.osteopathy.org.uk

Psychological therapy

Clinical psychology in pain management services

Clinical psychologists in pain management work across inpatient and outpatient settings. Generally they are closely integrated into multidisciplinary/interdisciplinary teams and their role is primarily to help patients to live life to the full despite their pain difficulties.

Pain is 'an unpleasant sensory and emotional experience, associated with actual or potential damage or described in terms of such damage' (IASP).[1] Therefore tackling it from a purely physical perspective is unlikely to be wholly successful for those who have been experiencing intractable pain for some time. Chronic pain reduces individuals' emotional and physical capabilities, challenges coping, often leads to behaviour change and relationship difficulties (marital, social, and work), and can lead to loneliness, isolation, and a sense of loss. People are often anxious, avoidant, fearful, and depressed.

Clinical psychologists work with patients to increase their ability to accept and work with their condition rather than battling against it. They aim to help patients regain a sense of control, reduce anxiety, improve memory and concentration, and improve self-esteem. They will encourage people to establish their priorities in life and to recognize and work with the historical and current factors which may inhibit effective pain management.

The pain clinical psychologist

Clinical psychology training is a doctoral training. Over the 3 years of the course, trainees will be working both academically and clinically in a variety of settings including child and adolescent, older adult, learning difficulties, mental health including severe and enduring mental health conditions, and a specialist placement which will be negotiated with their course directors. Placements usually require that students are away from home and occasionally specialist placements are overseas. During training, students will attend lectures, complete service evaluations and case studies from a variety of different therapeutic perspectives, and will be continually assessed on their performance during their clinical placements. In their final year, students continue to work at their clinical placements whilst completing and writing up their research projects for final examination and viva.

Following qualification, clinical psychologists will often go on to further study in specialist areas, such as chronic pain management. All clinical psychologists are required to undertake supervision throughout their careers, and will be subject to continuing professional development (CPD) scrutiny through their professional body (British Psychological Society and Health Professions Council) in addition to their annual appraisal. Their training develops skills in teaching, research and therapeutic modalities, and the development of their interpersonal skills lends itself well to team building, management, and negotiation.

Assessment

A clinical psychology assessment will be comprehensive. It will seek to:

- Identify behavioural changes at work and home, alterations to marital and social relationships, changes in sleep patterns and medication usage.
- Explore beliefs and attitudes in relation to pain, expectations of outcome, and current coping skills.
- Evaluate emotional state (anxiety and depression) and any impact of post-traumatic stress disorder (PTSD) on pain experience.

Treatments

Include:

- Individual psychotherapy: to increase understanding of emotional and behavioural responses to pain and how to modify them to improve pain experience.
- Pain Management Programmes: to learn self-management strategies (including those listed for 'Individual psychotherapy').
- Stress management and relaxation therapy: to reduce the activity of the nervous system which responds to stress and thereby increases pain experience.

Referral to a clinical psychologist in pain management may be 'the most positive and effective treatment solution available' for an individual with intractable pain.

The British Pain Society states that a pain management programme team must include as a core member 'a Chartered Clinical Psychologist or BABCP registered cognitive behavioural therapist with appropriate training/supervision'. They add that Pain Management Programmes require 'high levels of competence in providing an effective service to patients and in training and supervising staff not formally trained in psychological techniques.[11] The lead psychologist must have adequate training in cognitive and behavioural techniques in psychology and physical health problems and experience of group work.'[2]

Other roles

In addition, clinical psychologists in pain services will be involved in service management and development, team building, teaching and training (medical students, GPs, etc.,) audit, evaluation and research, supervision and management of clinical trainees, psychology assistants, and other staff.

Clinical psychology in acute pain

In acute pain settings, clinical psychologists often work alongside the pain doctor/anaesthetists and may undertake some direct patient work on the ward, often preparing a patient for discharge or engaging them in the prospect of subsequent pain management intervention where appropriate.

References

1 Merskey H and Bogduk N (eds) (1994). *Classification of Chronic Pain, Second Edition*. IASP Task Force on Taxonomy. IASP Press, Seattle.
2 British Pain Society (2007). *Recommended guidelines for pain management programmes for adults*. p.18.

The psychological management of chronic pain

There are differences between acute and chronic pain. Chronic pain has to be understood in terms of both physical and psychological factors. The traditional medical model is inadequate when explaining chronic pain and disability and should be replaced by a more holistic illness model. Formulation of a patient's pain problem should be approached from a multidimensional perspective. Consultation and management must take into account the impact of physical, psychological, and socioeconomic factors. In addition, the practitioner's own ideas/beliefs about chronic pain will inform and impact upon their approach to treatment.

The Melzack and Wall (1965) gate control theory of pain was one of the first to relate, in a neurobiological model, the complex interplay between tissue damage and perceptual aspects of pain experience and to tackle questions concerned with individual differences in response to pain. There is now a widespread appreciation of the biological basis for the interaction between the detection of a noxious event and the multiple interacting factors that influence the subsequent perception of pain. This movement from medical to biopsychosocial models places emphasis on the importance of psychological factors.

Psychological factors have a significant influence on pain and disability and are stronger determinants of outcome than the biomedical factors.

The key dimensions are:
- Attitudes and beliefs
- Distress (particularly in relation to previous treatment)
- Pain behaviour and coping strategies.

Early intervention which takes psychological factors into account can reduce iatrogenic problems and chronicity.

There are a number of common psychological presentations associated with the chronic pain experience:

Anxiety

Patients with chronic pain are often specifically focused on anxieties in relation to the significance or meaning of their pain and the impact it has in their lives. Underlying themes may include a belief that hurt is linked with harm and that there will be progressive consequences of pain (impending disability, loss of job, etc.). Consequently, patients will take evasive action to avoid pain for these reasons, often limiting their lives to the extent that these outcomes are paradoxically more likely. Anxiety is understandably common in patients experiencing chronic pain.

Generalized anxiety disorder

Is characterized by excessive anxiety and worry, and for a diagnosis this has to have occurred on the majority of days for the preceding 6 months. It is also associated with:
- Restlessness
- Fatigue
- Difficulty concentrating

- Sleep disturbance
- Marked muscle tension.

The anxiety itself may cause significant distress or impairment.

Measures
- Hospital Anxiety and Depression Scale (HADS)
- Pain Anxiety Symptom Scale (PASS).

Interventions
- Education to help the patient understand that chronic pain (thoroughly investigated), does not indicate underlying pathology.
- Relaxation techniques, including diaphragmatic breathing, guided imagery, and a variety of other approaches.
- Working to challenge unhelpful or negative thoughts often using cognitive behavioural techniques (see ☐ Cognitive behavioural therapy p.258).

These interventions are integral to Pain Management Programmes and local pain management services.

Depression

The relationship between pain and depression
People suffering with chronic pain are often low in mood and may be depressed. 'Depression' may refer to anything from low mood to severely incapacitating mental illness where people are unable to function and go about their daily tasks. The levels of depression present in many pain patients would not be diagnosable as a psychiatric illness. Patients with a history of depression have a higher risk of developing pain, although conversely pain is actually a stronger predictor of depression.

In chronic pain depression may result from:
- Reduced opportunity to engage in activities or contacts which are positively reinforcing.
- More frequently exposed to aversive events (pain, treatments, etc).
- Many failed interventions and chronic unresolved stressors.

In chronic pain, depression is generally best tackled as an understandable psychological response to the pain condition and the resultant accompanying life changes. A multidisciplinary cognitive behavioural approach to the pain problem is usually the best way forward although sometimes depression can be severe and may require medication/intervention in its own right.

There are clear diagnostic criteria (see DSM IV) which distinguish low mood from depressive illness.

Measures
- HADS
- Beck Depression Inventory (BDI).

Interventions
- Working to challenge unhelpful thoughts.
- Education about chronic pain.
- Realistic goal setting.

- Engagement in the socially supportive setting of a Pain Management Programme.
- Encouragement to participate in other activities (work, hobbies, etc.).
- Support to improve quality of life.
- Graded and paced activity and exercise.

Again these interventions are integral to Pain Management Programmes and local pain management services.

Anger

Anger is often observed in chronic pain patients. It may be expressed toward clinical staff or close family members in a variety of contexts, and should be explored when patients are referred for Pain Management Programmes or other psychologically focused interventions.

Sometimes it is directed towards the self, often associated with perceived 'failure' or 'inadequacy'. Sometimes it is externalized and focused on others, for example the patient's view can be that their doctor has 'given up' on them or has dismissed their pain as 'all in my head'.

Anger can also be directed toward family members and can be affected by the response of family members. Family-based therapy or family involvement in treatment programmes can be of benefit (e.g. significant-other involvement in Pain Management Programmes).

Acknowledgement and normalization of these feelings can be a simple yet powerful intervention.

Pain behaviour

Can be verbal or non-verbal and can often be outside of the patient's own awareness. These behaviours are often situation/context-specific and influenced by culture/beliefs and are best understood as a means of communication, particularly in family/close relationship settings. They may include:

- Uncharacteristic behaviour or activity (long periods of rest, withdrawal from contact with others).
- Verbal expression (moans, sighing, and general complaints about pain)
- Physical gesturing such as holding/rubbing/protecting the affected limb/area.
- Unwillingness to move the part of the body affected by pain. Immobilizing limbs etc.
- Facial contortions.
- Use of supports, equipment (e.g. wheelchairs, sticks) when these are not necessary.
- Heightened/inappropriate reaction to physical examination.

Interventions

Intervention generally focuses on changing the conditions that evoke or maintain pain behaviours which may include:

- Financial/economic reward
- Attention and reinforcement at home
- Escape/avoidance of work or other pressures.

Patient–doctor relationships and familial relationships impact on patient pain experience and the likelihood of engagement with and benefit from treatment. Effective intervention may involve input from family and friends, clinical staff, employers, and colleagues.

Early Pain Management Programmes used behavioural analysis and behaviour modification and an understanding of this approach can still be useful in monitoring patient response to proposed treatments/ interventions. Consideration of maintaining factors still forms part of the overall Pain Management Programme and pain service approach as pain behaviour is known to impact on clinical treatment efficacy.

Post-traumatic stress disorder

PTSD can be identified during consultation by asking whether the patient continues to 're-live' the traumatic event, avoids situations which are associated with the event, and is experiencing emotional numbness or heightened arousal. PTSD will generally warrant specific intervention and referral to local mental health services or other appropriate agencies (e.g. National Phobic's Society) is recommended.

Unresolved or recent bereavement

Recent bereavement is likely to be a source of distress which will impact on an individual's pain experience and emotional state.

Unresolved bereavement is likely to require specific intervention and referral to relevant agencies is recommended (e.g. CRUSE bereavement counselling service).

Abuse—physical, emotional, and sexual

Referral to specialist agencies (e.g. local mental health services or local services such as Sexual Abuse Centres) is recommended prior to reassessment by the pain service if appropriate.

Cognitive behavioural therapy

Cognitive behavioural therapy (CBT) is a psychological intervention originally developed for depression. The principles have been applied to a wide range of other psychological problems (including anxiety, panic, hypochondriasis, substance misuse, insomnia, etc.) and to the distress and disability associated with medical problems including chronic pain. Although supported by an evidence base, and the most widely available psychological intervention, it is not successful or suitable for everyone with chronic pain.

Applying cognitive behavioural model to managing chronic illness

The cognitive behavioural model proposes that people react to, and manage, their illnesses in ways which are consistent with their beliefs about their illness, themselves and their world.

Examples:

Belief: 'back pain is a sign of ongoing damage'.
Coping strategy: avoid activities which aggravate pain.
Thoughts: 'I've really hurt myself. This time it might not get better.'
Emotion: anxiety.

Belief: 'having any difficulty is a sign of weakness'.
Coping strategy: push self harder to cope, don't admit problems
Thoughts: 'Other people cope with their problems, I must keep going.'
Emotion: frustration, stress, depression.

CBT attempts to address these thoughts, feelings, and behaviours, and the underlying beliefs.

Assessing beliefs about pain conditions

Asking people in detail about their understanding of, and views about, their condition often helps make sense of their emotional reaction, coping strategies, and use of health care. The following provides a framework for assessing beliefs about illness.

- **Identity:** 'You've had these symptoms for some time and seen different doctors. Have any of them been able to explain what is wrong? What do *you* think is wrong? Do you ever think the doctors have missed something?'
- **Cause :**'Why do you think you have developed this pain problem? What do you put it down to?'
- **Control/cure:** 'Do you think there is any further treatment which would help? How much are you hoping for a cure?'
- **Timeline:** 'What do you think will happen to your pain in the future?'
- **Consequences:** 'What are the most important ways in which this problem is affecting your life?'

Common beliefs about pain which may be unhelpful

Each person has a set of idiosyncratic beliefs; however the following are common amongst people with chronic pain:
- My pain is a sign of ongoing damage.
- My back is crumbling/weak/fragile.
- It's going to get worse and worse until I am in a wheelchair.
- Nobody knows what's wrong with me. Something serious has been missed.
- In this day and age, it *must* be possible to cure my pain.
- There are treatments which would help if only I could find the right doctor/the NHS had more money/people would take me seriously.
- Nothing will help. Nothing I do makes any difference.
- People think I am mad/making it up/have a low pain threshold/lazy.

Components of cognitive behavioural therapy

CBT is individualized for each patient based on an assessment and for- mulation of their presenting problems. The following interventions are commonly used to address unhelpful patterns of thinking, develop better coping strategies, and tackle underlying beliefs:
- Education (about pain and the accompanying emotional problems).
- Keeping records of thoughts, identifying unhelpful patterns of thinking, and learning to challenge unhelpful thoughts.
- Setting goals and breaking them down into small manageable steps.
- Building confidence through testing out thoughts such as 'I'm bound to fail'.
- Setting up 'behavioural experiments' in order to test beliefs such as 'Without my tablets my pain will be unbearable' or 'If I don't vacuum every day my friends will think my house is dirty.'
- Coping skills training (including relaxation, assertiveness, sleep strategies, etc.).

Who provides cognitive behavioural therapy?

CBT is an intervention provided by staff with specialist training. This intervention is offered at various levels of skill by nurses, psychologists, or counsellors. Some pain service teams include staff with CBT skills who are familiar with the range of difficulties which accompany chronic pain. Others are based in NHS mental health services which may have restrictive referral criteria. There is a nationally recognized shortage of CBT provision.

Psychodynamic approaches to chronic pain

Psychodynamic therapeutic approaches to chronic pain are generally more long-term interventions and not the mainstream treatment of choice for all individuals experiencing chronic pain.

In psychodynamic language, pain can be explained as a defence against psychic conflict. Early trauma and/or abuse embed a set of 'expectations, autonomic nervous system responses and behaviours'.[1] These can be activated by a sufficiently painful emotional or physical stimulus.

There have been no prospective controlled studies of psychodynamic psychotherapy with chronic pain patients. However, some patients may not respond to the more usual short-term psychological interventions (e.g. CBT), particularly if their pain is linked to trauma or loss related to early experiences.[2]

The main focus of the approach is:

- Early relationships (especially family)
- Current relationships (particularly family and friends)
- The therapeutic relationship in the context of a patient's pain.

Relationship patterns formed in the early years may change when they are re-enacted in the context of the therapeutic encounter. The therapist aims to respond with empathy, understanding, and support—generating an experience of 'positive transference'.

Individuals learn to see how their previously adaptive expectations, responses, and behaviours—or survival strategies, now affect their current pain experiences and are no longer relevant or helpful to them as an adult dealing with chronic pain.

Unhelpful experiences of the health-care system can generate 'negative transference'. The patient may bring similar expectations to the therapy, acting as if the therapist is the 'foe'. Treatment would focus on revealing these expectations to the patient and exploring the underlying fears which motivated their responses.

Although psychodynamic interventions are not generally the focus of pain management, elements of the approach are often integrated into more short-term main stream psychological interventions, e.g. CBT, enabling patients to better understand pain experience as the culmination of many factors involving both mind and body.

References

1 Schofferman, Anderson, Hines and White (1992). *Spine* **17**: S138–144.
2 Turk DC *et al.* (1983). *Pain and Behavioral Medicine: A Cognitive-Behavioral Perspective.* New York: Guilford Press.

Acceptance

Developing a significant chronic pain condition usually goes together with a range of other problems which might include:

- Loss of employment and financial stability
- Strained or broken relationships
- Changes to valued roles
- Loss of other valued activities such as hobbies and loss of self-esteem
- Insomnia, low mood, etc.

People may also have to give up on or adjust some of their hopes or expectations for the future. All of this contributes to major life change and triggers the need for a process of adjustment, acceptance or accommodation.

The word 'acceptance' means different things to different people. One definition that is useful in this context:

Acceptance of pain is 'acknowledging that one has pain, giving up unproductive attempts to control the pain, acting as if pain does not necessarily imply disability, and being able to commit one's efforts toward living a satisfying life despite pain'.

People often mistakenly equate 'acceptance' with 'giving up'. The essence of acceptance is more positive. In coming to accept their pain people may abandon a fruitless, frustrating, and expensive search for a cure and refocus their energies on what they can achieve despite pain.

Why is acceptance important?

People with long-term pain who are accepting of it show better scores on a wide range of indicators of function. These include improvements in psychological state, and physical functioning. Although greater acceptance is associated with lower pain levels, pain levels do not explain acceptance.

Indicators of difficulty with acceptance

Patients may say:

- Why me? If only…
- I can't get my head around it.
- In this day and age we can put a man on the moon…surely this pain can be cured? If you can't treat me who should I go to see now?
- I used to be able to….
- My tablets aren't strong enough. I need something stronger.
- If only I could … find the right doctor/persuade someone to take me seriously/get an MRI scan if only the NHS had more money … I would be cured.
- I can't go on like this; my pain has taken everything in my life away.

Health professionals can sometimes struggle to accept:

- That patients may have pain despite clear scans, or when the reported pain appears out of proportion to physical findings.
- That despite their every effort the patient shows no improvement.

What helps or hinders the development of acceptance?

Clinical experience suggests the following factors may influence the acceptance of chronic pain.

Factors hindering acceptance

The person has:
- No idea what is wrong, or is confused by different diagnoses or inconsistent explanations, or the suggestion that their pain is 'all in my mind'.
- An unrealistic expectation of cure, or beliefs that a cure *could* be found, e.g. by searching out the right therapist/treatment.
- No hope that they can do anything about the problem themselves.
- Lost all sight of themselves other than through the lens of their pain.
- Battling to persuade others the pain is real, or having to pretend they do not have pain in order to avoid disapproval or disbelief.

Factors helping acceptance

The person has:
- An understanding of the reasons that their pain persists.
- An appreciation of the limitations of existing treatments, and why further treatments will not cure the pain.
- Confidence that they can make changes which will improve things.
- A sense of identity which is not entirely tied up with the pain.
- Support from health professionals, family, friends, employers, etc. in acknowledging the pain is real, but which also helps the person to make changes to the way they manage it.

Treatments that facilitate acceptance

It is important to explain carefully about the reasons that pain persists despite appropriate medical treatment (see 📖 Interventions p.255), and why further treatments might be unsuccessful or not recommended. Where there is little or no hope of success, persisting with further referrals, investigations, and treatments reinforces patients' unrealistic expectations of cure. This can make it more difficult for people to accept the likely long-term nature of their pain.

Psychological interventions such as CBT and Pain Management Programmes can facilitate acceptance. New treatments such as Acceptance and Commitment Therapy are being developed which address acceptance more directly. This therapy is not yet widely available.

Stress management in chronic pain

Diagnosing and managing symptoms of anxiety and stress is important in effective chronic pain management. There are physiological and psychological implications associated with distress and it is rare to encounter someone who has been in pain for any length of time that has not experienced considerable frustration, anger, fear, feelings of despair, and loss of role and identity as a result of their ongoing pain. These sequelae often contribute to a chronic stress response which may lead to increased pain, compromised immune system, and fear-avoidant behaviour.

Anxiety can range from a slight feeling of uneasiness through to full-blown terror. It is important for an individual to learn to recognize their earliest signs of nervous tension because it is more likely any techniques utilized at this stage will be more effective.

Signs of anxiety

Physiological
- Increased heart rate
- Increased muscle tension
- Sweating
- Shaking
- Choking feeling/dry mouth
- Dizziness
- Increased pain.

Cognitive
- Worrying, negative, or racing thoughts
- Negative predictions for the future
- Problems with decision-making
- Clouded thinking.

Behavioural
- Avoidance of activities
- Keeping 'safe', checking more frequently.

A cognitive behavioural perspective (see 📖 Cognitive behavioural therapy p.258) proposes that an individual's thoughts and feelings about their pain and associated experiences will impact on their physiological state. If those thoughts are distressing, e.g. 'I am useless, I can't do anything, it will never get better' then the feelings generated are likely to be stressful and lead to release of stress hormones, increased body tension, and heightened pain experience. Conversely, if thoughts are more constructive/realistic, e.g. 'I have got through bad days before and I know how to help myself by…' or 'Even though I may not be able to do everything, today I can do…', then the feelings generated are more likely to be accepting and calm. As a result of this body tension is reduced and pain is not augmented.

Anxiety provoking thoughts often include:
- All or nothing thinking.
- Over generalization, using words like 'always' or 'never'.
- Jumping to conclusions (usually negative).
- Catastrophizing: amplifying the negative aspects of one's mistakes.

- 'Should' thinking e.g. 'I *should* be able to clean the whole house, so I am useless because I cannot'.

An important aspect of CBT intervention in chronic pain management is relaxation training to augment the cognitive work on stress. Relaxation aims to reduce muscle tension and interrupt the negative thought cycle.

Approaches to relaxation may include:
- Breathing techniques (e.g. diaphragmatic breathing).
- Exercise such as t'ai chi or yoga.
- Attentional techniques to reduce tension in parts of the body (progressive muscle relaxation).
- Guided imagery relaxation exercises (relaxation CDs).
- Listening to sounds from nature.
- Being somewhere comfortable or soothing (e.g. a garden).
- Meditation on a candle or image.

Instructions for diaphragmatic breathing
- Sit or lie comfortably, with loose garments.
- Put one hand on your chest and one on your stomach.
- Slowly inhale through your nose.
- As you inhale, feel your stomach expand with your hand. If your chest expands, focus on breathing in the area of your diaphragm.
- Slowly exhale through your mouth.
- Rest and repeat.

Participants should not aim to breathe more deeply than normal; the emphasis is on locating the breath in the region of the diaphragm.

Guided imagery/progressive muscle relaxation/natural sounds/meditation

Patient instructions
On a daily basis take 20–30min for a relaxation session. There are many CDs available on the market and also online so searching for something that works for you is time well spent. Meditation on an object of your choice (e.g. candle) is fairly simple to organize.

Make sure that you are warm and comfortable and that you will not be disturbed. Remember that taking time for you is an important part of your daily treatment plan. If you find that you struggle to allow yourself to do this then focusing on the thoughts that get in the way and replacing them with more constructive thoughts is a good starting point.

▶ Caution: relaxation is generally beneficial for most people. However if a patient has untreated PTSD, a history of severe mental illness (e.g. psychosis), or an acute medical condition it may be wise to seek further advice before suggesting any new relaxation technique.

Hypnosis in chronic pain management

During the last 3 decades the biopsychosocial conceptualization of chronic pain has become more sophisticated, and a variety of psychologically-based treatment approaches have been developed and empirically validated for helping people to better manage their pain. These approaches to pain management have much to offer individuals with chronic pain in terms of reducing pain intensity, psychological distress and disability, and enhancing overall quality of life. Hypnosis has been used for longer than any other psychological method of analgesia and providing hypnosis and self-hypnosis training alone, or in conjunction with CBT and other psychological therapy, is becoming a commoner practice.

Definition of hypnosis

Hypnosis is a social interaction during which one person (designated as the patient) is guided by another (designated as the health-care professional) to respond to suggestions for changes in subjective experience, alterations in perception, sensation, emotion, thought, or behaviour. Individuals can also learn self-hypnosis, which is the act of administering hypnotic procedures to oneself. Hypnosis typically involves an introduction to the procedure during which the patient is told that suggestions for imaginative experiences will be presented. The hypnotic induction is an extended initial suggestion for using one's imagination, and may contain further elaborations of the introduction. A hypnotic procedure is used to encourage and evaluate responses to suggestions. Procedures traditionally involve suggestions to relax, though relaxation is not necessary for hypnosis and a wide variety of suggestions can be used including those to become more alert.[1]

The hypnotic session

The multifaceted and complex nature of chronic pain requires elaborate and comprehensive hypnotic interventions. Details of these interventions will differ depending on the exact nature of the problem, the purposes of the clinical endeavour, the goals of the health-care professional, and the abilities and preferences of the patient. In the *Handbook of Hypnotic Suggestions and Metaphors*,[2] the following hypnotic strategies and techniques for managing pain are described in detail: unconscious exploration to enhance insight or resolve conflict, creating anaesthesia or analgesia, cognitive-perceptual alteration of pain (and pain behaviour), and decreasing awareness of pain (distraction technique). Other useful hypnotic approaches to pain management include self-suggestions for relaxation, ego strengthening, decreased tension and emotional suffering, and Rossi's[3] mind-body healing approach. In this last approach, hypnotic suggestions can be given during the session for the patient to regress and access past learning, memory, and experience and use them as therapeutic resources for pain management. Table 10.1 shows an example of a hypnotic session for chronic pain management.

Table 10.1 Example of a hypnotic treatment session for chronic pain management

Induction and deepening suggestions	*As you sit there, very comfortable and very relaxed ... you become aware of a staircase ... a beautiful staircase with a polished, ornate banister running down alongside and a deep, rich carpet underneath your bare feet ... As you look down the stairs you notice that there are ten steps leading gently down ... these are the steps that will lead you deep into dreamtime—deep into relaxation ... and in a moment I'd like you to walk down those steps with me and I will count them off for you one at a time, and you will find that the deeper down you go, the more comfortable and the more relaxed you will become ... and as you reach the bottom step you can let the stairs and the ordinary, everyday world, further and further down—as you go deeper and deeper ... You are now standing at the bottom of the steps and feeling very comfortable, very relaxed and at peace with the world ...*
Analgesic suggestions	*You dive into a magical pool ... the water temperature is pleasant ... your body relaxes ... any discomfort that you maybe experiencing is leaving your body ... dissolving into the water ...*
	Imagine going back in time ... to a time long ago, before any pain or discomfort, when you were full of energy and had a sense of complete well-being ... when you come back to the here and now you will feel again the same sense of well-being ... Now see the pain ... what shape is it? ... see its colour? ... feel its texture? ... now change the shape, colour and texture ...
Ego-strengthening	*... you are going to feel physically stronger and fitter in every way ... you will feel more alert ... more wide awake ... every day ... you will become so deeply interested in whatever you are doing ... in whatever is going on around you ... that your mind will become completely distracted away from yourself and your difficulties ... you will be able to think more clearly ... you will become emotionally calmer ... every day ... you will feel more and more independent ... every day ... you will feel a greater feeling of well-being ...*
Posthypnotic suggestion	*From now, each and every time you feel these sensations (pain) in your back, you will immediately take in a deep breath, and as you breathe out your whole body will relax ...*
Termination	*Now I would like you to count backwards from 5 to 1 ... 1 you are feeling refreshed and alert and ready to continue with whatever you were doing before...*

How effective is hypnosis in chronic pain management

There is a body of research suggesting that hypnosis is an efficacious treatment for acute procedural pain[4] and chronic pain conditions.[5] Studies of acute pain often demonstrate that hypnosis is superior to other psychological interventions for pain management. However, this is in contrast to the findings in the chronic pain literature. In chronic pain management, hypnosis generally has a significantly greater impact on pain reduction as compared to no treatment, analgesic medication, physical therapy, and education/advice. However, the effects of self-hypnosis training on chronic pain tend to be similar, on average, to progressive muscle relaxation and autogenic training, both of which often include hypnotic-like suggestions. None of the published studies so far have compared hypnosis to an equally credible placebo. Consequently, conclusions cannot yet be made about whether hypnotic pain management has a specific effect over and above the effect of patient expectancy. Component analyses indicate that labelling versus not labelling hypnotic interventions as hypnosis has relatively little short-term impact on therapeutic outcome, although the hypnosis label may have a long-term benefit. Predictor analyses suggest that 'hypnotizability' and ability to experience vivid images are associated with good treatment outcome in hypnosis treatment.

References

1 Green JP et al. (2005). Forging ahead: the 2003 APA division 30 definition of hypnosis. *Int J Clin Exp Hypn* **53**:259–64.
2 Hammond DC (ed) (1990). *Handbook of Hypnotic Suggestions and Metaphors*. WW Norton, New York.
3 Rossi E (1993). *The Psychobiology of Mind-Body Healing: New Concepts of Therapeutic Hypnosis*. WW Norton, New York.
4 Liossi C (2002). *Procedure-Related Cancer Pain in Children*. Radcliffe Medical Press, Oxford.
5 Patterson DR and Jensen M. (2003). Hypnosis and clinical pain. *Psychol Bull* **129**:495–521.

Pain Management Programmes

Aims of Pain Management Programmes

Pain Management Programmes are a treatment approach for people with chronic pain who suffer distress and disability associated with their pain. The primary aim of Pain Management Programmes is not to relieve pain, but to enable people to cope or manage pain better with the aim of reducing distress and disability, and improving quality of life. They usually adopt a cognitive behavioural approach (see 📖 Cognitive behavioural therapy p.258), although increasingly programmes are incorporating acceptance/mindfulness-based models (see 📖 Acceptance p.264).

Staffing

Programmes are run by a multidisciplinary team which usually includes a physiotherapist and a psychologist, and may include an OT, nurse, and a doctor.

Format

Pain Management Programmes are usually offered on an outpatient basis with a course of sessions totalling about 25–40 contact hours spread over 6–10 weeks. A few specialist centres offer Pain Management Programmes on an inpatient basis. These are suitable for people with the greatest level of distress or disability, or with particularly complex presentations.

Pain Management Programmes are delivered in a group format, with 8–14 patients attending each group. Advantages of the group format include the opportunity to find that their experience of coping with pain is shared with others, and learning coping strategies from others.

Availability of Pain Management Programmes

The service is not available in every area. A list of UK services is maintained by the British Pain Society (🕭 http://www.britishpainsociety.org).

Issues commonly addressed

Programmes vary, although there is a common core of issues addressed:
• Understanding the nature and causes of chronic pain, and pros and cons of further medical interventions.
• Appropriate use of medication.
• Addressing common unhelpful beliefs/misconceptions about pain (e.g. 'I am going to get worse and worse until I end up in a wheelchair').
• Graded exercise programme and pacing activities.
• Relaxation.
• Improving sleep.
• Communication and relationships, including sex.
• Posture.
• Managing everyday activities including work.
• Managing depression, anxiety, frustration, anger, guilt, etc.
• Setting realistic goals, and working towards them successfully.

Referral

• Referral routes and inclusion criteria do vary from service to service so check the nature of the local service before referring.

- Many services are limited to adults with chronic benign pain, although a few specialist services are available for children and adolescents.

Preparation for referral

- Preparation for referral is important as patients are often sceptical about the potential benefits of the Pain Management approach (see FAQs).
- In order to be ready to make changes it helps if people have reached some acceptance that the pain is longstanding and unlikely to be cured by further treatment (although medical interventions with the aim of ameliorating the pain may continue). Where appropriate it is helpful if this message is delivered consistently and clearly by health professionals, and not undermined by further referrals, investigations, or treatments with the aim of curing the pain.
- Some pain management services offer 'information' or 'introduction' sessions to give people more information (see FAQs).

Frequently asked questions

Will a Pain Management Programme make my pain better?

No, Pain Management Programmes won't cure your pain *but* it might help you have a better life. Some people say their pain is a bit better, or they have fewer bad days, but usually their pain stays about the same.

But I've had my pain now for 20 years; I know how to cope with pain

Perhaps you are right. 20 years is a long time. However, you have nothing to lose by seeing the pain management team. Go and find out more before you decide whether pain management is for you.

Are you saying my pain is all in my head … I'm making it up?

No, your pain is real. By referring you to the Pain Management Programme I am hoping you will find some new ways of coping with this problem, and fine-tune your existing ways of dealing with it.

If you are sending me to see a psychologist, do you think I'm mad? Will they read my mind?

No you're not mad. Most people find that pain affects them physically, but also gets them down. It's frustrating, stops them sleeping, makes them more irritable, and lots of other problems. Equally, being stressed or low affects the amount of pain you experience, and how well you can tolerate it. For all these reasons psychologists can help—alongside other staff like nurses and physiotherapists … and no, they cannot read your mind.

Sitting around talking about my pain won't make a blind bit of difference

No. I agree. Talking makes no difference on its own. However, getting fitter and changing how you manage your pain might.

Specific clinical situations

Chronic low back pain

- LBP can be defined as pain arising from in the posterior area between the lower costal margin and the inferior gluteal folds.
- Chronic back pain is a single attack of back pain that persists for >3 months.

Anatomy, aetiology, and pathophysiology

Vertebrae

- Bone pain: periosteal irritation can be caused by an inflammatory source or space-occupying lesion. Fractures may induce pain from ligaments by excessive strain or stress. Osteoporotic pain arises from compression fractures of the spine.
- Facet joint pain: these synovial joints are innervated by medial branches of lumbar dorsal rami (see facet joint injections p208). The incidence of lumbar or lumbosacral facet joint pain in patients presenting with back pain can be 10–40%. The cause is unclear.
- Sacroiliac joint pain: the sacroiliac joint is a synovial joint with surrounding fibrous tissue and ligaments. Incidence of sacroiliac joint pain among chronic back pain suffers is 12–20%.

Intervertebral disc

- The disc contains an outer annulus fibrosus and an inner nucleus pulposus.
- Discogenic pain arises from intervertebral discs.
  - Found in an estimated 40% of mechanical back pain.
  - Annulus fibrosus disc nerve supply from sinuvertebral nerve and gray rami communicantes.
  - Nucleus pulposus has no sensory innervation.
  - Pain can be triggered by leakage of internal disc contents of nucleus pulposus via disruptions of the annulus.

Nerve roots

These exit via the vertebral foramen. The spinal nerve is formed at the lateral aspect of the foramen by the fusion of the anterior motor root with the dorsal sensory root.

- Nerve root pain: commonest cause is prolapsed disc causing pressure on one or more nerve roots. This leads to pain as nerve is compressed and stretched. Pain in the distribution of a nerve root is called radicular pain.
- Arachnoiditis: chronic inflammation between pia and arachnoid membrane. This is most commonly seen after surgery.

Ligaments

The anterior and posterior ligamenta flava, interspinous, and capsular ligaments maintain integrity of the spine. Ligamentous strain may be a cause of mechanical back pain.

Muscles

- Extensor muscle: erector spinae.
- Lateral and anterior flexors: iliopsoas and quadratus lumborum.

- Other muscle groups involved in the normal function of the spine are the anterior abdominal muscles and those of the lower limbs (mainly gluteal, quadriceps, and hamstrings).

Epidemiology of chronic low back pain
- The lifetime prevalence of LBP is 70–85%.
- 90% of episodes will settle spontaneously within 3 months.
- Those with a previous history of back pain are twice as likely to present with a new episode.
- These patients create an enormous demand on health-care resources.

Clinical presentation
Identification of causative pathology can be made in only 15% of patients.

History and examination
Triage
- Serious spinal pathology (red flags) (1%)
- Nerve root (radicular) pain (4–5%)
- 'Simple' musculoskeletal back pain (95%).

Investigations
These are dictated by history and examination. Plain radiographs of the lumbosacral spine are used to look for tumours and fractures. Blood tests (e.g. ESR, WBC, etc.) are used to screen for inflammatory disorders, infection, and malignancy.

Simple musculoskeletal pain
This is typically mechanical and 'nociceptive' in nature. Peak incidence in the 20–55-year age group. The pain normally occurs in the lumbosacral area and the buttocks but it may radiate to the thigh and is typically described as a dull ache varying with physical activity. This patient group are normally physically well. 40% of mechanical back pain is discogenic, 20% is from sacroiliac joints, and 10–15% from lower lumbar facet joints.

Investigations
Plain radiographs, CT, or MRI have no role in investigation as they do not alter the treatment plan. Diagnostic nerve blocks can be used (e.g. lumbar medial branch nerve blocks). Some believe that such diagnostic blocks can be predictive of the benefit from subsequent longer-term RF lesioning.

Nerve root pain
This is well-localized to the lower limbs in a dermatomal pattern. The pain normally radiates from the knee to the foot. It is a sharp, electric shock-like pain. Coughing and straining may exacerbate the pain and it can also be associated with paraesthesia.

Examination: may reveal sensory, motor, and reflex abnormalities.

Causes
- Posterior disc herniation causing direct compression by herniation into central canal or intervertebral foramen. Peak incidence is between 30 and 55 years. The pain arises from compression of nerve roots and also from inflammatory changes secondary to herniated disc material.

- Spinal stenosis—typically after age of 55 years due to bone and ligament hypertrophy. Causing compression and chronic inflammatory changes of the nerve roots along with adhesions.

Features
Neurogenic claudication is seen after 10–20min walking and settles on brief rest. Pain is exacerbated by spinal extension and flexion normally relieves it.

Investigations
Plain radiographs are of no benefit. MRI is the investigation of choice for soft tissue assessment. MRI is more useful than CT for nerve root pain. It should be noted, however, that these investigations reveal many false positives so results should always be reviewed in the context of clinical presentation. Nerve conduction studies can be useful to distinguish between a peripheral neuropathic and radicular pain.

Serious spinal pathology (red flags)
Serious spinal pathology (e.g. infection, cancer, instability) occurs in <1% of patients with LBP. However, there should be a high index of suspicion and its presence is suggested by 'red flags' listed in the box. These patients should be referred with some urgency as the condition may be progressive and irreversible (see 📖 p.147).

> ⚠ **Red flags: risk factors for serious spinal pathology**
> - Patient aged <20 or >55 years
> - History of significant trauma
> - Structural deformity
> - Drug abuse
> - Widespread neurological signs
> - Fever
> - Constant progressive pain
> - History of cancer or HIV infection
> - Use of steroids
> - Marked restriction of lumbar flexion (<5cm)
> - Unexplained weight loss and systemically unwell.

Epidural adhesions/arachnoiditis
These may occur following spinal surgery, chronic inflammation from leakage of nucleus pulposus, or the introdution of intrathecal drugs. The pain is continuous and independent of activity. The distribution can be mono- or multisegmental, and unilateral or bilateral.

Management
The general aims of treatment are to improve pain and optimize physical, psychological, and social functions.

Drugs
- Evidence supports the use of NSAIDs and opioids in back pain.
- Initial management is regular paracetamol and NSAID ± weak opioid.
- Strong opioids may be prescribed but should follow the recommendations produced by the British Pain Society.
- TCAs and anticonvulsants for neuropathic pain.

- There is little evidence for the use of methocarbamol, baclofen, or benzodiazepines for muscle spasm.

Psychology

Psychological approaches, e.g. CBT, have some evidence to support their use. These reduce pain and disability-related behaviour and improve function. The use of Pain Management Programmes and back schools address education about pain and the distinction between acute and chronic pain and can support people in improving their quality of life and coping skills.

Physical therapies

Exercise improves pain and functional status. Specifically-graded exercise programmes are supported by strong evidence (see ☐ Physiotherapy in chronic pain p.234).

Interventional treatments

- There is currently no evidence to support the use of caudal or lumbar epidural injections or facet joint injections in the treatment of simple musculoskeletal back pain.[1]
- Facet joint injections can produce some short-term relief. There is some evidence to suggest that RF lesioning of the lumbar medial branch nerves reduces pain and improves physical function.
- Transforaminal nerve root injections have been to shown to be effective in reducing the need for disc surgery.

Transcutaneous electrical nerve stimulation

TENS has been shown to be more effective than placebo in reducing pain in the short term.

Spinal cord stimulation

This has been found to be useful in selected patients (particularly those who have failed with previous surgery with radicular symptoms—see ☐ Spinal cord stimulation p.218) but there is a lack of evidence regarding efficacy.

Acupuncture: evidence has shown that it produces short-term pain relief.

Surgery

- Nerve root pain can be relieved by surgical discectomy
- Evidence for lumbar decompression/fusion surgery for degenerative conditions of the spine is of poor quality. These procedures are generally not recommended.

Reference

Yellow flags: risk factors for chronicity
- A negative attitude that back pain is harmful or potentially severely disabling.
- Fear avoidance behaviour and reduced activity levels.
- An expectation that passive, rather than active, treatment will be beneficial.
- A tendency to depression, low morale, and social withdrawal.
- Social or financial problems.

---

1 Cochrane Review.⌁ http://www.cochrane.org/reviews/en/a6001824.html

Failed back surgery syndrome

Definition

Failed back surgery syndrome (FBSS) can be defined as persistent back and/or leg pain after 1 or more lumbosacral spine operations.

Epidemiology

- Approximately 2,000 new cases in the UK each year.
- FBSS is reported in 10–40% of patients following low back surgery.

Aetiology

The major cause is that the lesion that was operated on is not in fact the cause of the patient's pain. Other reasons for failure in order of decreasing frequency:

Foraminal and spinal stenosis

Residual foraminal stenosis due to inadequate exploration of the nerve root during surgery or due to mechanical destabilization of the disc during enucleation with resultant foraminal disc bulge. Diagnosis is usually via MRI or CT scanning. Therapy is usually reoperation.

Painful disc disease

This condition is due to residual pain emanating from the discs above or below the fusion which still retain motion. Discography can help determine the presence of painful degenerative disc disease at segments on which surgery is contemplated, thereby helping avoid this complication.

Pseudoarthrosis

Inadequate fusion which leaves the disc with excessive motion or bone-on-bone contact across the 'fracture line' of the pseudoarthrosis. Treatment is by re-operation when absolutely necessary.

Neuropathic

This category includes peridural fibrosis which is diagnosed on MRI. In multiple revisions the incidence of fibrosis increases to >60%.

Recurrent herniated nucleus pulposis

This is much more uncommon than in the past due to surgeons removing part of the central nucleus during microdiscectomy or laminectomy/discectomy in order to prevent the recurrent herniated nucleus pulposis from occurring. Unfortunately, this may destabilize the disc complex leading to spinal instability. Treatment of this condition is via reoperation.

Spinal instability

Removal of too much of the central disc, removal of too many supporting ligaments, facets, or operation on multiple segments without fusion may lead to painful instability. Treatment is via fusion surgery.

Arachnoiditis

This is the inflammation of the meninges and subarachnoid space and can be due to non-specific scarring secondary to the surgery or the initial underlying pathology.

History and examination

- Risk factors.
- Clinical features.
- Symptoms and signs.
- Symptoms may occur in the immediate postoperative period or later and become chronic.
- Differential diagnosis.
- Acute symptoms may be due to epidural haematoma, recurrent herniated disc, and retained fragment.

Investigations

Despite the vast number of investigations that can be used for this condition, the diagnosis remains essentially clinical. MRI and CT are necessary to identify any lesions amenable to further surgical intervention. Unfortunately they cannot determine whether the intraspinal scarring is causing the symptoms. Neuropathic pain may not always have a burning quality, but other recognizable features are often present—e.g. delayed summation of pain after provocation, the extension of pain perception beyond dermatomal boundaries, and allodynia (pain resulting from touch alone).

Epidural endoscopy can also be used to view under direct vision the epidural space and some advocate its use to free adhesions or target drug deposits.

Management

A multidisciplinary approach is required, using the biopsychosocial model.

Treatment

Treatment options are mainly conservative, including exercise and manual therapy.

- Rehabilitation and Pain Management Programmes.
- Multimodal analgesia.
- More invasive options are spinal cord stimulators (recently approved by NICE) and/or implanted pump devices for analgesic delivery.

Peripheral neuropathies: aetiology

All components of the peripheral nervous system can be affected. This leads to various patterns of sensorimotor deficit and autonomic dysfunction.

Neuropathic pain

This is defined by the IASP as 'pain initiated or caused by a primary lesion or dysfunction of the nervous system'—thus pains resulting from peripheral neuropathy are, by definition, neuropathic.

Epidemiology

Peripheral neuropathy is the most common neurological disorder with a prevalence of 2.5% in the general population, rising to 8% with increasing age.

Classification and causes

There are many different classifications. See Tables 11.1–11.4. They can be grouped by anatomical distribution and classified as symmetrical polyneuropathies or asymmetrical mono- or multiplex neuropathies. A mechanism based classification is used here:

Metabolic neuropathies

Diabetic neuropathy

- Commonest cause of neuropathy.
- Affects 50% of diabetic patients over time.
- Several different clinical syndromes.

Acute diabetic mononeuropathy

Due to infarction of the nerve.

Cranial neuropathy

Acute ophthalmoplegia due to 3rd nerve involvement is the most commonly seen. Abrupt onset with pain behind or above the eye.

Peripheral nerves

May involve any peripheral nerve but most commonly median, ulnar, radial, femoral, lateral cutaneous nerve of the thigh, and common peroneal.

Asymmetric neuropathy and radiculopathy

Diabetic amyotrophy is a painful, asymmetrical neuropathy. Pain initially in hip or back spreading down the leg. There is usually no sensory involvement. The pathological process appears to be the result of ischaemic injury from microscopic vasculitis affecting small epineural vessels.

Thoracoabdominal radiculopathy

This is seen in the elderly population. With uni- or bi-lateral girdle-like pain.

Distal symmetric sensorimotor polyneuropathy

This is the most common diabetic neuropathy. The main symptoms are numbness and tingling. Generally confined to lower limbs and is worse at night.

Table 11.1 Polyneuropathies (painful) symmetrical

Metabolic or nutritional	Infective or post-infective
Diabetic	Autoimmune
Hypothyroid	HIV
Alcoholic	Acute or inflammatory polyradiculonephropathy (Guillain–Barré)
Beriberi	
Amyloid	
Burning feet syndrome	Borreliosis
Cuban neuropathy	
Tanzanian neuropathy	
Pellagra	
Strachan's syndrome	
Hereditary	**Malignant**
Heriditary sensory/autonomic neuropathy	Myeloma
Amyloid neuropathy	Carcinomatosis
Fabray's disease	
Charcot–Marie–Tooth	
Drugs	**Toxins**
Ethambutol	Alcohol
Antiretrovirals	Arsenic
Ethanol	Mercury
Isoniazid	Thallium
Disulfiram	Ethylene oxide
Vincristine	Acrylamide
Cisplatin	Dinitrophenol
Thalidomide	Pentachlorophenol
Nitrofurantoin	
Other polyneuropathies	
Trench foot	
Erythemalgia	

Table 11.2 Asymmetrical (painful) traumatic mononeuropathies

- Post thoracotomy
- CRPS II
- Entrapment neuropathies
- Amputation stump pain
- Neuroma
- Morton's neuralgia
- Painful scars

Table 11.3 Other mononeuropathies and multiple mononeuropathies

- Trigeminal neuralgia
- Herpes zoster/PHN
- Connective tissue diseases/vasculitis
- Vascular compression syndromes
- Herpes simplex
- Diabetic amyotrophy
- Malignant plexus invasion
- Radiation plexopathy
- Borreliosis
- Plexus neuritis
- Peripheral nerve tumours

Table 11.4 Painless neuropathies

- Congenital insensitivity to pain
- Tangier disease
- Leprosy

Small fibre neuropathy
This presents with distal burning pain with cutaneous hyperaesthesia and autonomic dysfunction. This is an early feature in diabetic polyneuropathy.

Acute painful diabetic neuropathy
Presents as a burning pain, which is worse at night and is associated with profound weight loss. This is seen following episodes of ketosis or when tight glycaemic control is established. There is hyperalgesia but improvement is seen with weight gain and adequate diabetic control.

Treatment-induced neuropathy
Rarely paraesthesia and pain may develop with the institution of insulin therapy.

Hypothyroid neuropathy
Hypothyroidism is associated with higher incidence of carpal tunnel syndrome (CTS) and sensorimotor polyneuropathy. This manifests with lancing pains and dysaesthesies. The neuropathy tends to improve with thyroxine replacement.

Deficiency states
Neuropathy secondary to nutritional deficiencies is rare in the developed world but can be seen in alcoholism, malabsorption, and following GI surgery.

B1 deficiency (thiamine)—beriberi
Initially presents with painful paraesthesiae in the feet, and if not corrected, symptoms progress proximally with distal motor weakness. There is a good prognosis if treatment is instituted rapidly.

B6 deficiency (pyridoxine)
This is associated with antituberculous drug isoniazid and the hypertensive drug hydralazine. Symptoms are symmetrical tingling and pain.

Niacin

Pellagra is characterized by dermatitis, diarrhoea, and mental changes. Neuropathic symptoms are due to coexistent deficiency of pyridoxine.

Toxic neuropathies

Alcohol

This neuropathy is in part due to vitamin B1 deficiency. Diagnosis is one of exclusion and symptoms are often non-specific.

Arsenical polyneuropathy

In chronic poisoning, neuropathic symptoms develop slowly in the distal extremities. Initial symptoms are pain, which may be aching or burning, and tingling or numbness starting at fingers and toes. This is followed by motor symptoms in a similar distribution. Diagnosis is by demonstrating high levels of arsenic in hair or nails. It is associated with a slow recovery and duration depends on prior exposure.

Thallium poisoning

Mainly due to accidental or suicidal ingestion. A rapidly progressing painful sensory neuropathy develops. This may be associated with persistent pain with allodynia. Prognosis depends on the severity of peripheral nervous system involvement.

Mercury poisoning

Chronic poisoning affects the CNS. An early complaint is paraesthesia starting distally and moving proximally.

Cytostatic drugs

This is seen with chemotherapeutic drugs including vinca alkaloids, cisplatin, and taxols. Initial presentation is with distal paraesthesiae (and often cold hyperalgesia) but few other sensory signs. The motor abnormalities predominate.

Antiretroviral drugs

These are associated with a dose-limiting peripheral neuropathy seen in 1–10% of patients. It may develop within weeks of initiating therapy. It is a painful and predominantly sensory distal polyneuropathy.

Autoimmune neuropathies

Patients with acute inflammatory demyelinating polyradiculopathy and chronic inflammatory demyelinating neuropathy may suffer from pain, paraesthesia, and dysaesthesia.

Pain predominates in vasculitic neuropathies (polyarteritis nodosa, Churg–Strauss syndrome, RA, lupus erythematosis, systemic sclerosis, and Wegner's granulomatosis) with the extent of sensory and motor dysfunction depending on the nerves affected.

Primary amyloidosis presents with painful dysaesthesiae and numbness. Symptoms are more common in the lower limbs. Diagnosis is through biopsy.

Hereditary neuropathies

Hereditary sensory and autonomic neuropathy (HSAN) type I is associated with a spontaneous burning, aching, or lancing pain. It is inherited in an autosomal dominant pattern. It is seen in the 2nd–4th decades preferentially affecting the lower limbs.

Fabry's disease (X-linked disease) is associated with painful burning sensations in the hands and lower legs in boys and young men.

Congenital insensitivity to pain

HSAN type IV or V. Patients with Type IV is have an onset of symptoms in infancy with recurrent episodes of fever, anhydrosis, mental retardation, self-mutilation, and absence of reaction to painful stimuli. It is associated with normal sensory action potentials. Mutations of the TrkA gene have been seen in some families with HSAN type IV.

Intriguingly genetic mutations in the sodium channel gene (Nav1.7) which is found exclusively in the peripheral nervous system can cause either a painful neuropathy (primary erythromelagia) or a congenital insensitivity depending on whether the mutation causes channel function to be gained or lost.

HIV associated neuropathy

This may be complicated by various forms of peripheral neuropathy. The most common is distal symmetrical polyneuropathy. A similar neuropathy can result from antiretroviral drugs and vitamin B12 deficiency.

Nerve compression and entrapment neuropathies

These are isolated nerve injuries occurring at specific locations. The most frequent is compression of the median nerve at the wrist. Other sites include the ulnar nerve at the elbow and wrist; suprascapular nerve at the spinoglenoid notch; lateral femoral cutaneous nerve of the thigh at the inguinal ligament. In these cases it is important to exclude systemic diseases such as diabetes, hypothyroidism, and amyloidosis, and also pregnancy.

Neuralgic amyotrophy

This may be spontaneous or secondary to infection, injection of vaccine or antibiotic, surgical procedure, or childbirth. It presents as severe pain around the shoulder with rapid development of weakness and atrophy. It is usually unilateral but can rarely be bilateral. It can be restricted to one or two nerve territories and can present as an isolated phrenic nerve palsy. It is usually associated with a good recovery.

Paraneoplastic neuropathies

These present as a distal symmetrical sensory or sensorimotor polyneuropathy. Occasionally a purely sensory neuropathy is seen.

There are 3 main classes of paraneoplastic neuropathy:
• Ataxic syndrome
• Hyperalgesia–ataxic syndrome
• Ataxic/hyperalgesic–ataxic syndrome.

Peripheral neuropathies: clinical features

Symptoms
- Allodynia: pain following an innocuous stimulus.
- Hyperalgesia: pain of abnormal severity following a noxious stimulus.
- Hyperpathia: increased pain in an area with sensory deficit.
- Spontaneous pain which may be continuous or paroxysmal. This is described as arising from muscle or bone (throbbing, cramping, aching) or from skin (burning, prickling, stabbing).
- Weakness or wasting of affected muscles.
- Hypoaesthesia.
- Loss of or attenuated tendon reflexes.
- Impaired autonomic function.
- Pain or hyperalgesia in absence of neurological symptoms or signs.

Investigations

Nerve conduction velocity, electromyography, and evoked potentials
Neurophysiological testing is a key component of diagnosis, but these techniques are usually limited to assessing the function of large myelinated fibres which are not the source of neuropathic pain. These differentiate between demyelinating or axonal neuropathies or the presence or absence of conduction defects. Proximal lesions can be studied with somatosensory- or magnetic-evoked potentials.

Quantitative sensory testing and autonomic testing
Assesses function of classes of unmyelinated and myelinated afferent fibres. These tests are useful in patients with hyperalgesia/allodynia and hypoalgesia providing an objective assessment.

Skin biopsy
Quantification of epidermal nerve fibre density is objective, specific, and a sensitive method for documenting loss of unmyelinated nerve fibres.

Cerebrospinal fluid examination
Increased protein levels and cellular responses can indicate radicular or meningeal involvement.

Nerve biopsies
Diagnostic tool in established neuropathies but invasive and suitable for only a few nerves.

Magnetic resonance imaging
Used to exclude focal mass lesions or external compression and invasive muscle atrophy. Useful in the differential diagnosis of peripheral nerve disease.

Treatment
- Treatment of the underlying cause.
- Drug treatment initially follows the WHO analgesic ladder (see 📖 WHO analgesic ladder p.34) with early use of adjuvant drugs such as:

Antidepressants (e.g. amitriptyline)

These remain a front-line treatment because they are potentially the most effective. TCAs for example amitriptyline started at a dose of 10mg at night then titrated in 10–25mg increments every few days. Benefit may occur after 2 weeks but often requires 8 weeks. Side effects affect compliance (alternatives include nortriptyline). 1 in 3 patients will get >50% pain relief. Duloxetine has recently been licensed for use in diabetic peripheral neuropathy. In contrast the SSRIs are not useful.

Anticonvulsants (e.g. gabapentin, pregabalin)

Also first-line agents. Appear to suppress synaptic transmission through an action at the $\alpha 2\delta$ calcium channel subunit. Gabapentin and pregabalin have been shown in multicentre trials to be effective in diabetic peripheral neuropathy.

Opioids

They can help in approximately 1 in 8 patients. Morphine is the standard drug of choice but other opioids may be used. They are generally used for severe acute pain states and in pain secondary to malignancy.

Tramadol

Is a weak mu receptor agonist and inhibits the reuptake of noradrenaline and serotonin.

Antiarrhythmics (e.g. lidocaine)

Lidocaine may be trialled at 5mg/kg intravenously over 1h with CV monitoring. A few patients may find beneficial effects that outlast the infusion period by weeks in which case the infusions may be repeated.

NMDA receptor antagonists

Ketamine can be used alone, or to potentiate the effects of opioids. It is given as an IV or SC infusion at a dose of 0.1–0.5mg/kg/h. It can also be delivered orally and titrated from 20mg bd to 50mg qid. However, absorption is poor and unreliable and its use is associated with psychomimetic side effect so is not well tolerated.

Topical drugs

These have fewer side effects. Pain in delineated, accessible cutaneous areas is suitable for topical treatment.

Capsaicin

This inactivates pain C-fibres. It is applied 3–4× a day for up to 8 weeks for an effect to be shown. There are 2 strengths: 0.075% for neuropathic pain and 0.025% for arthritic pain. It has been used as a treatment in PHN and painful diabetic peripheral neuropathy.

Lidocaine patches

These have recently become available in the UK and are licensed for the treatment of postherpetic neuralgia. They may also be useful for other peripheral neuropathies.

Transcutaneous electrical nerve stimulation

Involves selective activation of large diameter fibres. It has been shown to be of some benefit in some neuropathic pain patients although individual trials are needed to identify responders. (See 📖 Transcutaneous electrical nerve stimulation p.216.)

Spinal cord stimulation

This is based on the gate theory of pain. Initially a trial period with temporary external stimulation is used. It can produce long-term analgesia in neuropathic pain patients. (See 📖 Spinal cord stimulation p.218.)

Pain Management Programmes

A programme using primarily psychological and physiotherapy techniques to help patients improve their ability to cope and function. The aim is to empower the patient to adapt and achieve as optimal a quality of life as possible (see 📖 Pain Management Programmes p.262).

Complex regional pain syndrome

CRPS types I and II are chronic pain syndromes characterized by vasomotor, sudomotor, and trophic changes together with allodynia and hyperalgesia. These syndromes were previously known as: reflex sympathetic dystrophy, Sudeck's atrophy, causalgia, and post-traumatic arthritis. They commonly affect the limbs but can occur anywhere and can occasionally present or generalize to multiple sites.

In CRPS type II the symptoms follow nerve damage. The symptoms and signs are identical in CRPS type I but follow local injuries such as fractures, sprains, surgery, or distant insults such as MI and stroke. In up to 25% of cases there is no obvious preceding event.

Clinical features

Pain

Pain is the dominant feature of CRPS. It presents usually as a burning, throbbing, or shooting pain but there is much variability between patients. The intensity fluctuates spontaneously and in response to both external (temperature) and internal influences (stress).

Allodynia and hyperalgesia are often found on examination. Temperature perception and proprioception are also altered.

Vasomotor changes

Affected areas can be red, cyanotic, or pale. They are often mottled and blotchy. These colour changes can occur at any time in the natural history of the condition and do not follow a predictable course. It used to be thought that affected areas were initially hyperaemic (red) then ischaemic (cyanotic leading onto pallor), but recently it has been realized these changes can occur at any time during the course of the condition and in any order.

Temperature changes are also common and variable. The affected site can be either warmer or cooler that the corresponding contralateral site and can change during the course of the disease.

Sudomotor changes/oedema

The affected area can be swollen with either increased or decreased sweating.

Motor abnormality

There can be reduced range of movement, weakness, impaired coordination, tremor, or dystonia. These usually present late in the condition. They are due to pain, trophic changes, and occasionally a neglect-like syndrome. The end result can be a useless, contracted limb.

Trophic changes

Abnormal hair and nail growth are the commonest trophic changes. There can also be atrophy of the skin, demineralization of bone, and vascular complications (thrombosis or spontaneous haematomas).

Pathogenesis

The pathogenic mechanisms underlying CRPS remain largely undetermined. There is autonomic dysfunction but whether this is a cause or a result of the pain is unknown. Animal studies have demonstrated aberrant interaction and coupling of the sympathetic and sensory nerves. There is peripheral and central sensitization which could explain the spontaneous pain, allodynia, and hyperalgesia but the cause of these changes remains obscure.

Diagnosis

The diagnosis of CRPS is in practice a clinical one and, in the past, there has been much confusion about the diagnostic criteria used to identify these conditions. The IASP has attempted to standardize the terminology and diagnostic criteria.

Diagnostic criteria for complex regional pain syndromes I and II

Continuing pain disproportionate to inciting event

1 symptom in each of the following categories:

- *Sensory:* allodynia or hyperaesthesia.
- *Vasomotor:* temperature asymmetry and/or skin colour changes and/or skin colour asymmetry.
- *Sudomotor/oedema:* oedema and/or sweating changes and/or sweating asymmetry.
- *Motor/trophic:* decreased range of motion and/or motor dysfunction (weakness, tremor, dystonia) and/or trophic changes (hair, nails, skin).

1 sign in 2 or more of the following categories

- *Sensory:* hyperalgesia (to pinprick) and/or allodynia (to light touch).
- *Vasomotor:* evidence of temperature asymmetry and/or skin colour changes and/or skin colour asymmetry.
- *Sudomotor/oedema:* evidence of oedema and/or sweating changes and/or sweating asymmetry.
- *Motor/trophic:* evidence of decreased range of motion and/or motor dysfunction (weakness, tremor, dystonia) and/or trophic changes (hair, nails, skin).

Treatment

Treatment is aimed primarily at preventing further loss of function and restoring normal function. It must be tailored to individual patients as response to the numerous methods listed here is variable and each patient will require a different combination of the various options.

- Physiotherapy: early and proactive physiotherapy is essential to functional restoration. Active mobilization along with other physical techniques (massage, hydrotherapy, and desensitization) prevents secondary changes due to disuse and altered autonomic function.
- Sympathetic blockade: can be useful diagnostically and can be repeated as treatments. This can be performed as sympathetic ganglion block (stellate or lumbar) using LA or phenol. It can be performed surgically as a sympathectomy or with RF ablation.
- Anticonvulsants: gabapentin, carbamazepine, lamotrigine, and sodium valproate are all used.

- Antidepressants: TCAs are well established. Side effects often limit their use in which case serotonin and noradrenaline uptake inhibitors (SNRIs) can be helpful.
- Analgesics: simple analgesics, such as paracetamol, may give some relief but it is often necessary to progress up the WHO analgesic ladder and add in weak opioids followed by strong opioids in resistant cases.
- NMDA antagonists: ketamine has been used in treating CRPS but there is little evidence to support its use and side effects often make it intolerable to patients.
- Other drugs: calcitonin has occasionally been used with some success.
- TENS: the success rate of TENS in CRPS had been found to be very variable in different studies. Nevertheless it is cheap and non-invasive so should be considered.
- SCS: some studies have reported very high success rates with SCS. However it should still be reserved for severe cases when all other modalities have failed.
- Amputation: no studies have demonstrated a beneficial effect of amputation for pain. Patients can develop phantom limb pain following amputation which may be more disabling than the original problem. Amputation should only be carried out for intractable infection or ulcers.
- Psychological therapy: see 📖 The psychological management of chronic pain p.254.

Conclusion

There are more controversies than agreements surrounding the optimal treatment for CRPS. The aim should be to be to restore function with a multidisciplinary approach within which early and aggressive physiotherapy plays a key role.

Chronic postsurgical pain

Definition

Pain that develops after a surgical procedure, lasts for >2 months, and is not an exacerbation of a pre-existing condition.

Epidemiology

Chronic postsurgical pain has been estimated to occur in 10–50% of all patients following surgery and is reported as being severe and interfering with daily activities in 2–10%. It has been estimated that 20% of all chronic pain clinic attendees attribute some of their pain to a surgical episode.

Aetiology

The causation is multifactorial but many of the persisting pains are neuropathic in origin and result from nerve injury sustained in the perioperative period. The presence of a neuropathic component may be indicated by reports of burning, shooting, stabbing, or electric shock-like pain.

Recognized syndromes

Breast surgery

This is probably the best recognized of the postsurgical chronic pains. The incidence of pain after breast surgery has been estimated at 20–49% with a higher incidence after reconstruction. These pains start within weeks of surgery and are thus distinguishable from the pains associated with subsequent radiotherapy or tumour spread. There are several sources/types of pain including: scar, arm, chest wall, and phantom pains.

Thoracic

That chronic postoperative pain is common after thoracotomy is perhaps not surprising given the surgical retraction, rib resection, and proximity of the intercostal nerve to the rib. Indeed, severe pains can result from injury to the intercostal nerve to give rise to classical neuropathic pain symptoms. The incidence of chronic pain following thoracic surgery has been linked to the intensity of acute postoperative pain and analgesic consumption. However, as yet, it has not been shown that the incidence of chronic pain can be reduced by particular analgesic strategies, e.g. regional blocks.

Postlimb amputation

Pain following limb amputation can be split into stump pains (originating from the limb remnant) and phantom pains (identified as originating in the amputated tissue). Stump pains appear to be the result of a variety of pathologies: scar, neuroma, and ongoing inflammation. The quoted incidence of stump pain varies widely from 5–62%. It is influenced by surgical technique and can be reduced by appropriate prosthesis fitting. There is little evidence that surgical revisions, scar/neuroma excision, or further amputation improve pain in the longer term. Phantom pains (see 📖 eafferentation and phantom pains p.296) are common with an incidence of 50–80%. They represent a type of neuropathic pain and seem to originate from discrepancies in CNS remapping following amputation. The incidence is higher if the patient had pain before amputation and may be reduced by early fitting of a correct prosthesis.

Inguinal hernia repair

The surgical outcomes after inguinal hernia repair have been extensively investigated and chronic pain is relatively common (63% at 1 year). This incidence is increased by the use of mesh and decreased by laparoscopic approaches.

Management

The management of postsurgical pain syndromes is similar irrespective of the cause (once pre-existing complaints and other inciting conditions have been excluded). In essence, a distinction needs to be drawn between pains that are nociceptive/inflammatory and those that are neuropathic in origin. This distinction will often be guided by the history and findings on examination. The therapeutic options then follow from this distinction (see previous sections).

There is often a considerable emotional overlay associated with postsurgical pains with a history of blame, guilt, denial, and recrimination on both sides of the therapeutic alliance. This may be addressed through normal clinical discussions but may also be an indication for a psychology-based pain management approach.

Prevention

As the treatment options for postsurgical chronic pain are limited, attention has been focused on prevention. There is evidence that 'nerve sparing' surgical approaches reduce the incidence of neuropathic pains for operations such as mastectomy, herniorrhaphy, and thoracotomy. There is also interest in the use of multimodal analgesic regimens (combinations of conventional analgesics, LA, and drugs such as ketamine or gabapentin) that might prevent central sensitization, hyperalgesia, and the subsequent development of chronic pain.

Central pain syndromes

Definition

'Pain resulting from damage to the central nervous system.'

Central pains (CPs) seem almost paradoxical because they originate from damage to the brain, an organ with no intrinsic nociceptive innervation. However, there is growing appreciation that a large number of insults at all levels of the neuroaxis can produce pain syndromes. This is thought to occur via interruption of the normal pain matrix, especially those involving disruption of the spino-thalamo-cortical tracts. There is a common association between altered sensation (particularly thermal) and pain.

Epidemiology

CPs can result from a heterogeneous set of conditions including poststroke pain, MS, syringomyelia/bulbia, spinal cord injury, and metastatic tumours or infections. The most common is central poststroke pain (>90%, CPSP, either infarcts or haemorrhage) especially those involving the sensory thalamus, internal capsule, and parietal territories. The pain frequently develops during the weeks and months following the infarct, often as the motor symptoms improve. This may explain why the incidence of post-stroke pain has been underestimated in the past. An estimated 2–8% of all stroke patients develop CP with much higher proportions if the affected territory includes the sensory thalamus. This compares to around 30% of all MS and spinal cord injury patients.

Aetiology

CP typically presents with classical neuropathic pain symptoms with regional (sometimes hemibody) dysaesthesiae, mechanical and thermal allodynia, shooting and lancinating pains alongside continuous burning or freezing sensations. This is often accompanied by the loss of normal tactile or thermal sensation and proprioception. Although the common neuro-anatomical thread through this mix of signs and symptoms is interruption of the spino-thalamo-cortical pathways, there is debate as to why this pro-duces rather than obtunds pain. Competing theories invoke maladaptive reorganization, disinhibition, or denervation hypersensitivity or indeed a mix of all three to explain the observed phenomena. To date there is little evidence upon which to base targeted therapy.

Management

The key first step is correct diagnosis and education of the patient about their condition. Many patients will have found their symptoms inexplicable and may have received little prior medical support.

Many therapeutic options have been explored but only a few have been shown to be of any benefit. Rational trials of conventional neuropathic pain medications such as tricyclics, anticonvulsants, or even opiates are appropriate but the response is often modest. Patients with spinal pathology may benefit from intrathecal baclofen or clonidine infusions. Similarly the treatment of associated muscle spasm with oral baclofen may be associated with reduced pain. Specifically for MS pains there is some evidence supporting the use of cannabinoids as analgesics.

There is little logic to the use of SCS in a syndrome characterized by loss of spinothalamic transmission (particularly for supra-tentorial lesions) nor for neurosurgical ablative procedures. Interestingly some refractory patients have been reported to benefit from DBS. Physical therapies are usually ineffective but there is a strong rationale for psychological interventions aimed to help patients cope with ongoing symptoms. There is also a recognized increased risk of self-harm and suicide in this patient group.

Conclusions

CP syndromes are relatively common in patients with lesions of the CNS and may be associated with severe neuropathic pain symptoms. Their aetiology is incompletely understood and they are often refractory to current neuropathic pain treatments.

Deafferentation and phantom pains

Definition
Painful sensation originating from an amputated or deafferented body part.

Epidemiology
An estimated 50–80% of patients after amputation will, if asked, report phantom limb pain (PLP). Although it is most commonly reported after loss of a limb, there are also reports of phantom breasts, teeth, testicles, penis, and rectum. An analogous phenomenon is also reported following denervation injuries (e.g. brachial plexus avulsion) where there is no amputation. Patients with a history of pain in the body part prior to amputation appear more likely to develop a painful phantom. PLP typically occurs soon (within weeks) following amputation and although there is a tendency for the symptoms to improve with time there are many patients who experience years of unrelieved pain.

Aetiology
PLP represents a classical neuropathic pain and may in part depend upon activity from sensitized peripheral nerve fibres whose original territory was the amputated tissue. However, it is thought that the major component of the pathology results from discordant reorganization of CNS sensory maps. Phantoms are common following amputation but not all are associated with pain, indicating that there are differences in the underlying changes in neural processing. Patients may report pains that are stabbing, cramping, burning, or throbbing which are often localized to the distal part of the amputated tissue.

Management
In taking a history it is important to distinguish between phantom pains and stump pains that may both be reported as coming from the amputated limb. In particular, there may be some reluctance on the part of the patient to report phantom pain for fear of being considered 'of unsound mind'. Thus an important therapeutic role is to reassure the patient that phantom pain is a common consequence of amputation.

Many therapeutic options have been explored but few have been shown to be of benefit. In particular there is no evidence of benefit for surgical revisions or more extensive amputation. Similarly there is little support for the use of repeated LA blocks, regional techniques, or sympathectomy, except possibly for the use of LAs to decrease ectopic activity originating from neuromas.

Conventional neuropathic pain treatments have a place in the treatment of PLP with some evidence of benefit being obtained from either anticonvulsants or TCAs. There are also some small randomized trials indicating benefit from opioids, ketamine, and calcitonin.

Some more novel treatment approaches have been developed over the last decade that can be grouped under the heading biofeedback. The starting point for this approach came from the observation that the use of well-fitted limb prostheses appears to reduce the incidence of PLP.

This lead to the suggestion that 'appropriate' sensory and proprioceptive inputs from the limb might be helpful. This has been extended through the use of myoelectric prostheses that have been shown to both improve symptoms and reverse cortical reorganization (demonstrated using fMRI scanning). An analogous approach has been to use 'mirror boxes' or virtual reality software to create the illusion of movement of the phantom limb. Several case reports suggest that this has allowed phantom limbs to be repositioned into a less contorted position and thus relieved cramping pains.

Prevention

There has been a lot of interest in the possibility of preventing the development of PLP. The obvious first step in prevention is to encourage tissue conservation and, in particular, avoid amputation solely for pain control as this is especially likely to result in the development of painful phantoms.

The association between pre-existing pain and the development of a painful phantom led to interest in providing pre-emptive analgesia prior to amputation to prevent central sensitization. This was examined in a number of studies using continuous epidural or regional blocks for days prior and following amputation but after some initial hopeful findings, larger, better controlled studies have failed to show any evidence of benefit. It remains to be seen whether the multimodal combination of extended-duration LA techniques with drugs that may reduce central sensitization, such as ketamine, baclofen, or gabapentin, will be any more effective.

Acute herpetic neuralgia (shingles)

Definition
Acute pain associated with an attack of herpes zoster.

Epidemiology
- 0.5–3:1,000 incidence.
- The risk is age dependent.
- >1% over the age of 75 years.
- The lifetime risk is estimated at 10–20% and is thus one of the most common neurological conditions.
- Shingles most commonly affects truncal dermatomes and the ophthalmic division of the trigeminal nerve.
- Pain often precedes rash appearance (prodromal).

Aetiology
- Herpes zoster occurs after recrudescence of virus that has lain dormant in dorsal root ganglia following varicella zoster (chickenpox) infection earlier in life.
- Viral reactivation appears to depend on waning cell-mediated immunity, hence the association with old age and immunosuppression (e.g. after chemotherapy/steroids).
- Virus is transported to the skin along the axons of primary afferents to cause the characteristic blistering rash.
- The presence of virus in the dorsal root ganglion triggers a cell-mediated immune response which causes inflammation, cell loss, and axonal demyelination and degeneration.

Symptoms
- The rash and pain are typically dermatomal.
- The area is often exquisitely sensitive to touch and patients commonly report deep aching, superficial burning and itching, or electrical shock-like pains.
- These pains often outlast rash resolution but the majority (90%) have settled by 3 months after rash onset.

Diagnosis
- The diagnosis is usually fairly clear from the history, and examination reveals the characteristic rash.
- Blister fluid may be sent to confirm the identity of the virus but this is seldom clinically needed.
- There is a recognized rash-free variant (zoster sine herpete) in which dermatomal pain is not accompanied by a rash.
- Patients presenting with zoster affecting the ophthalmic division of the trigeminal should be referred for specialist eye care.

Management
The management of acute herpetic neuralgia has two main aims: inhibition of viral replication and provision of symptomatic analgesia.

Inhibition of viral replication

The use of antiviral agents (e.g. aciclovir) is supported by evidence in patients with risk factors for worse prognosis:

- Age >50 years.
- Immunocompromised.
- Involvement of ophthalmic division.
- Severe pain or large area.
- These treatments:
  - Reduce the duration of the rash.
  - Can reduce the severity of the pain.
  - In patients aged >50, shown to reduce the duration of the pain and reduce the incidence of PHN (see 📖 Postherpetic neuralgia, p.300).
- There is some evidence that adding an oral steroid to the antiviral can hasten resolution of symptoms.

Symptomatic analgesia

A significant proportion of patients will have moderate to severe pain associated with shingles. This may require combinations of:

- Enteral opiates
- Neuropathic medications such as amitriptyline/gabapentin.

It has been suggested that that treatment of the acute pain with amitriptyline can reduce the subsequent incidence of PHN. Some centres advocate the use of epidural steroids for severe shingles to reduce the incidence of PHN but this remains controversial.

Postherpetic neuralgia

Definition
Pain persisting 120 days after the onset of acute herpes zoster rash.

Epidemiology
Around 20% of patients over the age of 50 will have pain at 6 months following an episode of shingles. The risk of PHN following acute zoster is greater in the elderly, in ♀, in patients with worse rashes and more severe acute pain, and in those that experienced a prodrome.

Aetiology
The primary pathology is destruction of primary afferent neurons in the dorsal root ganglia consequent on viral reactivation; thus it is a neuropathic pain. Following this deafferentation there may be subsequent changes in the neural circuitry of the spinal DH. The origin of the pain can therefore be both peripheral and/or central.

Symptoms
The pain is typically dermatomal and can be described as sharp, burning, stabbing, or throbbing. The pains may be spontaneous or provoked. This is a classical neuropathic pain syndrome and patients may present with evidence of allodynia, hyperalgesia, hyperpathia, and hypoaesthesia.

Diagnosis
The diagnosis is usually by history and examination to confirm the chronology with respect to an episode of zoster and the dermatomal distribution of the affected area.

Management
The management of PHN is as per other neuropathic pain conditions with trials of conventional analgesics such as opiates along with TCAs and anticonvulsants. Good evidence exists from RCTs for the specific efficacy of gabapentin, pregabalin, and amitriptyline for PHN.

Therapies specific to PHN include:
- Topical capsaicin: acts to deplete C-fibre afferents in the affected dermatome and may reduce burning pain with repeated application.
- Topical lidocaine patches: may be particularly effective in patients with a prominent peripheral component to pain.
- Topical aspirin in acetone.
- For particularly severe cases there are reports of successful excision of the skin of the affected dermatome and the use of epidural or intrathecal steroids although these treatments remain controversial.

There are some reports of benefit from antiviral therapy, steroids, SCS, TENS, or nerve blocks.

Prevention

The use of antivirals and analgesics such as TCA drugs in the initial acute zoster attack can reduce the subsequent incidence of PHN.

The introduction of a vaccination program against varicella zoster in the USA has reduced the incidence of chickenpox and presumably will reduce the incidence of shingles and PHN. Furthermore, administering the same vaccination to patients >60 years who have been exposed to varicella reduced the incidence of shingles and PHN by over half.

Outcomes

The natural course of PHN is favourable with a majority of patients reporting resolution of symptoms within a year. However, a significant minority of patients are left with severe neuropathic pain that remains refractory to treatment.

Trigeminal neuralgia

Trigeminal neuralgia (TN) is a condition characterized by severe, unilateral, paroxysmal facial pain. Management of TN involves establishing the diagnosis, investigating for a possible cause, instituting appropriate first-line drug therapy, and knowing what to do if this fails. Surgical treatment is reserved for cases refractory to medical management or where the side effects of medical treatment outweigh the risks of surgery.

Incidence

TN is rare and has an incidence of about 4.5 per 100,000 people per year. ♀ are affected nearly twice as often as ♂. The mean age of onset is about 50 years with the peak incidence in the 6th and 7th decades. The lifetime prevalence in the primary care population is about 0.7/1,000.

Diagnosis

TN presents with severe, unilateral, facial pains. These pains last from seconds to a couple of minutes and recur many times daily. They are often evoked by trivial stimulation in the offending trigeminal nerve distribution. The paroxysms are stereotyped for each individual. The pain is often in the maxillary and mandibular divisions of the trigeminal nerve and rarely (5% of cases) affects the ophthalmic division. The right side is more often involved that the left.

In 'classical' TN there is no associated trigeminal sensory loss or any background pain between paroxysms but this is not the case in 'atypical' TN. The importance of 'atypical' TN lies in the fact that it is more likely to be both refractory to medical or surgical management and to be associated with pathological abnormality of the trigeminal nerve root.

Differential diagnosis

The differential diagnosis of TN presents 2 main challenges: the closest mimics of TN are rare and may evade consideration, whilst less convincing mimics are abundant. Dental pain is the commonest mimic and patients with TN often present first to dentists. If the pain is dull, bilateral, and/or constant then persistent idiopathic facial pain and temporomandibular joint pain should be considered.

Of the rare mimics there are 2 conditions where the pattern of attacks is especially similar to TN. Both of the conditions affect the forehead, which is the case in only about 5% of TN attacks:

- Idiopathic stabbing headache, or ice pick headache, consists of brief stabs of forehead pain usually lasting a second or less, but probably never >10s.
- SUNCT (Short lasting Unilateral Neuralgiform headaches with Conjuctival injection and Tearing) is the briefest of the trigeminal autonomic cephalalgias. Attacks typically last 5s–5mins but can be differentiated from TN as the pain is accompanied by profuse, ipsilateral, trigeminal autonomic overactivity including tearing, nasal stuffiness, and conjuctival injection.

Pathogenesis

In 80–90% of TN a blood vessel—usually an artery—is found to be compressing the trigeminal nerve root and is probably causative. <10% of TN will be caused by underlying non-vascular compression (e.g. neoplasms) or MS. In a small number of patients no cause will be identified.

Investigations

MRI is mandatory to exclude secondary causes such as neoplasms and MRA can identify vascular compression prior to surgical exploration.

Natural history and treatment

The severity of the pain necessitates intervention so there is no untreated natural history data. The available evidence suggests that the average episode of TN lasts nearly 2 months (range 1 day to 4 years) and 70% of patients will go on to have further episodes after a variable period of remission.

Management

Initial management of TN is pharmacological and around 70% of patients get benefit from carbamazepine which is therefore the drug of first choice. Other treatment options include trials of drugs for neuropathic pains such as anticonvulsants (e.g. gabapentin), TCAs, and adjuncts such as baclofen or opioids. Unfortunately, a significant proportion of patients either obtain little benefit from medical management or are troubled by the side effects of the drugs. For these medical non-responders, surgical intervention or neurolytic blocks should be considered (see 📖 Trigeminal Nerve Blocks p.190).

Headache

- 60–75% of adults have at least 1 headache/year.
- These can be very disabling and this has an impact on both the individual and on society.
- The mechanism of a headache may be due to traction, distension, inflammation, or direct pressure on intracranial vessels or meningeal structures.
- Extracranial contraction of muscles or diseases of local organs may be a factor.

Classification

Primary headaches (no other causative disorders)
- Tension
- Migraine
- Cluster.

Secondary headaches (caused by another disorder)
- Trauma or injury
- Vascular disorder
- Intracranial lesion
- Infection (e.g. meningitis)
- Disease of sinuses, neck, ears, teeth, eyes, or mouth
- Central causes (e.g. after stroke).

Warning signs

⚠ Headache could be indicative of a possible serious underlying organic cause such as: subarachnoid haemorrhage (SAH), tumour, meningitis, encephalitis, temporal arteritis, idiopathic cranial hypertension, cerebral venous thrombosis.

Consider further investigation if:
- Worsening headache over a short period (check neurological examination).
- New or different headache.
- Sudden onset ('thunderclap headache'—SAH).
- New headache in >50 year-old (temporal arteritis).
- Associated systemic disorders (e.g. fever, weight loss, scalp tenderness, stiff neck).
- Associated neurological signs.
- Seizures, confusion, loss of consciousness.

⚠ Need to remain vigilant for secondary causes of headache particularly when there is a previous established primary headache disorder.

Tension headache
- Most common primary headache, caused by contraction or tensioning of facial and neck muscles resulting in referred pain.
- ♂:♀ ratio 1:1.5; onset commonly in teens, peaks in 40s.
- Treat with simple analgesics. Tricyclics may reduce severity.

- Other therapies include acupuncture, biofeedback, CBT, relaxation, manipulation, and TENS.

Migraine

- Most common of the vascular headaches.
- Symptoms appear to be due to changes in blood flow, although their aetiology is still debated. Can be precipitated by various triggers.
- Onset most commonly in 20s and 30s, more common in ♀.
- Prevalence of 10–20%.

Characteristics

- Severe pain in one or both sides of the head.
- Nausea and/or vomiting with photophobia, phonophobia, and osmophobia.
- Trigger agents (⚠ one or a combination may provoke an attack)—environmental/lifestyle/hormonal/emotional/medication/dietary.

Treatment

Depends on severity, disability, and frequency of attacks—aim for early intervention:

- Simple analgesics: aspirin, paracetamol, NSAIDs, and antiemetics for nausea.
- $5-HT_1$ agonists (triptans): specific antimigraine, treatment of choice for acute attacks unresponsive to simple analgesics.
- Ergot alkoids: rarely used due to side effects of vasospasm.
- Stronger analgesic, e.g. opioids.
- Oestrogen replacement in 'menstrual associated migraine'.
- ⚠ Excessive use of any of the analgesics, can itself lead to 'medication overuse headache'.

Prophylaxis

- Needs to be individualized depending on the side effects.
- Patients need to have realistic goals and expectations of treatment.
- Avoid provoking factors (stress, lifestyle, chemicals—alcohol, oral contraceptive pill).
- Consider preventative medication if:
  - >2 attacks/month.
  - Increasing frequency of headaches.
  - Significant effect on quality of life.
  - Intolerant of treatment for acute attacks.
- Treatment options include: propranolol (B-blocker), pizotifen (antihistamine, $5-HT_{1\&2}$ antagonist), sodium valproate, topiramate, TCAs, cyproheptadine ($5-HT_2$ antagonist) and clonidine.

Cluster headache

- Affects <0.5% of population, more common in ♂.
- Repeated short duration, but excruciatingly intense attacks of unilateral periorbital pain associated with local autonomic signs and symptoms.
- Typically daily or nightly attacks over a period of weeks or months.
- Acute treatment with high-flow oxygen can give relief within 15min.
- SC sumatriptan or ergotamine with antiemetics (metoclopramide).

Orofacial pain

The vast majority of patients developing orofacial pain will have an acute pain originating from the teeth. Treatment of the underlying dental problem will lead to resolution of the symptoms in most cases. This chapter is concerned with pain persisting for >3 months which has not responded to identification and treatment of any underlying pathology.

The aetiology of chronic orofacial pain is complex and not well understood. This has led to a number of different ways of classifying the condition. One classification places patients into 3 groups on the basis of the tissue of origin:

- Musculo-ligamentous/soft-tissue
- Dento-alveolar
- Neurological/vascular

Another classification is based upon the presumed cause of the orofacial pain. Possible causes include infection, trauma, neuropathic, vascular, neoplastic, psychogenic, idiopathic, and referred pain.

This chapter uses the clinical presentation to classify different forms of orofacial pain.

Dental pain

Dental pain is pain that originates from the teeth or their surrounding structures. Pain may be due to physical defects of the teeth or surrounding structures, inflammation of the pulp, infection, or can be idiopathic (atypical odontalgia). All of these patients should be referred to a general dental practitioner or dental hospital for definitive treatment.

Temporomandibular joint pain

There are numerous different terms to describe the pain associated with the temporomandibular joint (TMJ). The most commonly accepted and currently used terms are: temporomandibular pain and dysfunction syndrome, oromandibular dysfunction, and facial arthromyalgia.

The symptoms of TMJ pain include severe pain on chewing, restricted jaw movement, a change in the muscles of mastication and clicking or popping sounds.

There is very little evidence on which to base specific treatment for TMJ pain and the American Dental Association recommend only conservative, reversible forms of treatment. Reassurance, exercise, physical therapy, relaxation, biofeedback, splints, and psychological interventions have all been used. Drug therapy following the WHO analgesic ladder can be tried particularly with NSAIDs. Arthroscopy and other surgical procedures have been used and are sometimes successful but there is little good supporting evidence.

Sinusitis

Inflammation can occur within any of the facial sinuses leading to pain. It is usually a result of retention of secretions caused by either a restriction to the drainage or a change in the viscosity of secretions. The most common cause is a bacterial or viral infection. Diagnosis is usually made on plain X-ray or CT scanning.

Most patients will improve spontaneously or with the use of decongestants. There is some evidence to support the use of antibiotics.

Some patients may develop chronic sinus pain but there is no way to predict which patients will do this. These patients will require a multidisciplinary team approach to their treatment.

Burning mouth syndrome

Burning mouth syndrome is defined as a burning pain in the tongue or other oral mucous membranes with no obvious medical cause. Possible medical causes include: bacterial or fungal infection, allergy, oesophageal reflux disease, folate and vitamin B12 deficiency, iron deficiency, and diabetes. 70% of patients have associated anxiety and depression.

There is limited evidence for the use of CBT, otherwise treatment is empirical.

Atypical facial pain

The International Headache Society defines atypical facial pain as 'persistent facial pain that does not have the characteristics of the cranial neuralgias and is not associated with physical signs or a demonstrable organic cause. Pain may be initiated by an operative procedure or injury to the face, teeth or oral tissues.'

At the outset, pain is often confined to a limited area, but then spreads becoming poorly localized. It is usually severe, continuous, and persists from weeks to years. Laboratory tests and scans do not reveal any pathological abnormality. There is some evidence to support the use of TCAs as treatment of atypical facial pain. Psychological intervention should be considered, particularly when associated with anxiety and depression.

Atypical odontalgia

Atypical odontalgia is defined as severe pain in a tooth without pathology. The aetiology is unclear but it has been suggested that this is a neuropathic pain due to deafferentation secondary to dental treatment. The pain is confined to the teeth, or sites of extraction, and is usually continuous, lasting from weeks to years. There is little evidence to guide treatment, but TCAs may be useful.

Trigeminal neuralgia

Trigieminal neuralgia is discussed on ☐ Trigieminal neuralgia, p.302.

Ophthalmic postherpetic neuralgia

see ☐ Postherpetic neuralgia p.300.

General principles of management

A biopsychosocial approach to the management of these patients is essential. There is limited evidence on which to base specific treatments for the various orofacial pain conditions. It is vital to take a thorough history of the pain condition, the psychological consequences, and to establish realistic treatment aims. Most patients will value the opportunity to tell the story of their pain problem and will be more likely to accept a reduction in their pain, rather than a complete cure if they are listened to empathetically. Involving patients in discussions about the diagnosis and possible treatment plans is important from the very beginning. Agreeing the goals of treatment and negotiating a management plan with the patient is likely to improve the outcome.

The range of treatments available which may be of benefit in orofacial pain is similar to treatments for most other chronic pain conditions. These include:

• Pharmacological
• Physical
• Psychological
• Surgical
• Self-management strategies.

Summary

Chronic orofacial pains are a heterogenous group of conditions that cause considerable personal morbidity and are relatively refractory to conventional treatment approaches. For the majority of cases the best results are obtained from a biopsychosocial management approach.

Further reading

Zakrzewska JM and Harrison SD (eds) (2002). *Assessment and Management of Orofacial Pain*. Elsevier, London.

Whiplash

Definition
Collection of symptoms produced as a result of soft tissue injury of the cervical spine.

Epidemiology
- Road traffic rear-end collision most common (2x).
- Frequently low velocity impact (<10km/h) with little vehicular damage.
- 110 million working-days lost/year; 7% never work again.
- Annual cost to UK society of £3 billion.

Incidence
- Increased since introduction of compulsory seatbelts in UK (1983).
- Head restraints reduce incidence.
- 300,000 new cases per annum (UK).
- 5% of UK population will be involved in a rear-end collision.

Pathology
- Hyperextension of neck due to fixed trunk and unsupported head.
- Muscle tears, ligamentous disruption, retropharyngeal haematoma, disruption of sympathetic chain, facet joint haemarthrosis, posterior disc herniation, cartilage plate clefts.
- Long-term pain linked to facet joint injury.

History and examination
- Neck pain (98%) radiating to occiput, shoulders, and upper limb within 48h.
- Delayed presentation in 35% of patients.
- LBP often overlooked.
- Visual, auditory, and vestibular symptoms.
- Symptoms often disproportionate to physical signs of:
  - Stiffness (87%)
  - Tenderness (64%)
  - Neurological deficit (17%)
  - Postural abnormality (12%).

Classification
- Impact on lifestyle (see Table 11.5)[1]
- Information on prognosis (see Table 11.6).

Investigations
- No diagnostic test.
- Poor correlation between symptoms and findings on X-ray, scintigraphy, and MRI.
- Radiographs only indicated for high-velocity injury.
- MRI for neurological compromise.

Table 11.5 Gargan and Bannister grading of whiplash severity (1990)[1]

Grade A	No symptoms
Grade B	Nuisance symptoms. Do not interfere with occupation or leisure
Grade C	Intrusive symptoms requiring intermittent analgesia, orthotics, or physical therapy
Grade D	Disabling symptoms. Requiring time off work and regular analgesia, orthotics, and repeated medical consultation

Table 11.6 Quebec classification of prognosis (1995)[2]

Grade 0	No symptoms or signs
Grade I	Symptoms of neck pain or stiffness but no signs
Grade II	Neck symptoms and objective stiffness and point tenderness
Grade III	Neck symptoms and neurological deficit
Grade IV	Neck symptoms and fracture/dislocation

Treatment

Controversial as 50% of rear-end road traffic collisions are asymptomatic.

Acute

'Active rehabilitation' most effective approach:
- Promote early return to usual activities.
- No evidence for collar immobilization.
- Physiotherapy probably useful in early stages.
- Zygapophyseal joint pain may be treated by LA injection or percutaneous RF neurotomy.
- Analgesia/NSAIDs limited role.
- 0.5% require surgery (poor results).
- High-dose methylprednisolone may decrease number of symptoms and length of sick leave—controversial.

Chronic

- Multidisciplinary team approach including rehabilitation and Pain Management Programmes.
- Chiropractic treatment may help long-term symptoms.
- Must address psychological response to pain.
- Use of antidepressants effective if PTSD apparent.
- CBT may be of benefit.

Outcome
- Best assessment after 3 months following injury.
- Patients attending Emergency Departments for treatment of whiplash have a 33% risk of developing chronic whiplash syndromes.
- Final state is reached by 97% at 2 years.
- 93% asymptomatic patients at 3 months postinjury will still be asymptomatic at 2 years.
- 86% symptomatic patients at 3 months postinjury will still be so at 2 years.
- The more severe the initial symptoms, the more likely they are to persist.

Risk factors for worse prognosis
- Rear-end road traffic collision
- Front seat passenger
- Headache
- Radicular symptoms and signs
- Severity of initial symptoms
- Previous whiplash injury
- Neck tenderness
- Muscle pain
- Pre-injury axial pain
- Anxiety and depression
- Frequent GP attendance.

Behaviour, psychology, and litigation
Biopsychosocial model applies:
- Biological component of whiplash is significant in the acute phase, but chronic symptoms appear to be attributable to psychological effects of symptoms and social factors.
- Patients rarely exhibit symptoms for financial gain.
- 10–40% have psychological symptoms (still present at 15 years).
- Psychological distress is probably caused by pain.
- Resolution of psychological distress can follow resolution of pain.
- Litigation probably does not affect outcome.

References
1 Gargan MF, Bannister GC (1990). Long term prognosis of soft-tissue injuries of the neck. *Journal of Bone and Joint Surg (Br).* **72**: 901–3.
2 Spitzar WO, *et al* (1995). Scientific monograph of the Quebec Task Force on Whiplash associated disorders: redefining 'Whiplash' and its management. *Spine.* **85**: 1–73.

Chest pain

Pain arising in the thorax is a common experience for patients, but despite this there is a lack of reliable chest pain prevalence data. One study in the USA showed a prevalence of 12% for chest pain occurring for more than a whole day within the previous 6 months.

Many patients with chest pain are referred to specialist chest pain clinics run by cardiologists. The majority of patients attending such clinics will not have a cardiac cause for their symptoms.

Aetiology

Chest pain can either be visceral, somatic, or neuropathic in origin.

Visceral pain arises from:
- The heart, pericardium, or great vessels
- The lungs and pleura
- The upper GI tract, mainly the oesophagus.

Somatic pain is musculoskeletal in origin and arises from:
- Cervical and thoracic spine
- Joints (mainly costochondral)
- Muscles
- Periosteum.

Neuropathic pains can arise from damage to intercostal nerves following trauma, neoplasm, or surgery.

⚠ Assessment of chest pain

Some conditions presenting as chest pain are life threatening if not treated adequately and promptly. A thorough history and examination can often lead to the correct diagnosis. For example, central crushing chest pain precipitated by exercise and relieved by rest is indicative of myocardial ischaemia. Sharp stabbing pain brought on by deep inspiration and accompanied by breathlessness suggests a pleural or lung cause for the symptoms. Depending on the history the appropriate investigation should confirm or refute the diagnosis, allowing the patient to receive prompt treatment.

Cardiac chest pain

The most important diagnostic distinction to make when assessing a patient with chest pain is whether or not the pain is arising from the heart. Any underlying, organic, treatable pathology of the heart, pericardium, or great vessels must be identified and referred to cardiological services to prevent unnecessary suffering and possible premature death.

Angina pectoris

Angina pectoris is pain due to myocardial ischaemia. It is usually due to reduced blood supply secondary to coronary artery disease (CAD) but can also be due to increased myocardial oxygen demand (e.g. with left ventricular hypertrophy). The symptoms associated with myocardial ischaemia show considerable interindividual variation. They can include:

- Central chest tightness, heaviness, pressure, burning, or pain
- Fear and anxiety
- Suffocating breathlessness.

However, many episodes of myocardial ischaemia are entirely symptom-free.

Patients suspected of suffering with CAD or having any other cause of angina pectoris should be referred to and investigated by a cardiologist. Once the correct diagnosis has been made appropriate treatment will be instigated. Treatment for CAD is either prognostic, i.e. expected to prolong the patient's life, or palliative, i.e. expected to improve the quality of the patient's life.

Interventional prognostic treatments available to cardiologists and cardiothoracic surgeons include coronary artery bypass grafting (CABG) and percutaneous coronary intervention (PCI) with either balloon angioplasty or stenting or both. These treatments are only prognostic when disease in the coronary arteries is in the left main stem, when there is 3-vessel disease with ventricular dysfunction, or 2-vessel disease with proximal left main stem stenosis and ventricular dysfunction.

Pharmacological prognostic treatments include the use of antianginal drugs designed to reduce myocardial ischaemia and antiplatelet drugs designed to reduce the likelihood of a subsequent MI.

The palliative treatments offered by the majority of cardiologists and cardiothoracic surgeons are identical to the prognostic treatments.

There are many patients who benefit from this ischaemia-based model of management—their lives are lengthened and the quality of their lives is improved. However, there are also many patients who still suffer with angina pectoris despite appropriate interventions and optimal medical/surgical management.

Chronic refractory angina

Chronic refractory angina (CRA) is defined as: chronic stable angina that persists despite optimal medical therapy and when revascularization is either unfeasible or where the risks are unjustified.

It is a complex pain condition caused by myocardial ischaemia and results not only in pain, but severe psychological consequences for the sufferer, their relatives, and friends. Many patients with CRA believe that each episode of angina represents a small heart attack and causes more damage to the heart. Most believe it is important to avoid anything that precipitates an attack of angina. These beliefs are maladaptive and are likely to increase the risk of subsequent MI rather than to reduce it. There is evidence that short periods of ischaemia both promote new vessel growth and protect the myocardium from further ischaemic insult (pre-conditioning).

Patients with CRA attend and are admitted to hospital on a regular basis due to their symptoms. It has been acknowledged by both the American College of Cardiology and the European Society of Cardiology that patient education and rehabilitation are important at the outset of angina management. Both societies admit that these areas are often neglected.

A recent audit has shown that a multidisciplinary pain management approach to the treatment of patients with CRA results in a reduction in the rate of hospitalization.

Treatment model

The aim of treatment is to improve quality of life by improving both psychological and physical function. Ideally treatments should be delivered by a multidisciplinary team comprising a cardiologist, pain physician, psychologist, clinical nurse specialist, and specialist physiotherapist.

The diagnosis of chronic stable angina where revascularization is no longer considered feasible should be established at the outset of treatment. Anti-anginal medication should be optimized. Treatment then follows the stepwise approach outlined here.

Patient education and counselling

The most important element of the treatment process for patients with CRA is education and counselling about their condition. As noted earlier, many patients with CRA have unhelpful beliefs about angina and the best way of managing it. A thorough explanation of the condition and an exploration of patient beliefs are vital at the beginning of any treatment programme. It is also useful to agree realistic and achievable goals of treatment at the outset of the programme with both patient and their family.

Rehabilitation

The importance of rehabilitation for patients following a MI is well recognized and programmes are widely available. Rehabilitation for patients with CRA should follow a similar regimen, including risk factor reduction, exercise, lifestyle advice, relaxation training, and psychosocial support.

Multidisciplinary Pain Management Programmes

It has been demonstrated that a cognitive behavioural chronic disease management approach to patients with angina has a significant impact on their symptoms. This improves frequency and stability of angina, quality of life, and reduces anxiety and depression.

Transcutaneous electrical nerve stimulation

There is some evidence to suggest that 40–70% of patients will report significant symptom reduction with the use of a TENS machine. There have been concerns that TENS may predispose to dysrhythmias, but this has proved unfounded. The usual treatment method is to stimulate for 1h 3x daily as prophylaxis and then use the machine on demand should angina occur.

Sympathetic blockade

Left stellate ganglion block with LA is sometimes useful in the treatment of CRA, but there is limited supporting evidence. If effective this usually only provides temporary relief, lasting weeks to months at best.

Spinal cord stimulation

There is good evidence to support the clinical effectiveness of SCS in reducing the frequency of angina and improving the quality of life. There is also evidence to support the safety of the technique. However, these improvements have taken place in a clinical trials environment and when used outside of this environment the effectiveness is questionable. NICE recently reviewed the use of spinal cord simulators and concluded that there was insufficient evidence on survival and benefits in terms of quality of life to recommend the routine use of SCS in the treatment of patients with CRA. They did condone the use of SCS in the context of research as part of a clinical trial.

Opioids

Opioids have been used in the treatment of CRA when the earlier discussed measures have failed to adequately control symptoms. There is anecdotal evidence of their effectiveness but little in the way of controlled trials.

Syndrome X

Patients with Syndrome X have typical angina symptoms induced by exercise and a positive exercise stress test with normal coronary angiograms and normal left ventricular function at rest. It is more common in women and is associated with a normal life expectancy.

CBT has been shown to improve symptoms, quality of life, and social activities. A variety of pharmacological interventions, including β-blockers, ACE inhibitors, TCAs, calcium channel blockers, nitrates, adenosine antagonists, are all used with limited supporting evidence. There is also limited evidence for the use of spinal cord simulators, TENS, and pain management programmes.

Pericardium

Recurrent pericarditis can give rise to disabling symptoms similar to angina. There are 2 clinical syndromes: incessant pericarditis and intermittent pericarditis. Initially these may present with an effusion, cardiac tamponade, heart failure, or arrhythmias but these are rare during relapses when chest pain is the predominant symptom. Treatment is symptomatic with NSAIDs and colchicine.

Upper gastrointestinal tract

Pain from the upper GI tract can mimic angina pectoris. Thus a cardiac cause must first be excluded. Subsequently a cause–effect relationship between the pain and a GI abnormality must be established and treatment of the problem should result in relief of the pain.

The most common cause of chest pain originating in the upper GI tract is gastro-oesophageal reflux disease (GORD). A trial of PPIs is often successful in treating the symptoms and can remove the need for further investigations.

Pain due to GI motility dysfunction is difficult to diagnose due to a lack of correlation between pain and positive findings in oesophageal motility tests. There is also no gold standard treatment for these disorders. Botulinum toxin injection at the gastro-oesophageal junction has been reported to be effective in some cases.

Musculoskeletal chest pain

Musculoskeletal problems are the third most common cause of chest pain after cardiac and upper GI causes. These patients tend to have pain on palpation of the chest wall and pain following certain movements or in certain postures.

Costochondritis is the most common cause of musculoskeletal chest pain. Recreational drug abuse, diabetes, infection, and cardiac surgery all predispose to costochondritis. Many different treatments are used including NSAIDs, steroid injections and very occasionally, more invasive surgery.

Tietze's syndrome is costochondritis with swelling of the affected costochondral joint.

Note - referred musculoskeletal chest pain can arise from either the thoracic or cervical spine. Diagnosis is by exclusion and treatment is identical to that for mechanical LBP.

Chronic abdominal pain

Abdominal pain is one of the most common reasons patients present to health care services. Acute abdominal pain is usually due to underlying organic pathology which must be identified and treated appropriately.

Causes of acute abdominal pain include:
- Infection or inflammation
- Musculoskeletal problems
- Neoplasm
- Gynaecological conditions
- Neurological disorders.

A medical history, physical examination, and the appropriate investigations must be carried out in order to identify treatable organic pathology.

Chronic abdominal pain is frequently not associated with any identifiable organic pathology and is often referred to as 'functional gastrointestinal disorder'. Organic causes of chronic abdominal pain include pancreatitis, carcinoma of the pancreas, and inflammatory bowel disease.

Chronic pancreatitis

Chronic inflammation of the pancreas results in permanent cell death, calcification, and ductal fibrosis. Excess alcohol consumption is the primary aetiological factor in 70–80% of cases. The majority of the remainder are said to be idiopathic.

The symptoms of chronic pancreatitis include:
- Severe epigastric pain: with frequent exacerbations and spontaneous resolution
- Steatorrhoea: due to pancreatic insufficiency
- Malnutrition: if associated with excess alcohol.

There is little good evidence on which to base the treatment of pain associated with chronic pancreatitis. The following options are generally recommended:
- Abstinence from alcohol
- Opioid analgesics
- NSAIDs
- Endoscopic treatment of blocked ducts and stones
- Oral pancreatic enzyme treatment
- Neurolytic coeliac plexus blocks (see 📖 Coeliac plexus block p.210)
- Surgical diversion or resection
- Pseudocyst drainage.

Evidence to support the use of coeliac plexus blocks in non-malignant chronic pancreatitis is conflicting. If blocks are effective, their duration of action is often limited, requiring retreatment. There is also the potential for side effects such as chronic diarrhoea and rare but potentially catastrophic neurological sequelae.

Care must be taken when treating alcoholic pancreatitis with opioid medication due to the potential for opioid misuse and addiction. Due to the difficulty in achieving adequate analgesia in these patients, a biopsychosocial approach is essential.

Carcinoma of the pancreas

70% of pancreatic tumours originate in exocrine tissue in the head of the pancreas. ♂ predominate with an incidence of 2:1, it is more common in black people and in those from developed countries. The most common presentation is with abdominal pain, weight loss, and jaundice.

The pain of pancreatic cancer is usually located in the central upper abdomen and often radiates through to the back. It is severe in 20–30% of patients at presentation and in 80% of patients with advanced disease.

Treatment of pain secondary to carcinoma of the pancreas involves use of the following modalities:
- Opioid analgesics
- NSAIDs
- Curative surgery
- Palliative surgery
- Neurolytic coeliac plexus blocks
- Psychological support
- Palliative medicine involvement.

The evidence for coeliac plexus blocks in malignant pancreatic pain is far better than that for non-malignant pain. Several studies show a reduction in opioid requirements and improved quality of life.

Inflammatory bowel disease

Ulcerative colitis and Crohn's disease are the commonest GI inflammatory disorders that present with pain as one of their initial symptoms. The medical and surgical treatment of these conditions is beyond the scope of this handbook. There is no specific treatment for the pain associated with these inflammatory bowel disorders.

Functional gastrointestinal disorder

A diagnosis of functional gastrointestinal disorder (FGID) can only be made once underlying organic pathology has been excluded. Characteristic symptoms include pain and alterations in GI function such as diarrhoea, constipation, and dysphagia. Only conditions where pain is a predominant feature will be discussed.

The underlying mechanism for pain in FGID has not been fully identified but it seems likely that there is an alteration in the perception of visceral afferent stimuli (visceral hypersensitivity).

Irritable bowel syndrome

Irritable bowel syndrome (IBS) is the most common FGID. It is a diagnosis of exclusion based on accepted diagnostic criteria (Rome II).[1]
- No identifiable organic cause
- 12 weeks of continuous or recurrent symptoms of pain or discomfort within any 12 months:
  - Relieved by defecation
  - Or associated with a change in stool consistency
  - Or with a change in stool frequency.

The prevalence of IBS has been reported to be 4–14%. Up to 70% of referrals to gastroenterologists are for symptoms compatible with the diagnosis of IBS. It is approximately twice as prevalent in women compared to men.

IBS is commonly associated with psychiatric disorders such as:
- Generalized anxiety disorder
- Panic disorder
- PTSD
- Depression.

IBS is also commonly associated with other chronic pain conditions:
- Fibromyalgia
- Chronic fatigue syndrome
- Migraine
- Interstitial cystitis.

There is no specific treatment for IBS. The following have some evidence to support their use:
- Patient education
- Dietary modification
- Pharmacological therapy:
  - TCAs
  - SSRIs
  - Antispasmodics
- Psychological therapy.

Functional dyspepsia

Functional dyspepsia (FD) is also a diagnosis of exclusion. It is defined as persistent or recurrent upper abdominal pain with no detectable underlying organic pathology. Diagnostic criteria include 12 weeks of persistent or recurrent dyspepsia which is not relieved by defecation or associated with change in bowel habit.

There is considerable overlap with IBS. Many patients exhibit symptoms compatible with both diagnoses at different times. Treatment options are similar to those described for IBS.

Functional abdominal pain syndrome

The diagnostic criteria for functional abdominal pain syndrome (FAPS) include 6 months with the following features:
- Continuous pain
- No relationship with physiological events such as eating or defecation
- Loss of daily functioning
- No evidence of malingering.

FAPS is less common than IBS or FD, the prevalence being around 2%.

Health care utilization and health-related absence from work are more common in patients with FAPS. Treatment options are as described for IBS.

Reference

1 Drossman DA (2006). *Gastroenterology*. **130**: 1377–90.

Chronic pelvic pain

Definition
Intermittent or constant pain in the lower abdomen or pelvis persisting for >6 months.

Epidemiology
A common problem affecting up to 1 in 6 of the adult ♀ population and accounting for up to 50% of gynaecological laparoscopies performed.

Aetiology
- Secondary to gynaecological, urological, GI, and musculoskeletal pathology.
- Also occurs in individuals with no signs of disease, 'CPP without obvious pathology'.
- Pain often multifactorial, many different components need to be addressed during assessment and management.
- Due to overlap in the sensory innervation of pelvic structures, symptoms can be difficult to relate to specific organs or systems, causing difficulties in diagnosis.

History
- A full history must be taken focusing particularly on the genitourinary, GI, and musculoskeletal systems.
- Pain tools (e.g. questionnaires, VAS, and pain diaries) can be used to gain an accurate pain assessment and symptom-based tools detect psychological comorbidity.

Examination
Thorough physical examination (including gynaecological, rectal, and neurological) should be performed by appropriate specialists.

Investigations
Results of all previous examinations, investigations, and surgery must be collated. Multidisciplinary input is required to enable appropriate investigation.

Initial tests may include
- Blood investigations (FBC, U&E, ESR)
- Urine, cervical, urethral, and possibly stool cultures
- Radiological investigations such as US and perhaps CT and MRI
- Further investigation depends on individual presentation.

Gynaecological causes
Cyclic pelvic pain (dysmenorrhoea)
Pain typically suprapubic, cramping with radiation to the back, normally lasting 48h after onset of menses.
   Affects up to 50% of women of reproductive age:
- Primary (no underlying disease state present)
- Secondary (e.g. to endometriosis or fibroids).

Treatment options
- NSAIDs and oral contraceptive pill (OCP)
- TENS and acupuncture
- Neuroablative treatment.

Adhesions (secondary to surgery, infection, endometriosis)
- Pain typically associated with sexual intercourse—dyspareunia.
- Found in up to 50% of patients undergoing laparoscopy for investigation of pain, but the role of adhesions in pelvic pain is uncertain.

Treatment
- Adhesionolysis controversial (some studies show a successful outcome only in patients with bowel obstruction or dense vascular adhesions).
- Meticulous surgical technique is the only recommended method to prevent further adhesions secondary to surgery.

Endometriosis
Characterized by dysmenorrhoea, dyspareunia, and CPP. May present as an incidental finding at laparoscopy. There is generally poor correlation between clinical symptoms and extent of disease.

Medical treatment
- Hormone analogues/OCP
- Simple oral analgesia.

Surgical treatment
- Laparoscopy (+histology) enables definitive diagnosis and treatment opportunities (e.g. laser ablation or resection).
- Total abdominal hysterectomy and bilateral salpingo-oophrectomy.

Ovarian pain
- Mittelschmerz (mid-cycle pain at the time of ovulation).
- Cysts (pain through torsion or compression of nearby structures).
- Ovarian remnant syndrome (ovarian cortical tissue left *in situ* during surgery can become cystic and functional causing cyclic or constant pain).

Treatment
- Remnant suppression with gonadotropin-releasing hormone (GnRH) analogues, OCP, and danazol.
- Removal of remnants—laparotomy (rather than laparoscopy) is favoured as it reduces the risk of complications secondary to extensive adhesions which are often present.

Pelvic congestion
Ovarian dysfunction can lead to excessive production of local oestrogen, causing dilatation and stasis in the pelvic veins. Pain is typically dull and aching, aggravated by activities increasing intra-abdominal pressure (e.g. standing). Can be diagnosed on US or CT, venography enables definitive diagnosis.

Treatment
- Medroxyprogesterone acetate as an ovarian suppressant
- Ovarian vein ligation or embolization
- Hysterectomy and bilateral salpingo-oophrectomy.

Salpingo-oophritis
Normally a cause of acute pain but may lead to adhesions and chronic pain if untreated.

Malignancy
Ovarian tumours or uterine leiomyoma cause poorly localized lower abdominal discomfort associated with fullness and a mass on palpation.

Urinary causes

Interstitial cystitis
A clinical syndrome characterized by:
- Urinary urgency, frequency, and nocturia
- Pelvic pain (localized to the abdomen, pelvis, groin, or perineum).

Diagnosis
Cystoscopy may reveal mucosal ulcers or glomerulations, urothelial disruption, and exposure of bladder sensory nerves in severe cases. May show normal appearances.

Treatment
No treatment is universally accepted for interstitial cystitis, options include:
- Initially antihistamines, TCAs, and antispaspodics.
- Intravesical glycosaminoglycan (e.g. hyaluronidase).
- Opioids (controversial).
- Diet changes (avoiding acidic foods).
- TENS.
- Sacral nerve stimulation (good for urinary symptoms but less for pain) or hypogastric plexus blocks.

Recurrent infectious cystitis
Dysuria, frequency, urgency, suprapubic pain + positive urine cultures.

Treatment
- Appropriate antibiotics (sometimes prophylactic).
- Vaginal oestrogen creams may be of use in peri- and postmenopausal women.

Urethral syndrome
- Lower urinary tract symptoms in the absence of obvious infection or urethral abnormality.
- May be due to chronic inflammation of the periurethral glands secondary to subclinical infection.

Treatment
- Antibiotics
- Urethral dilatation
- Vaginal oestrogen creams.

Carcinoma
- Often presents as asymptomatic haematuria.
- Pain may result from metastases or urinary obstruction.

Treatment
- Chemotherapy, radiotherapy, surgery as appropriate
- NSAID and opioid analgesia.

Gastrointestinal causes
- Endometriosis affecting bowel
- Hernias (inguinal, femoral, incisional, umbilical) leading to small bowel obstruction
- Inflammatory bowel disease
- IBS
- Diverticular disease of colon.

Neurological causes
- Neuroma, e.g. scar pain following surgery (e.g. incidence of chronic pain after Pfannenstiel incision is 3.7%)
- Neuralgias of ilioinguinal, iliohypogastric, genitofemoral nerves secondary to injury, surgery, or due to muscular impingement.

Musculoskeletal causes
- Fibromyalgia
- Lumbar, thoracic, sacral spinal disorders
- Musculoskeletal pain may result from postural changes secondary to pain.

Chronic pelvic pain without obvious pathology
- A diagnosis of exclusion when investigation has not identified pathology.
- The diagnosis does not assume that pain is psychological in origin.
- Management is as for other chronic pain syndromes and should be multidisciplinary.

Vulvodynia
Definition
- Burning vulval discomfort with dyspareunia, stinging, irritation, and soreness.
- Commonest form is idiopathic (vulval vestibulitis syndrome) but can be secondary to definite pathology (candidiasis or vulvitis, vulvar papillomatosis).

Management

Treatment aims

The multifactorial nature of pelvic pain should be discussed with the patient from the start and a management plan agreed to aim for near normal functioning, rather than a cure. Referral to a specialist pain clinic should be considered.

Medical treatment

Large randomized studies evaluating different analgesics are lacking; however the following have been used successfully:

- NSAIDs
- Opioids, (the use of opioids for non-cancer pain remains controversial and requires regular follow-up, see 📖 Opioids for chronic non-cancer pain p.162)
- Antidepressants (e.g. low dose tricyclics)
- Anticonvulsants
- OCP, GnRH agonists etc. for cyclic pelvic pain.

Surgical treatment

Diagnostic laparoscopy/adhesionolysis

Laparoscopy for evaluation ± treatment of CPP remains controversial, as pathology identified at laparoscopy doesn't necessarily account for pain experienced. It is potentially of benefit in patients with known dense adhesions or endometriosis.

Hysterectomy

Indicated for women with cyclic pelvic pain or dysfunctional uterine bleeding uncontrolled with medical management, with no identifiable pathology. Importantly, pain may persist following hysterectomy (up to 1 in 4 patients).

Presacral neurectomy (superior hypogastric plexus transaction)

The superior hypogastric plexus carries pain afferents from the upper vagina, cervix, uterus, and proximal fallopian tube as well as the bladder and bowel. Transection (via laparotomy or laparoscopy) is used for midline pelvic pain not responding to medical management. Potential complications include long-term constipation and urinary retention.

Nerve blocks and trigger point injections

LA blocks (including caudal epidurals) may provide relief from neuralgic pain and can be both diagnostic and therapeutic.

Alternative therapies
Small studies have shown improvement in pain with acupuncture, hypnosis, and chiropractic treatments.

Psychological management
CPP may be associated with underlying psychological issues such as depression, relationship problems, and abuse. Assessment and appropriate management by experts is an important part of the multidisciplinary approach to CPP.

Patients with CPP require psychological input (e.g. CBT, relaxation, and psychotherapy) for management of potential underlying psychological disorders and to help them overcome the effects of the condition.

The multidisciplinary approach
Studies have shown improved results when a team approach is adopted. Referral to pain clinics should be considered as pain centres generally achieve better results than those seen with efforts within a single specialty.

Non-obstetric pain in pregnancy

Pain management principles

Uncontrolled non-obstetric pain occurring in pregnancy presents a problem for conventional pharmacotherapy because of placental drug transfer and the potential for congenital malformation. With the exception of heparin and insulin, nearly all medications reach the fetus to some extent. The most critical period for minimizing maternal drug exposure is the phase of organogenesis from the 4th to the 10th week of pregnancy. Neonates receive 1–2% of the maternal dose of most medications through breastfeeding.

Drug treatment

Epidemiological studies have shown that:

- *Paracetamol* is safe in recommended doses.
- *NSAIDs*: miscarriage risk unproven. Stop 8–6 weeks prior to delivery to reduce risk of persistent fetal circulation, impaired renal function, and bleeding tendency in neonates.
- *Opioids*: no evidence of teratogenicity.
- *LAs*: lidocaine and bupivacaine pose no significant developmental risk to the fetus. No studies of mexiletine.
- *Steroids*: single maternal doses of depot steroid in regional anaesthetic techniques are of low risk to the fetus.
- *Diazepam*: studies have confirmed an association with congenital inguinal hernia but not cleft palate.
- *Antidepressants*: amitriptyline is not associated with birth malformation. Maternal imipramine use linked to neonatal CV defects.
- *Anticonvulsants*: carbamazepine, valproate, and phenytoin use in epilepsy may cause fetal neural tube defects. Continuation of therapy requires monitoring of serum drug levels, folate supplementation, and maternal α-fetoprotein screening for neural tube defects. Their use should be avoided in the management of non-obstetric pain in pregnancy.

Back pain

Back pain is experienced by 50% of mothers during pregnancy. It is more prevalent in young mothers and multiparous women. Biomechanically pain correlates with the relative change in centre of gravity and increase in abdominal girth. Pain may be low lumbar-reducing with gestation or sacroiliac-increasing as pregnancy progresses.

Symphyseal pain

Symphyseal pain is less common than back pain and usually associated with sacroiliac pain. US evidence of symphyseal widening may be present but pain intensity and duration is unrelated to the degree of widening. Pain is usually limited to the gestational period.

Symphyseal diastasis

Incidence: 1:300–30,000 deliveries.

Clinical features
- Antepartum: nil or audible crack, pubic/groin/leg pain in 2nd stage of labour.
- Postpartum: pubic swelling and pain, sacroiliac pain, waddling gait.

Associated factors
- Multiparity
- Fetal macrosomia
- Pathological joint laxity
- Exaggerated abduction of thighs
- Masked by epidural anaesthesia.

Treatment
- Bed rest
- Abdominal binder
- Mild analgesics
- Intrasymphyseal injection of lidocaine and depot steroid, cryoanalgesia, and epidural analgesia have been successful in severe cases.

Recovery
- Typically complete in 4–6 weeks postpartum.

Bone marrow oedema syndrome

Definition
Transient osteoporosis of the hip in pregnancy.

Clinical features
- Pain on weight bearing
- Gait disturbance
- Onset usually in 3rd trimester.

Diagnosis
- MRI shows evidence of bone marrow oedema and joint effusion.

Treatment
- Limitation of weight bearing, bed rest
- Oral analgesia.

Recovery
- Early postpartum
- MRI changes may persist until after cessation of lactation.

Visceral referred pain

The acute abdomen in a pregnant patient may present with an atypical pattern of pain because the anterior abdominal wall is separated from the viscera by the enlarged uterus. Acute appendicitis is the most common emergency (1:1500–1:6600 deliveries), followed by bowel obstruction and cholecystitis. Ectopic pregnancy can present as a painful inner thigh, caused by a tubal pregnancy compressing the obturator nerve.

Mononeuropathies of pregnancy

Spontaneous persistent neurogenic or neuropathic somatic pains associated with pregnancy and recurring in subsequent pregnancies are uncommon. Their aetiology may be related to the water retention associated with pregnancy or simple stretching of neural tissue by the gravid uterus. The differential diagnosis must always include consideration of visceral referred pain.

Carpal tunnel syndrome

1:20 pregnant women experience symptoms of CTS. The majority recover spontaneously immediately postpartum.

Clinical features
- Painful nocturnal paraesthesiae of the palmar surface of the hands
- Severity related to manual activity
- Sensory blunting in territory of the median nerve
- Rarely motor signs.

Treatment
- Night splint, wrist neutral/slight extension
- Steroid injection to carpal tunnel.

Meralgia paraesthetica
- Greek 'meros'—thigh, 'algos'—pain.
- In mild form a common affliction.

Cause
- Inguinal compression of the lateral cutaneous nerve of thigh
- 50% cadavers show nerve enlargement/pseudoganglion.

Clinical features
- Burning sensation/numbness anterolateral thigh.
- Worse on standing, walking, hip extension, relieved by sitting, lying.
- May present postpartum and be falsely attributed to epidural block.

Treatment
- Reassurance, usually resolves spontaneously postpartum.
- Avoid tight belts, standing for long periods.
- For persistent burning/paraesthesiae—LA ± depot steroid injection.

Iliohypogastric neuralgia

Incidence 1:3000–5000 pregnancies, 2nd or 3rd trimester.

Cause
- Nerve stretching with uterine enlargement; anterolateral entrapment by abdominal musculature.

Clinical features
- Severe pain in lower abdominal quadrant, over iliac crest or flank.
- Hyper or hypoaesthesia in nerve distribution.

Differential diagnosis: renal colic, perforated appendix, diverticulitis, volvulus, ovarian cyst/torsion, abruptio placentae.

Treatment
- Iliohypogastric nerve block ± depot steroid medial to anterior superior iliac spine. Cryothermy may be used for persistent pain.

Intercostal neuralgia

Limited to case reports.

Cause

- Probable stretching of lateral branch of intercostal nerve as it emerges through muscle layers in the midaxillary line to become subcutaneous.

Clinical features

- Neurogenic pain anteriorly in an intercostal dermatome distribution.
- Altered sensation over the same area.
- Usually T 7–11 unilaterally.
- Pain ↑ with gestational age.
- Spontaneous recovery postpartum.
- Re-occurrence in subsequent pregnancies.

Differential diagnosis: cholecystitis, duodenal ulceration, threatened abortion, premature labour, pre-eclamptic pain.

Treatment

- Intercostal nerve block at point of pain origin in midaxillary line—LA ± depot steroid injection.
- In late pregnancy, continuous low-dose epidural analgesia.

Bell's palsy

♀ of reproductive age affected 2–4x more often than ♂. Pregnant women are 3x more at risk than non-pregnant. The majority of cases occur in the 3rd trimester.

Cause

Unknown. Possible link with development of hypertensive disorders.
Clinical features:
- May begin with acute otalgia.
- Ipsilateral 7th cranial lower motor neuron palsy.
- Hyperacusis through involvement of nerve to stapedius.
- Decreased taste anterior 2/3 of tongue (chorda tympani).

Treatment

- Supportive care, analgesia.
- Use of oral corticosteroids is controversial in pregnancy. Benefit is maximal when used within 48h of onset.

Recovery

- Slow but satisfactory for those with incomplete paralysis.
- The prognosis for recovery of complete paralysis is poor.

Sciatica

True sciatica occurs in 1:10,000 pregnancies.

Myofascial pain/fibromyalgia

- Myofascial pain is a common cause of pain affecting most people at some stage in their life, as skeletal muscle can make up 50% of body weight.
- Muscular spasm/myofascial pain accounts for a large part of chronic ongoing pain for many patients.
- About 10% of the population has a chronic widespread muscular pain.
- Fibromyalgia is more common in ♀, age 40–50 years. There is no racial or social predisposition identified.

Definition

Myofascial pain

Is associated with taut bands of muscle fibres called myofascial trigger points (MTrP).

Clinical characteristics of MTrP include:

- Compression causes local or specific referred pain in the area where the patient normally experiences pain.
- Rapid compression across the fibres may elicit a 'local twitch response'.
- Restricted range of stretch may cause tightening of the muscle group.
- Muscle weakness without significant atrophy.
- There may be associated autonomic phenomena (e.g. sweating, tinnitus).

Abnormal stress on muscle groups are thought to be common causes for MTrP. Perpetuating factors can be structural (e.g. scoliosis, joint laxity), mechanical (e.g. poor posture), or metabolic.

Fibromyalgia

(both diagnostic criteria need to be satisfied)[1]

- History of widespread pain of 3 or more months' duration:
  - Pain in at least 2 contralateral quadrants of the body and
  - Axial skeletal pain.
- Pain in 11 of the 18 trigger points (Fig. 11.1) on digital palpation with a force of 4kg (sufficient to blanch a finger nail).

Associated with sleep disturbance. (EEG studies have shown reduced deep (non-REM) sleep).

Differential diagnosis

Exclude reversible causes for myofascial pain:

- Hypothyroidism: TFTs.
- Systemic lupus: FBC, ESR, plasma viscosity, anti-nuclear factor.
- Inflammatory myopathy: creatinine kinase.
- Hyperparathyroidism/osteomalacia: Ca^{2+}, alkaline phosphatase, vitamin D.

⚠ The symptoms of fibromyalgia can occasionally be a presentation of an underlying pathology, e.g. cancer.

Management

Education and reassurance is the key in helping patients to manage their condition. This requires a multidisciplinary team approach.

- Identification and correction of the perpetuating factors (e.g. improving poor posture).
- Trigger point therapy:
  - Self-massage (requires awareness of their MTrP and education on technique)
  - Dry needling
  - Stretch and spray (use of vapocoolant spray to temporarily relieve pain to allow stretch of the affected muscle group)
  - LA ± steroid injection
  - Acupuncture.
- Paced gradated exercise to improve fitness.
- Restoration of normal sleep pattern (medication, exercise).
- Relieve stress:
  - Relaxation techniques
  - Counselling
  - Biofeedback.
- Medication: low-dose TCAs, e.g. amitriptylline.

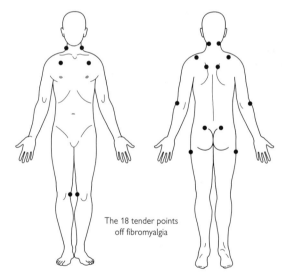

The 18 tender points off fibromyalgia

Fig. 11.1 Tender point location.

Reference

1 Wolfe F et al. (1990). The American College of Rheumatology 1990 Criteria for the classification of Fibromyalgia. *Arthritis and Rheumatism* **33**, 160–72.

Chronic fatigue syndrome/myalgic encephalopathy

- Classified by WHO as a neurological disorder (ICD 10, 1969).
- Population prevalence of 0.2–0.4% (NICE 2006).
- Chronic fatigue syndrome/myalgic encephalopathy (CFS/ME) is often misunderstood.
- Pain is one of the most debilitating symptoms of this condition.
- 70% of CFS/ME patients have widespread pain and trigger points that are comparable to fibromyalgia.
- Aetiology unclear.

Diagnostic criteria

CFS/ME is a diagnosis of exclusion; Fukuda criteria (1994), recommends the following tests to exclude alternative pathologies: FBC, ESR/CRP, U&E, Ca, liver/thyroid, creatinine kinase, glucose, urinalysis, and consider autoantibody tests to rule out other differential diagnoses.

Referral criteria to specialist services may vary in relation to recommended clinical tests, but it is imperative that any other causes of fatigue are excluded.

Clinical features

Clinical features may include:

- Pain and fatigue causing significant functional impairment
- Muscle wasting due to loss of activity (often rapid)
- Deconditioning—as a result of increasing pain and fatigue
- Light and chemical sensitivity
- Frequent infections
- Impaired concentration span and cognitive impairment
- High levels of distress
- Withdrawal from exposure to others.

25% of sufferers will have significant disability.

Fatigue

Often confused with persistent tiredness but unalleviated by rest, presenting as lethargy and malaise:

- Triggered by physical exertion (mild to vigorous).
- Sleeping throughout or regularly during the day to compensate for unrefreshing sleep. This can lead to sleep reversal patterns, and disrupted bodily rhythm that is challenging to realign.

Pain

This is variable dependent on several factors including exercise, activity, physical condition, and general symptom presentation. Not all individuals with CFS/ME experience pain, but for others, pain is their primary cause of distress. Pain can take the form of:

- Joint pain without swelling
- Muscular pain comparable to fibromyalgic symptoms.

In the initial 'flare-up', muscular and joint pain may be experienced as well as fatigue; the convalescing period of illness and consequent inactivity leads to deconditioned muscles which can contribute to pain when resuming exercise (especially if resuming too quickly). The knock-on effect of this experience may be a routine devoid of 'pain inducing activities', i.e. exercise (see Fig. 11.2). This avoidance feeds into the cycle of deconditioning and consequent pain and, after a time, pervasive pain can be triggered by relatively short periods in any fixed position. It is also possible that pain is experienced independently of this cycle but it cannot be easily differentiated, formulated or understood: It can be pervasive and widespread and often goes untreated.

CFS/ME can also present with other clusters of overlapping symptoms such as hyperventilation and hypermobility, causing increases in both fatigue and joint pain.

Cognitive difficulties

Memory and concentration/attention span is a source of difficulty for individuals with CFS/ME. These areas seem to be:

- Subjectively impaired.
- Often without a clear and consistent pattern.
- Exacerbated by high levels of fatigue and inactivity.
- Often referred to as 'brain fog'; CFS/ME can cause:
  - Feelings of confusion.
  - Inability to concentrate.
  - Headaches, dissimilar to those prior to onset and triggered by exertion, light sensitivity and noise, can also present independently.

These symptoms are often considered the most debilitating, as impact on interaction and daily functioning can be severe. This can be extremely anxiety provoking and can lead to social anxiety, low mood, and difficulties around self-esteem and confidence.

Management and treatment

Treatment is primarily aimed at

- Increasing levels of daily functioning
- Improving subjective quality of life
- Improving sleep (medication may be prescribed)
- Reducing pain (medication may be prescribed)
- Tackling bacterial infections (medication may be prescribed)
- Improving mood or addressing anxiety.

Due to chemical sensitivity, some individuals may be unable to regularly take medication. Currently there is no drug treatment of choice that has an overarching effect on symptomatic presentation of CFS/ME.

Questions remain regarding aetiology and there is no universal understanding of the cause, so attention is turning toward a biopsychosocial approach, already adopted in the management other chronic conditions, including pain. The focus is on managing symptoms and experience, taking account of the social and psychological impact of the condition.

For example, an individual who suffers increased pain and fatigue whilst standing for prolonged periods wishes to be able to clean dishes as they previously did. Due to the difficulty in adapting to change, they may push on through the pain and fatigue to do so, precipitating a flare-up/exacerbation of their symptoms.

Many individuals who feel disabled by an 'invisible' illness such as CFS/ME feel forced to choose between managing the pain and discomfiture of performing everyday tasks they were quite capable of pre-onset, and the guilt and embarrassment they experience when having to ask for help or failing to complete the task.

Strong emotions such as loss, anger, and fear are often experienced due to the dramatic course that CFS/ME can sometimes take.

Fear of increased symptoms or the possibility of decline cause some to avoid physical or challenging activities due to the perceived potential for relapse or worsening of symptoms. Others push on through at the cost of high levels of pain and fatigue. This can be the beginning of a 'boom and bust' cycle that prevents physical reconditioning and symptom management.

The boom and bust cycle represents the pattern of activity which is found in pain-related conditions; individuals do more than usual on a good day and then suffer the 'pay-back' of a flare-up and increase of symptoms. Symptoms abate and the cycle may repeat on the next good day. This can link into other cycles such as activity avoidance or continuing activity through pain and fatigue.

These cycles can become well established and difficult to break, so early intervention is imperative.

Learning to exercise and pace is often experienced as unachievable and too challenging, whilst struggling with a change in health status and the transition to a life that is multidimensionally changed.

Aim of interventions
- Address the 'boom and bust' cycle
- Develop skills in activity pacing
- Encourage self-management.

As illustrated in Fig. 11.2, continued activity during a flare-up period can cause rebound and increased symptoms. On the other hand, avoidance of activity due to pain and fatigue and the consequential physical deconditioning can also cause a rebound effect.

Individuals with CFS/ME often suffer repeated flare-ups. Prior to the implementation of activity pacing and finding baselines to work from, it is important to highlight the potential rebound effects of both inactivity and activity, aiming to shift the flow into 'recuperative rest'. From this point, pacing, goal settings, rest, and baselines become fundamental in managing this condition when in a flare-up period.

Pacing

Pacing involves:

- Setting realistic targets and goals.
- Breaking down goals into manageable chunks.
- Breaking down difficulties into small goals.

Breaking down goals into manageable chunks gives a sense of achievement and encouragement, and also dispels the fear related to focusing on getting completely 'better' all at once. Breaking difficulties down into small goals involves challenging thinking patterns and belief systems, from ideas like 'I have to do this, I have to get better' to taking a more measured, realistic, and practical approach to symptom management and improving quality of life. This is the basis of goal-setting and working from baselines.[†]

This approach also aims to equip service-users with the necessary skills to manage their sleep patterns, pace exercise and troubleshoot everyday tasks.

Emphasis is placed on identifying coping strategies that no longer work and finding more adaptive strategies around managing a chronic health condition.

Importance should also be placed on tailoring routines of activity and rest to accommodate symptoms and also activities with high levels of personal enjoyment. These routines can be adjusted as individuals improve and move away from the 'boom and bust' pattern.

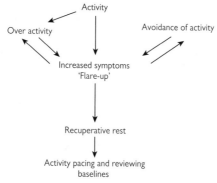

Fig. 11.2 The possible cycles of CFS/ME.

Rest

A significant aspect of this approach is scheduling appropriate recuperative rest. In the 'boom and bust' cycle, resting is often omitted but is an essential component to managing energy levels.

A good guide for the moderately affected is 10min every 1–2h. It is imperative that rest is used to recuperate and reduce the amount of pressure the body is under. 'Rest' represents a period without any stimulation which does not lead to sleep.

Activity schedules

Activity scheduling is a very effective behavioural intervention that highlights the amount of rest and physical or mental energy that activities demand: high, medium, or low. This should

- Indicate if a boom bust cycle exists.
- Identify if an individual is overdoing high and medium level activities.
- Enable an individual to plan energy management and rest in advance.
- Provide a strategy to prevent and manage relapse.
- Enable an individual to adopt a self-management approach to their condition.

Sleep hygiene

A primary intervention used in treating CFS/ME which encourages a move towards 'regular' sleeping hours and away from daytime napping. This is difficult to implement as symptoms often increase in severity during the period of change with positive effects not being immediate.

Scheduling more regular rests can assist throughout this transition although patients may struggle not to accidentally fall asleep, being used to sleeping in the daytime.

When successfully implemented there is often a definite shift in quality of life towards feeling able to lead a 'normal' life in relation to levels of social functioning and daily activities, and a subjective significant improvement in sleep quality and levels of pain and fatigue.

Reference

1 Gladwell P (2006). Practical guide for goal setting. In: Gifford L(ed). *Topical issues in pain 5*. CNS Press, Falmouth.

Pain in survivors of torture

This section covers specific issues concerned with pain arising as a result of torture: other chapters on assessment and treatment apply.

Torture

The World Medical Association *Declaration of Tokyo* (1975)[1] defines torture as 'the deliberate, systematic or wanton infliction of physical or mental suffering …' Torture is usually carried out to intimidate and destroy the individual and in doing so to intimidate others; to punish individuals and communities, and to divide and fragment communities. Most survivors are civilians; politically active or bystanders.
- Prevalence of torture is estimated to be up to 30–60% in refugees.
- Survivors have a high incidence of physical disability, e.g. amputation, as well as psychological and emotional difficulties.

Exile and asylum
- It is very difficult to arrive in the UK by legal means.
- Detention is common in countries of origin and of exile, and both are detrimental to physical and mental health.
- The asylum process is bureaucratic and confusing.
- Welfare support is meagre and work is usually forbidden.

Presentation
- Persistent pain is one of the most common effects of torture.
- Symptom reporting may be partial due to:
  - Impaired memory after psychological trauma, head injury, or loss of consciousness.
  - Shame and distress on remembering and disclosing torture, anticipation of disapproval, or disbelief from health-care worker.
  - Stigma associated with sexual torture in ♂ or ♀.
- Pain and health problems may be less urgent than welfare and legal ones.

Pain
- Ask sensitively about experiences of exile, imprisonment, torture, other forms of violence, and loss.
- Acknowledge torture, which others may have doubted; establish trust.
- Some of the commonest problems are:
  - Musculoskeletal and joint pains from beating, forced positions (oil drums, standing, etc.).
  - Pain and neurological deficits in limbs, from suspension by arms or legs.
  - Headache, ear pain, neuropsychological problems from beating to head.
  - Pain, sexual dysfunction, HIV, and STD from rape and sexual assault.
  - Pain in feet and lower legs, at rest or weight bearing, from falaka.
- Relationships between the type and severity of torture and subsequent persistent pain are frequently not straightforward.

- Consider ongoing causes of pain such as malunited fractures or pelvic infection.
- Multiple mechanisms may produce pain: for instance
  - Falaka may produce neuropathic pain in the feet, vascular insufficiency, damage to periosteal membrane, thickening of plantar fascia, secondary pain from gait disruption.
  - Suspension by the arms may produce total or partial lesion of the brachial plexus, damage to joint structures, overload injuries to soft tissue, secondary pain from adaptations to pain and weakness.
- Pain should be properly investigated and not simply attributed to 'somatization' of psychological distress.
- Chronic pain which has no obvious explanation may in some instances be associated with undisclosed sexual torture.
- Symptoms may be exacerbated by isolation, racist attacks or bullying.

Forms of torture
- Beatings
- Breaking limbs
- Burning
- Chaining
- Cutting and mutilation
- Cutting off limbs or organs
- Damage to teeth
- Deprivation of food or water
- Drowning
- Electrical assault
- Simulated execution
- Extreme heat and cold
- Extreme pressure to part of body
- Falaka (beating soles of feet)
- Forced positions
- Hooding
- Rape and sexual assault
- Removal of clothes
- Sensory deprivation or overload
- Sleep deprivation
- Solitary confinement
- Suffocation
- Suspension
- Whipping
- Witnessing or forced participation in torture of family members or compatriots (including children).

Distress

- Expression of distress is diverse and subject to cultural, personal, and situational influences; effects of torture depend on the specific nature of torture endured and its meaning and context.
- Cultural differences may limit the applicability of psychiatric diagnoses.
- Survivors may describe severe and disabling experiences of nightmares, intrusion, and avoidance; there is no single 'torture syndrome' and the diagnosis of PTSD should be used judiciously.
- Distress is exacerbated by conditions in the UK, particularly lack of social support and poor physical health.
- Psychological distress worsens the experience of pain and its impact on life.
- People may describe distress mainly in somatic terms owing to lack of appropriate language, the stigma of mental health problems, or the belief that health workers are more interested in physical problems.
- As well as treating physical pathology it can be useful to explore the meaning and context of symptoms, particularly where they persist.

Examination and investigations

- Torturers may try not to leave marks; it may be hard to attribute scars to torture with certainty.
- Persistent pain can neither be confirmed nor refuted by examination.
- Absence of physical signs does not mean that torture has not taken place.
- Investigations which require undressing should be done sensitively and only where necessary (the person may have undergone forced removal of clothing as a form of torture).
- A thorough and skilful examination of the body, including an assessment of the head and eyes, mobility of the back and affected joints, may help to reassure.
- Some survivors are particularly averse to examination because of:
  - Nakedness having been used to humiliate and in torture.
  - The type of torture, or similarity of instruments or setting.
  - The involvement of health-care professionals in torture or detention.

Providing a service for survivors of torture

- Make the service accessible by:
  - Recognizing torture survivors when they present to clinic.
  - Providing proper interpretation services, and briefing and debriefing interpreters for whom the work can be distressing.
  - Avoiding early appointments for those for whom insomnia is a problem, or appointments on relevant religious festivals.
- Establish trust through continuity, offering choice of gender of health worker and interpreter.
- Share control: be sensitive about the person having been rendered passive during torture.
- Identify, acknowledge, and, where possible, explain the pain and any interventions which may help.

- Describe identified damage and its implications; document carefully and impartially.
- Be aware that certain treatments may have associations with past traumatic experiences, e.g. TENS and electrical torture; this is not necessarily a contraindication but should be fully described and discussed.
- Massage is a common musculoskeletal treatment in some cultures (e.g. Middle Eastern). It may also be used to help overcome fears of being touched; full consent is essential and anxiety should be monitored.
- Encourage independence and support resilience, although refugees may require assistance to access services.
- Group work on pain management techniques can be helpful.
- Counselling can help to address underlying adjustment issues, but it may be outside cultural norms to share distress with a stranger rather than with kin.
- Liaise with torture survivor organizations—in UK the Medical Foundation for the Care of Victims of Torture.
- Be aware of the impact of social and legal problems; particularly isolation, poverty, poor housing, and anxiety about the asylum claim.
- Children may need individual help and support as well as family intervention.

Prescribing

- Medication may help in some circumstances, but is unlikely entirely to resolve persistent pain.
- Antidepressants may help symptoms of clinical depression, if used in conjunction with practical and social support.
- Sleep problems are often due to pain or nightmares. Offer sleep management (sleep hygiene) advice. Mirtazapine 15mg nocte or trazodone 100–200mg may help if insomnia is marked. In children it is generally not advisable to use antidepressants or sedation at night.
- When prescribing, liaise with the GP and ensure that information about the drug and its possible side effects are clearly understood.

Looking after yourself

- Work with asylum seekers is both rewarding and challenging.
- Hearing survivors' experiences and dealing with their current situation can arouse strong emotions.
- Do not set up unreal expectations of effectiveness of pain treatments.
- Be aware of your own health needs: don't become isolated or attempt to take on too much; ensure adequate support, rest and recuperation.

Training and audit

- Where possible, collaborate with torture survivor and refugee organizations to offer teaching and training on pain and to improve pain clinicians' understanding of refugee and torture issues.
- Audit casework and write it up or use examples in teaching.

Further reading

Burnett A and Peel M (2001). The health of survivors of torture and organised violence. *BMJ* **322**:606–9.

Burnett A (2002). *Guidelines for health workers providing care for asylum seekers and refugees.* Medical Foundation, London. Available at: http://www.torturecare.org.uk/articles/bibliography/344

Burnett A and Fassil Y (2002). *Meeting the health needs of refugees and asylum seekers in the UK: an Information and resource pack for health workers.* London Directorate for Health and Social Care/Department of Health, London.

Gorst-Unsworth C and Goldenberg E (1998). Psychological sequelae of torture and organised violence suffered by refugees from Iraq, trauma related factors compared with social factors in exile. *B J Psychiatry* **172**:90–4.

Health for Asylum Seekers & Refugees Portal: online health information for work with minority populations. http://www.harpweb.org.uk

Medical Foundation for the Care of Victims of Torture website: http://www.torturecare.org.uk

Peel M (ed.) (2004). *Rape as Torture.* Medical Foundation for the Care of Victims of Torture, London.

Silove D et al. (2001). Detention of asylum seekers: assault on health, human rights and social development. *Lancet* **357**:1436–7.

Thomsen AB et al. (2000). Chronic pain in torture survivors. *Forensic Sci Int* **108**:155–63.

Williams ACdeC and Amris K (2007). Topical review: pain from torture. *Pain* **133**:5–8.

Reference

1 World Medical Association (1975). *Declaration of Tokyo.* http://www.wma.net/en/30publications/10policies/c18/index.html

Chronic pain in children

Introduction

Paediatric chronic pain represents a biopsychosocial condition influenced by many different factors (age, sex, previous experiences, cognitive, behavioural, social and family factors, environment, culture).

- Children may present to any medical or surgical discipline.
- They pose a diagnostic challenge—it may take months to exclude a remediable cause for the pain.
- Referral to pain management clinics often occurs late (if at all).

The consequences of untreated or poorly managed chronic pain in children include:

- Decreased physical, psychological, and social functioning
- Depression
- Fear
- Anxiety
- Family stress
- School absenteeism
- Social isolation.

However, if the condition is recognized early and managed correctly, in an interdisciplinary manner, children can improve and go back to functioning normally with or without pain.

Chronic pain is a dynamic process due to a myriad of pathophysiological changes in the peripheral tissues and CNS in response to disease, injury, or loss of function. Initially these changes are reversible but tend to become fixed depending on the nature and duration of the original cause, as well as the emotional state, cognitive capacity, and genetic susceptibility of the patient. The nervous system of a child is considered inherently more adaptable and plastic than the adult nervous system. So central sensitization may be more dominant in the developing child. Hence, failure to prevent or manage pain in infants, children, and adolescents may have long-term consequences.

Epidemiology

Recurrent or persistent pain has been reported in 5–10% of children sampled randomly, but overall prevalence may be as high as 25%. The prevalence increases with age.

There are no sex differences in young children but as they enter school-aged years, girls are more willing to express their pain compared with boys. Hence the prevalence is reported to be significantly higher for girls, particularly girls aged between 12–14 years. There are gender differences in site of chronic pain (headache and abdominal pain in girls, back and limb pain in boys).

Aetiology

The causes of chronic pain in children fall under 4 categories:

Pain that persists beyond normal healing time for the disease or injury

- Following minor or major trauma
- CRPS

- Poorly managed acute pain—particularly after orthopaedic corrective surgery, amputation, and thoracotomy.

Pain that occurs and recurs without a remediable cause
- Chronic headaches
- Recurrent abdominal pain
- LBP
- Chest pain
- Limb pain
- CRPS.

Pain related to chronic disease
- Juvenile RA
- Sickle cell disease
- Haemophilia
- Cerebral palsy.

Pain associated with malignancy
- Tumour invasion
- Painful procedures (e.g. venepuncture, lumbar punctures, bone marrow aspirates)
- Related to adverse effects of chemotherapeutic drugs and radiation.

Risk factors

It is not known what causes some children to embark on a downward spiral of decreased physical and social functioning and not others. Psychological testing of children with chronic pain commonly, but not universally, reveals recognizable psychological factors such as:
- Perceptual distortions (suggesting extreme stress and/or neurological impairment)
- Poor problem solving skills
- Excessive use of denial and repression to cope with life events
- Active avoidance of strong and aversive emotions
- Anxiety disorders
- Learning disorders
- Communication disorders.

History

It is important to believe the child has pain. A full history should include:
- Pain history
- Past medical history
- Social history
- Family history.

Pain assessment is essential to gauge the magnitude of the pain and to determine the effectiveness of therapy. Self-report is the gold standard for pain assessment in children and includes interviews, questionnaires, pain diaries, and pain rating scales.

The Varni–Thompson Paediatric Pain Questionnaire is designed to assess chronic or recurrent pain. It includes a VAS, a colour-coded scale and body outline, specific pain descriptors, and questions about family history and socioenvironmental factors. There are versions for children (designed for children >7 years of age), adolescents, and parents.

The Children's Comprehensive Pain Questionnaire has also been used to assess chronic and recurrent pain in children. The BAPQ assessment tool is specifically for adolescents with chronic pain.

A focussed examination is required to exclude organic disease and to direct the pain management team to the most appropriate therapeutic modalities.

Clinical features/symptoms and signs

Will depend on the aetiology of the chronic pain.

Differential diagnosis

Always be aware of a potential organic cause for pain. Especially in the presence of:
- Night pain
- Thoracic pain
- Pain in a dermatomal distribution
- Pain in a younger patient
- A past medical history of oncological disease.

Investigations

Check that investigations to exclude organic or remediable pathology have been performed.

Once they have been completed it is useful to explain that no more will be performed so the family is more accepting of symptomatic treatment.

Treatment

Treatment is aimed at preventing further loss of function and restoring normal function and empowering the child and family to take control of pain + pain behaviours. It must be tailored to individual patients. The key message is to keep it simple and do no further harm. Response to the various methods listed next can be unpredictable and must be tailored to effect with accurate and repeated assessment of the chronic pain.

Pain management

The interdisciplinary approach involves a team which may include:
- Paediatricians/neurologists
- Anaesthetists
- Chronic pain nurses
- Physiotherapists
- OTs
- Psychologists/psychotherapists.

Delivering an interdisciplinary service has a number of advantages:
- Immediate assessment of each individual child's needs.
- Definitive action plans for treatment by all the team members.
- Easier integration of the specialists with the child/family.
- Reduced number of hospital visits and therefore reduced disruption to the child and family life.

Reassurance and explanation

Children with chronic pain become disillusioned and angry at the differing diagnoses they may have received. Reassurance is extremely important and will need to be re-emphasized throughout the time of the child's care.

A simple diagram that allows them to understand pain pathways as well as the development and maintenance of chronic pain is a vital part of the explanation.

Physiotherapy

Early and aggressive physiotherapy is essential for functional restoration. Active mobilization along with other physical techniques (hydrotherapy and desensitization) prevents secondary changes due to disuse.

Transcutaneous electrical nerve stimulation

TENS can be very effective for some children. It is patient-directed, cheap, non-invasive, and associated with few side effects. It is can be used in school, and often confers some 'street credibility' for the child.

Analgesic drugs

Simple analgesics such as paracetamol in combination with NSAIDs may give relief. Tramadol can be a useful adjuvant analgesic although nausea can limit its usefulness in some children. Opiate-based drugs are best avoided in non-organic pain due to side effects especially in those children attending school and /or working for exams.

In children with cancer or severe nociceptive pain, opiates will be the mainstay of treatment following the algorithm of the WHO analgesic ladder (see 📖 WHO analgesic ladder p.34).

Anticonvulsants

Gabapentin, carbamazepine, lamotrigine, and sodium valproate.

Antidepressants: TCAs.

Other drugs: clonidine. Lidocaine patches and/or infusions.

Interventional nerve blocks

Blocks used in children include:
• Peripheral nerve blockade
• Rectus sheath block
• Central nerve blockade
• Caudal
• Epidural
• Guanethidine block
• Sympathetic block.

Interventional blocks are useful for some children with chronic pain but only a few chronic pain conditions are helped by them. They can be useful diagnostically and can be repeated as part of the treatment plan; however they are only a small part of the whole package of therapy and should not be viewed as magic wands but as bridges to aid restoration of function.

The indication for interventions depends on the type of pain and the findings on clinical examination.

A plan needs to be drawn up and agreed with the child and their family so that the criteria for repeated interventions are clear.

Improve sleep profile

The child may have difficulty getting off to sleep, can be woken from sleep, or both. When getting off to sleep is difficult then different types of relaxation techniques should be adopted. Strict control of the day/night routine (with no daytime 'cat naps') is necessary to regain the normal sleep pattern.

Melatonin can be useful to help re-establish the day/night routine.

Psychological therapy

This vital part of the interdisciplinary approach utilizes a number of strategies including CBT and psychoeducation. It should run in parallel with, and complement, the medical, physical, and mental health therapies. Psychological therapy aims to:

- Promote self-management/empowerment for the child and their family.
- Reduce illness and anxiety-related thoughts and behaviours.
- Encourage positive coping and control strategies.
- Promote paced activity.
- Promote functional adaptation based on acceptance of pain.
- Encourage increased physical/social functioning in the presence of pain.
- Provide continued reassurance and support.

Adjuvant therapies

- Homeopathy
- Massage
- Aromatherapy
- Hypnosis
- Acupuncture
- Yoga.

Prevention

Prevention of chronic pain in children requires an understanding of the multifactorial aspects of the problem and addressing the following issues:

- Adequate treatment of acute pain.
- Pre-emptive treatment of chronic disease-related pain.
- Recognition of chronic pain with no remedial cause.
- Early institution of appropriate therapy.
- Prevention of the downward spiral of decreased functioning.
- There is a need for high quality multicentre studies to redress the lack of evidence in paediatric chronic pain.

Chronic pain in the elderly

The prevalence of persistent pain increases with age. It peaks in the 7th decade at approximately 14% in ♂ and 23% in ♀. Persistent pain interferes with activities of daily living and quality of life, yet detection and management of chronic pain remain inadequate in the elderly population.

Causes for inadequate pain management in the elderly

Patient factors

- Reluctance on the part of elderly patients to report pain.
- Belief that pain is an essential part of the ageing process.
- Difficulty in communication.
- Fear of being negatively judged for having pain.
- Fear that pain portends serious illness or death.
- Belief that their pain cannot be alleviated.
- Fear of addiction and dependence on pain-killers.

Physician factors

- Belief that pain is an essential part of the ageing process.
- Inadequate assessment strategies.
- Difficulty in communication with elderly patients.
- Belief that elderly patients have a higher threshold for pain.
- Fear of prescribing drugs to the elderly.

Common painful conditions in the elderly

- Musculoskeletal pain: joint pain and back pain are most commonly reported.
- Non-articular pain in the limbs, e.g. leg pain at night.
- Soft tissue disorders: myofascial pain, fibromyalgia.
- Neuropathic pain: PHN, painful diabetic neuropathy, entrapment neuropathies.

Assessment of pain in the elderly

A comprehensive assessment should include history taking, physical examination, evaluation of psychosocial and cognitive function and diagnostic tests when indicated for identifying the precise aetiology of pain. Standardized geriatric assessment tools are available to assess function, gait, affect, and cognition. See table 11.7.

In patients with dementia and cognitive impairment, one should attempt to assess pain via direct observation or history from caregivers. Direct observation should include facial expressions, verbalizations, body movements, changes in interpersonal interactions, changes in daily routines, and changes in mental status. Various clinical tools are available for assessment of pain in demented and cognitively-impaired patients.

Regular reassessment should include evaluation of analgesics and non-pharmacological interventions, side effects, and compliance issues to ensure an optimal response.

Management of persistent pain in the elderly

Pharmacological treatment

General principles

- All older adults with functional impairment or diminished quality of life as a result of persistent pain are candidates for pharmacological therapy.
- The least invasive route of administration should be used first.
- Fast onset, short-acting analgesic drugs should be used for episodic pains and sustained-release preparations for continuous pain.
- Incident pain that can be anticipated should be pre-treated.
- Paracetamol should be the drug of choice for mild to moderate pain of musculoskeletal origin.
- NSAIDs should be used with extreme caution.
- Opioid analgesics have a definite role in moderate to severe pain.
- Titration of drug dosages should be done slowly and carefully, with close monitoring for side effects.
- Side effects such as constipation should be anticipated and prevented.

Non-opioid analgesics

These are generally the first-line drugs for treating pain, mainly of musculoskeletal origin. Round-the-clock paracetamol works well in the elderly population. NSAIDs should generally be avoided except in cases where inflammation is the cause of pain. Concomitant administration of PPIs or misoprostol should be considered to reduce the risk of GI bleeding.

Neuralgesic agents such as amitriptyline, gabapentin, pregabalin, and other anticonvulsants have a specific role in management of neuropathic pain. However, the dosage should be titrated with caution and drug interactions should be kept in mind.

Opioid analgesics

Age is not a contraindication to use of opioids. Physical dependency can occur and is managed by gradual dose reduction over several weeks. True addiction is rare in the elderly.

Certain opioids need to be prescribed carefully. Tramadol should be avoided in patients with history of seizures and renal impairment. Methadone has complex pharmacokinetics and can be difficult to titrate in the elderly.

Interventional procedures

Interventional pain-relieving procedures can offer substantial benefit in certain painful conditions that do not improve with less invasive measures. However, proper patient and procedure selection, coupled with an appropriate rehabilitative programme, is essential for optimum outcome. The evidence base is lacking for most of these treatments.

Non-pharmacological methods of pain management

Physical therapies

These include treatments like TENS, acupuncture, application of heat, and US. Active treatments include progressive strengthening and stretching exercises.

Cognitive behavioural therapy
There is increasing scientific evidence for efficacy of CBT in treating persistent pain in the elderly. Patients should be given opportunity to ask questions in order to dispel the misconception that psychology referral is akin to their pain not being considered 'real'.

Complementary and alternative medicine
Physicians need to be aware of potential interactions between medications and alternative modalities (herbal therapy).

Multidisciplinary Pain Management Programmes
There is increasing evidence that patients who attend Pain Management Programmes report improvements in physical functioning and quality of life. The focus is on restoration of physical and psychosocial function, rather than treatment of pain.

Table 11.7 Tools for pain assessment in older adults

Instrument	Pain dimension measured	Comments
Numeric rating scales: Scale range 0–5, 0–10 and 0–20	Intensity	Preferred by many older patients, requires abstract thought, vertical version more suitable
Verbal descriptor scales: 5- point verbal rating scale Pain thermometer Present pain inventory Graphic rating scale	Intensity	Most preferred by elderly, low failure rate even in cognitively impaired, requires abstract thought, limited number of response categories, thermometer adaptation may assist with understanding of tool
Pictorial pain scales Faces pain scale	Intensity	Language not a barrier, requires abstract thinking and not suitable for those with cognitive impairment
Visual analogue scales	Intensity	Not preferred by most elderly, requires greater abstract thought, higher failure rates
Short-form McGill pain questionnaire	Intensity Quality	Shorter form of MPQ, not suitable for cognitively impaired
Neuropathic pain scale	Quality	Distinguishes between neuropathic and non-neuropathic pain, sensitive to treatment changes
Pain disability index	Pain-related disability	Short and easy to use
Brief pain inventory	Intensity Interference	Well validated and a useful research tool

Index

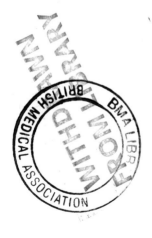